Tuberculosis

A Comprehensive Clinical Reference

Tuberculosis – A Comprehensive Clinical Reference

Publisher: iConcept Press Ltd.
Cover design: Pineapple Design Ltd.
Interior design: iConcept Press Ltd.
Typesetting and copy editing: iConcept Press Ltd. and Pineapple Design Ltd.

ISBN: 978-1-922227-94-2

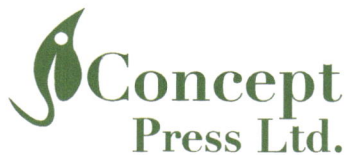

Concept
Press Ltd.

www.iconceptpress.com

Contents

Preface

Tuberculosis is a common, and in many cases lethal, infectious disease caused by various strains of *mycobacteria*, such as *Mycobacterium tuberculosis*. Tuberculosis typically attacks the lungs, but can also affect other parts of the body. The classic symptoms are a chronic cough with blood-tinged sputum, fever, night sweats, and weight loss. *Tuberculosis – A Comprehensive Clinical Reference* serves as a useful reference for individuals working in biomedical laboratories, and for clinical professionals. It provides the latest research you need to know about tuberculosis.

There are totally 10 chapters in this book. Chapter 1 highlights health systems weaknesses that are hampering diseases control efforts and proposes possible health system strengthening interventions that can easily be implemented. Strengthened health systems are essential for the control of tuberculosis. Chapter 2 proposes an original model for preparing and dispensing the drugs and monitoring of patients with tuberculosis under a direct observed treatment (DOT) program. It also includes the results and analysis of the model after the implantation. Chapter 3 shows the associated cost to an original program of Direct observed treatment (DOT) using the perspective of the Spanish Health Care System and comparing for each case of DOT, the cost of a Self-administered Treatment (SAT) based on a theoretical model. Chapter 4 reviews the present scenario of Multi-Drug Resistance Tuberculosis (MDR-TB) and the advantages of newer molecular approaches for the laboratory diagnosis of MDR-RB, with special reference to Rifampicin resistance as a surrogate marker for it.

Chapter 5 mainly focuses on the algorithmic approach in diagnosis of tuberculosis-related uveitis. It also gives key points in the pathogenesis, clinical manifestations and treatment of tuberculosis-related uveitis. Pulmonary tuberculosis can lead to various forms of complications. It can be categorized as parenchymal, airway, vascular, pleural lesions and general complications. Chapter 6 describes the pathogenesis, clinical manifestations, diagnostic criteria and management of complications of pulmonary tuberculosis. Chapter 7 discusses *Mycobacterium tuberculosis* complex in human beings. Tuberculosis in humans is caused mainly by two of the seven closely related bacteria within *Mycobacterium tuberculosis* complex (MTBC), namely *Mycobacterium tuberculosis* (MTB) and *Mycobacterium africanum* (MAF). Chapter 8 aims on difficulties of anti-TB chemotherapy, especially for Urogenital Tuberculosis, and discusses the way to minimise the side effects.

Chapter 9 aims on improving in-time diagnosis of extrapulmonary tuberculosis and particularly urogenital tuberculosis by making clear its features. Chapter 10 deals with the comparative genomics, bioinformatic analyses and genome-wide screening approaches for the better understanding of these immunologically important proteins, and summarizes that PEPPE domain from mycobacteria belongs to the family of serine hydrolase proteins and the phylogenetic analysis has shown that Mycobacterium tuberculosis is of recent decent

Editing and publishing a book is never an easy task. Each chapter in this book has gone through a peer review, a selection and an editing process so as to guarantee its quality. Without the supports and contributions of the authors and reviewers, this book can never be able to complete. We would like to thank all of the authors in this book and all of the reviewers who participated in the reviewing process: Jeffrey K. Actor, Douglas Allington, Myo Nyein Aung, Ibraheem Awowole, Subash Babu, Thomas Barry, Gaetano Caramori, Chih-Hao Chen, Alakananda Dasgupta, Sajal De, T. Eleftheriadis, Lígia Fernandes, José-María García-García, DrSurenderNikhil Gupta, Dorothee Heemskerk, Daud M. Ishaq Aweis, Kauser Jabeen, Shiwen Jiang, Theodoros Kelesidis, Kyeong-Hee Kim, G. Krishna Kumar, Chii-Wann Lin, Yecai Liu, Hongzhou Lu, Ibrahim M, Vikas Manchanda, C K Minija, Stellah G. Mpagama, V. Mukta, Noboru Nakata, Hoa Nguyen Binh, Albert Nienhaus, B. O'Shea, Carla Palma, Eric Walter Pefura Yone, Ernesto Prado Montes de Oca, Suraj B. Sable, Gursimrat K Sandhu, Krishna Kanchan Sharma, Matthias Stoll, José Torres Costa, Tibor Tot, Vishwanath Venketaraman, Miguel Viveiros, Reza Yaesoubi and Zhendong Zhao. We hope that you, the reader, will find this book interesting and useful. Any advices please feel free and are always welcome to tell us.

iConcept Press Ltd
September 2014

Tuberculosis Control in Resource Limited Settings: Health Systems Considerations

Juliet Nabyonga Orem, Joy Belinda Nabukalu
Health Systems and Services Cluster
WHO Uganda Country Office, Uganda

Abel Nkolo
Management Sciences for Health, Uganda

Miriam Nanyunja
Disease Prevention and Control Cluster
WHO Uganda Country Office, Uganda

1 Introduction

Tuberculosis (TB) remains a significant public health problem globally, with higher incidence and prevalence in resource limited settings in sub-Saharan Africa and South East Asia (World Health Organization, 2012). This is compounded by the high Human Immunodeficiency Virus (HIV) prevalence in some of the resource limited countries, especially in sub-Saharan Africa where HIV is associated with increasing TB incidence of 5 – 10% annually (De Cock & Chaisson, 1999). Globally about 8.7 million new cases of TB occurred in 2011, with about 60% of cases in South East Asia and Western Pacific World Health Organization (WHO) regions, 24% of cases in Africa, and 13% co-infected with HIV (World Health Organisation, 2012). About 1.4million deaths due to TB occurred in the same year, with about 430,000 of deaths co-infected with HIV (World Health Organisation, 2012). India and China together contribute about 40% of the global burden of TB while Africa has the highest rates of TB cases and deaths per capita (World Health Organisation, 2012). Resource limited settings in this chapter refers to low and medium income countries based on the World Bank classification of Gross National Income of US$1,035 or less and $1,036 - $4,085 respectively(World Bank, 2013,). In such settings, resources for health are quite limited and do not allow for access to the whole range of preventive and curative health care services for all their populations. These include Africa, South East Asia, Caribbeans, Eastern Europe, and some parts of Latin America, and Western Pacific region (World Bank, 2013,).

Efforts to control TB have been ongoing for centuries however; achieving global TB control remains a challenge. In 1993, WHO declared TB a global emergence and provided a five-point frame work for control of TB which included 1) political commitment, 2) diagnosing TB using sputum smear microscopy, 3) use of short course chemotherapy under direct observation, 4) regular supply of drugs and 5) a standardized recording and reporting system. In mid 1990s most countries had adopted this approach (World Health Organisation & Stop TB Partnership, 2006). However, with the emergence of new challenges like HIV and multi drug resistant TB (MDR-TB); some aspects of this framework, for example, the directly observed treatment, short-course (DOTS), where a patient is observed by a health worker or community member while swallowing medicines, was insufficient in controlling TB (De Cock & Chaisson, 1999; Harries, Hargreaves, Chimzizi, & Salaniponi, 2002). Currently the recommended strategy for TB care is the Stop TB Strategy which emphasizes expansion of quality DOTS, addressing HIV and MDR-TB, strengthening health systems, engaging all health care providers, empowering people with TB through partnerships and promoting research (World Health Organization, 2010). Although the 6th Millennium Development Goal (MDG 6) to halt and reverse the TB epidemic has been achieved at a global level with declining prevalence and incidence and a reduction in death rates (World Health Organisation, 2012), the burden of tuberculosis is still high. Furthermore, this global achievement conceals the picture in most sub-Saharan African countries which are not on track to achieve the global targets (World Health Organisation, 2012). Due to the inadequate coverage of TB control interventions, reductions in incidence of TB have been modest where they occurred with a global fall in incidence rate of about 2.2% documented between 2010 and 2011 (World Health Organization, 2012). In addition, inadequate coverage of effective treatment has resulted in emergence of multi-drug resistant (MDR) and extreme-drug resistant (XDR) TB in several countries, with India, China, Russian Federation, and South Africa reporting the highest numbers of MDR-TB globally in 2011 (World Health Organization, 2012). Many resource limited countries especially in sub-Saharan Africa are not reporting MDR-TB and XDR-TB due to inability to undertake confirmatory tests; hence the reported cases are likely to be an underestimate of the actual burden (World Health Organisation, 2012). Nevertheless, in the few sub-Saharan countries that have reported MDR and XDR TB, this poses special challenges where the second-line anti-TB drugs are largely not affordable, and the treatment lasts a long time (20 months) (World Health Organization, 2012).

Tuberculosis control in most countries has been guided and implemented by vertical national TB control programmes (World Health Organization, 2012).Although some successes have been achieved in some countries using the vertical approach (Atun, Bennett, & Duran, 2008) there is emerging evidence that without strong health systems, and a health systems integrated approach to TB control, meeting the TB control targets will remain a challenge, especially in the resource limited settings (Atun, Weil, Eang, & Mwakyusa, 2010). Several countries in the eastern part of the WHO European Region have noted the negative effects on effective management of TB posed by vertical programmes (Atun *et al.*, 2008).Some researchers have advocated for vertical programs in special circumstances like the need for rapid response, focusing on special groups and delivery of complex interventions among others. They however, caution that such approaches should be time bound and, linkages between vertical and horizontal elements of the system worked out (Atun *et al.*, 2008). A few resource limited countries have documented increased coverage through integrating TB interventions into primary health care, engaging non-governmental organizations, and the private sector in service provision (Atun *et al.*, 2010).

Through review of both published and grey literature and, verification of reported findings with TB and Health Systems Strengthening (HSS) experts in sub-Saharan Africa, this chapter highlights the health systems bottle necks to TB control. It further proposes health systems considerations and possible solutions for overcoming these bottlenecks in order to achieve TB control targets. These will however need to be tailored to the country context given the level of development of the different HSS building blocks, the TB prevalence and existing partnerships with the private sector. The health systems considerations highlighted in this chapter could guide TB control programmes in resource limited settings to address key bottlenecks and ensure that their programmes are more effective.

2   The Health System

In this chapter, we adopt the definition of a health systems as provided by the WHO defined as "all organizations, people and actions whose *primary intent* is to promote, restore or maintain health" (World Health Organisation, 2000). Using the framework of the six building blocks as provided by WHO namely; Service delivery, Health workforce, Information, Medical products, vaccines & technologies, Financing, Leadership & governance (World Health Organisation, 2007) - see figure 1 - we examine how each of the building blocks impacts on TB control efforts with specific reference to resource limited settings. We also underscore specific HSS issues for consideration by TB control programmes in low resource settings to enhance TB control.

3   Health Systems Considerations for Effective TB Control

3.1 Service Delivery

Good health services are defined as those that ensure delivery of effective, high quality, safe preventive, curative, and rehabilitation health care services to those that need them, when needed, with as minimal wastage as possible (World Health Organisation, 2007).

Health system building blocks   **Goals/Outcomes**

Service delivery
Health work force
Information
Medical Products, Vaccines& Technologies
Financing
Leadership/ Governance

Access
Coverage

Quality
Safety

Improved health (level & equity)
Social & financial risk protection
Responsiveness
Improved Efficiency

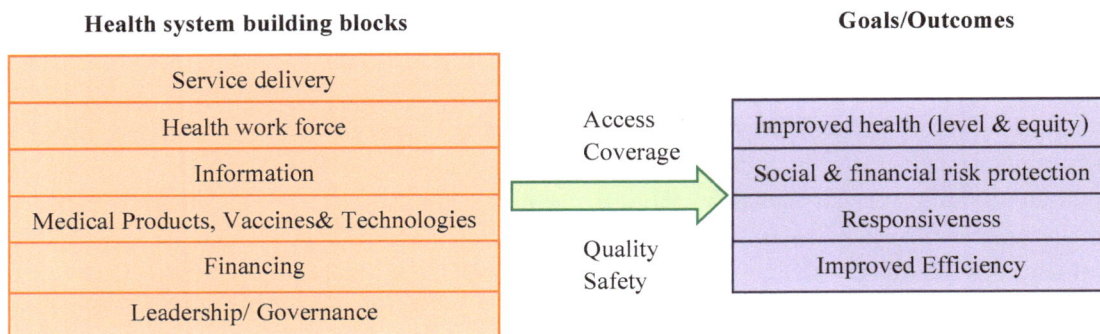

Figure 1: The WHO Health Systems Framework. Source: WHO: 2010, strengthening health systems: everybody's business (World Health Organisation, 2007).

These services may be delivered in health facilities, at home, at workplaces, or in the communities depending on the mode selected (Atun *et al.*, 2010). Although there are no standard modes of delivery of health care services, the mode selected for different diseases and communities; should put into consideration the community as well as the treatment characteristics of a given disease and ensure equitable access, quality, safety, and continuum of care (Malmborg, Mann, Thomson, & Squire, 2006; World Health Organisation, 2007). Preventive and curative services for TB control are delivered using different modes in different countries; integrated into Primary Health Care (PHC) in most sub-Saharan African and South East Asian countries, and vertically delivered in some Eastern European countries (Atun *et al.*, 2010). Furthermore, to ensure adherence, it is recommended that TB treatment is delivered as DOTS (Gabriel & Mercado, 2011; World Health Organization, 1994). To ensure DOTS, several modes of delivery have been adopted to deliver 1st and 2nd line anti-TB medicines by different countries including Health Facility-based DOTS (HF-DOTS), community-based DOTS (CB-DOTS), and a combination of the two. HF-DOTS is more effective where health facilities are within proximity, particularly for the poor and vulnerable patients (Malmborg et al., 2006). In several African countries, where access within 1km radius is still low, in addition to HF-DOTS, CB-DOTS was adopted that involves community health workers or treatment supporters observing patients' treatments daily (Adatu, *et al.*, 2003; Mafigiri, McGrath, & Whalen, 2012). This ensures continuity of treatment once an admitted patient is discharged; and also avoids unnecessary admissions for HF-DOTS (Adatu, *et al.*, 2003). Where this has been implemented very well, treatment adherence and treatment success rates have been enhanced (Gabriel & Mercado, 2011; Shargie & Lindtjorn, 2005). CB DOTS has been shown to be cost effective compared to the conventional management of TB where the patient spends the initial two months in hospital further constraining the already weak health system (Wilkinson, Floyd, & Gilks, 1997).

3.2   Service Delivery Bottlenecks for TB Control

The effectiveness of DOTS is being compromised by the high prevalence of HIV/AIDS in many resource limited countries and, some researchers have raised the need for TB control programmes to adjust to the realities of the HIV/AID era, calling for integrated service delivery (Corbett, Marston, Churchyard, & De Cock, 2006; De Cock & Chaisson, 1999). Lack of universal access to effective preventive, diagnostic and treatment services remains a big bottleneck for TB control in resource limited settings (He, *et al.*, 2011;

Malmborg, *et al.*, 2006; Parsons, *et al.*, 2011). This results in delays in diagnosis and starting of treatment and, incomplete treatments following which drug resistance has been reported (World Health Organisation, 2012). Other factors contributing to limited access to effective TB prevention and control services include inadequate coverage of routine immunization with the BCG vaccine, Isoniazid prophylaxis and, limited numbers of diagnostic and treatment centres (Atun *et al.*, 2010; Awofeso, Schelokova, & Dalhatu, 2008; Travis *et al.*, 2004). Lack of adherence or defaulting from treatment remains a challenge in some countries due to cost, access, lack of continuity of treatment after discharge from health facility, and lack of information on the importance of adherence (World Health Organization, 2012). This has contributed to emergence of MDR-TB and XDR-TB (World Health Organisation, 2013a). Emergence of MDR-TB has posed additional challenges in service delivery; the facilities required for effective treatment of MDR-TB patients are not available in many resource limited settings and the treatment is much longer. In addition, MDR-TB treatment is associated with higher rates of adverse drug reactions hence requires active monitoring and patient checkups (World Health Organization, 2012).

3.3   Health Systems Considerations

Integration of services: In order to ensure universal access to effective preventive, diagnostic, and treatment services for TB, TB services in resource limited settings should be integrated into the package of services delivered at the different levels of the health systems (Atun *et al.*, 2010). For example, at health facility level, BCG vaccination should be integrated into routine immunization services, TB diagnostics (laboratory and X-ray) should be delivered as part of the package of diagnostic services delivered by both private and public health facilities and, outreaches to communities from the health facilities should include TB services such as re-fill of the medicines of patients within the targeted communities (Atun *et al.*, 2010; Awofeso *et al.*, 2008). Tuberculosis services were being delivered integrated within primary health care in 20 of the 22 high-burden countries globally, and in 83% of 173 countries that were reporting progress in tuberculosis control to WHO in 2007 – 2008 (Atun *et al.*, 2010).

TB-HIV integration: Given the high TB incidence in HIV infected patients, there is need to integrate TB and HIV services, to ensure every TB patient is tested for HIV and treated for both if necessary, and every HIV infected patient is regularly screened for TB to enable early detection and treatment of TB (De Cock & Chaisson, 1999; Harries, *et al.*, 2002). This TB/HIV collaboration should be guided by appropriate policies and guidelines and, an environment favorable for integrated service delivery. Supplies to enable delivery of TB/HIV integrated services should also be availed at all health facilities providing the services. If this is to be realized, both TB and HIV control programmes must re-think their approach, considering their similarities and potential synergies (Harries *et al.*, 2010; Khan *et al.*, 2010). Whereas integration of TB and HIV services has been challenging, this is slowly improving; Kenya and Rwanda are countries that have successfully integrated TB and HIV services and are performing very well, indicating that this is achievable in resource limited settings (World Health Organization, 2012).

Pro-poor services: TB diagnosis and treatment ought to be considered a public health good and provided free or highly subsidized by the Governments to ensure access and continuity of treatment for those that need it. However, governments in resource limited settings are often not in position to deliver effective anti-TB services single handedly; there is need for collaboration with the private sector and Non-Governmental Organizations in service delivery to achieve universal access. This should be guided by a relevant public-private-partnership policy and guidelines, with clear guidance on roles, reporting, and supply chain management. In order to subsidize the cost of TB treatment in the private sector and ensure treatment completion, the Governments could consider providing free anti-TB medicines to recognized private providers and regulate the costs charged for consultations and service delivery. However, governments would have to regulate and supervise the private for profit providers of TB services to ensure that standards and quality are maintained, and that TB treatment is not too costly to encourage high default rate (Malmborg, *et al.*, 2006). In Myanmar, this model was implemented whereby Government signed a Memorandum of Understanding with Population Service International (PSI), and international non-governmental organization and the two agreed that in all private clinics affiliated to PSI, physician consultation fees would be $0.30 and anti-TB drugs would be provided free. The people that used the PSI affiliated clinics for TB treatment reported being very satisfied with the services (Saw, *et al.*, 2009).In many resource limited settings, the first line of health care consultations is the private sector due to several reasons including ease of access, short waiting periods, better client care, and convenient opening hours (Malmborg, *et al.*, 2006; Rutebemberwa, Pariyo, Peterson, Tomson, & Kallander, 2009). Effective TB control in the public health system will require adoption of some of these key factors that are attractive to the population.

Patient Tracking System: A system of follow up of patients started on anti-TB treatment to avoid defaulting should be established. Innovative technology such as mobile phone rapid short messaging service (SMS) could be used to remind patients of their re-fill and review dates. Ideally a multi-disciplinary approach involving physicians, nurses, social workers, and treatment buddies should be employed in anti-TB care initiation and follow up to enable them follow up on any person that is defaulting within 48hours of the appointment. This approach has been implemented in some research studies as well as anti-retroviral therapy clinics with success (World Health Organization, 2003). Cross notification between districts and between countries should also be done, supported by appropriate policy environment, to prevent international spread of TB, especially MDR-TB, in line with international health regulations. Active follow up of patients should be heightened when dealing with MDR-TB cases to avoid XDR-TB. The use of treatment buddies has enhanced adherence among patients on MDR TB treatment (World Health Organization, 2012).

4   Health Workforce

Effective service delivery requires adequate, well-trained and motivated human resources for health (HRH), working in a conducive environment. Inadequate HRH has been highlighted as one of the major challenges to attainment of MDGs in sub-Saharan Africa (Travis *et al.*, 2004).Globally, there are over 50 countries facing a human resource for health crisis and 36 of these are in the Africa Region. Other estimates show an average of 2.3 health workers per 1000 inhabitants in Africa (Awofeso *et al.*, 2008). Health workers are essential in tuberculosis control given fact that they determine the quality and efficiency of provision of TB control interventions.

4.1   Human Resource for Health Bottlenecks for TB Control

National Tuberculosis Programme (NTP) managers from 18 of the 22 tuberculosis high-burden countries; ranked human resource as a major constraint to attainment of TB targets (Figueroa-Munoz *et al.*, 2005). They highlighted challenges affecting performance of the health workforce as; inadequate and over-worked staff, lack of carrier growth, low incentives and low morale.

Bottlenecks	Health Systems Considerations
High prevalence of HIV/AIDS compromising TB control, calling on interventions beyond DOTS	*TB-HIV integration* whereby HIV screening and treatment is fully integrated in TB care and TB screening and treatment fully integrated in HIV care. *Appropriate policy environment and guidelines* for TB-HIV integration
Lack of universal access to effective preventive, diagnostic, and treatment services remains	*Integration of effective TB preventive, diagnostic, and treatment services* in the package of services delivered at different levels of the health systems, and in primary health care *Pro-poor services whereby* TB diagnosis and treatment services are a public health good and provided free or highly subsidized by the Governments. *Partnership in TB control* with government subsidizing TB care in the private sector
Lack of adherence or defaulting from treatment	*Establishment of a patient tracking system* for follow up of patients started on anti-TB using innovative technology such as, mobile phone rapid short messaging service (SMS) to identify and follow up defaulters within 48 hours *Multi-disciplinary approach* involving physicians, nurses, social workers, and treatment buddies in anti-TB care initiation and follow up *Use of treatment buddies* to enhanced adherence. *Enhanced follow up MDR-TB cases* on treatment to avoid XDR-TB. *Cross-border notification of MDR-TB cases* that move across district and/or national borders

Table 1: Bottlenecks and health systems considerations in the Service delivery building block for TB control in resource limited settings.

Key Bottlenecks	Health systems considerations
Inadequate numbers of HRH to provide TB services	*Addressing HRH gaps* where the TB program supports resource mobilization; harmonization of donor support for HRH and ensuring linkages with relevant stakeholders involved in training, recruitment and deployment of HRH. *This must be within the broader HRH development.* *Partnerships with the private sector* where the government provides subsidies including seconding staff to the private sector. *This must be within a formal agreement framework.* Use of *community health workers* to extend TB services to the community level. *Need for linkages with the formal health systems and supervision by qualified health workers.*
Inadequate skills among health workers	*Enhancing health worker skills for TB control* through in-service training. *Must be implemented as part of an integrated in-service training strategy.* *Capacity building opportunities should be extended to the private sector as well.* *Strengthening pre-service curriculum* should be implemented alongside to minimize the need for in-service training in the medium to long term.
Attrition of HRH	*Improving retention of health workers* through provision of incentives. *Should however be incorporated in the overall remuneration package to minimize distortions in service delivery.* *Motivational packages adopted will be country specific given the context and resources available.*

Table 2: Bottlenecks and health systems considerations in the HRH building block for TB control in resource limited settings.

Health workers at various services levels lack skills to manage TB and this is coupled with high attrition rates (Figueroa-Munoz et al., 2005). Majority of low income countries also face additional challenges of mal-distribution where majority of qualified staff are in urban areas, migration to other countries as well as from the public to the private sector within the country (Nunn et al., 2002). Inefficiencies in HRH management have also been documented, for example, a study conducted in Uganda showed that the country lost close to US$12M per year due to health work absenteeism (World Bank, 2009).The need to enhance skills of health workers in TB control has been highlighted, however, investment by developing countries in this areas are suboptimal. NGOs have in the past taken up this role although in a disruptive way. Allowances and incentives provided to health workers while undertaking in-service training have tended to sidetrack large numbers of human resources away from front-line tuberculosis control duties for a substantial period of time (Figueroa-Munoz et al., 2005).

4.2   Health System Considerations

Addressing HRH gaps: The WHO HRH action framework for implementation of the Stop TB Strategy highlights several roles to be played by the National TB programs in improving HRH among which is resource mobilization; harmonization of donor support for HRH and ensuring linkages with relevant stakeholders involved in training, recruitment and deployment of HRH (World Health Organisation, 2013,).This however must within the overall HRH development plan of the country. The private sector is a significant player in health service provision in majority of countries in sub- Saharan Africa (Malmborg et al., 2006; Nabyonga-Orem, Mugisha, Kirunga, Macq, & Criel, 2011; Rutebemberwa et al., 2009). Forging partnerships with the private sector and provision of subsidies, including seconding of health workers, can alleviate the HRH crisis to some extent (Rangan et al., 2004; Ssengooba, Cruz, Yates, Murindwa, & McPake, 2006). This could be through formal agreements where user fee reductions are negotiated given subsidies received, to enable a higher percentage of the population access services from the private sector. Community health workers can also contribute significantly to improving access to TB care especially at village level but, these must have linkages with the formal health systems and need to be supervised by qualified health workers (Atun et al., 2010; Saw et al., 2009).

Enhancing health worker skills for TB control: Skills of health workers must be enhanced to pro-vide TB services. This however calls for a coordinated way of skills enhancement through development and implementation of integrated in-service training strategies, whilst ensuring continued provision of services. Capacity building opportunities should be extended to the private sector as well. Strengthening pre-service curriculum should be implemented alongside to minimize the need for in-service training in the medium to long term.

Improving retention of health workers: Provision of incentives improves retention of health work-ers, however, this should not be programs based but incorporated in the overall remuneration package to minimize distortions in service delivery. Evidence has shown that health workers tend to concentrate on provision of services to which incentives are attached (Oxman & Fretheim, 2009). Other documented motivational factors include, good HRH management,career development, continuing education, and recognition/appreciation and the TB program can contribute to these (Willis-Shattuck et al., 2008). Some countries have tried earmarking local and internationally funded tuberculosis training slots to applicants from geographical regions with high tuberculosis prevalence and after training, work in particular regions for a specified period (Awofeso et al., 2008).The decision as to which motivational package is adopted will be country specific given the context and resources available. The important issue to note is a mainstreamed approach where incentives are part of the overall HRH development as opposed to a program based approach.

5 Health Information

Generation and use of information is an integral component of a good health system and effective disease control programme. "A well-functioning health information system is one that ensures the production, analysis, dissemination and use of reliable and timely health information by decision-makers at different levels of the health system, both on a regular basis and in emergencies" (World Health Organisation, 2007).Data are needed to monitor the trends of TB cases and deaths, the population at risk, the prevalence, detection and cure rates of TB, the number requiring re-treatment, the number of MDR and XDR-TB cases, number co-infected with HIV, number on both anti-TB and antiretroviral drugs, among others(World Health Organisation, 2012a). In addition, these data are needed for monitoring performance and coverage of the programme, effect of the programme interventions, and progress towards national and international targets (World Health Organisation, 2012a). Generation of these data and related information routinely requires development of standardized tools, instruments, and guidelines; strengthening the health information and surveillance systems to collect and report the data; build capacity at different levels for analysis and use of the data to direct programme improvements where necessary (World Health Organisation, 2012a). In many countries TB data is collected vertically, and often with the programme and partners using parallel reporting systems (Atun *et al.*, 2010). Standardized tools developed by WHO and adopted by most countries have enabled collection of comparable data from different countries (World Health Organisation, 2012a). Most resource limited settings use paper-based reporting, however a few have introduced electronic reporting of health information including TB and HIV data using computers or mobile telephones (World Health Organisation, 2012a). In Uganda, mobile telephone rapid SMS based reporting (mTrac) has been rolled out to all districts for immediate and weekly reporting of notifiable conditions including MDR-TB and tracer drugs consumption; and a computer based reporting system (DHIS 2) has been rolled out for monthly electronic reporting from all districts. In the African region, since the adoption of the integrated disease surveillance and response (IDSR) approach in 2007 (Perry *et al.*, 2007), more countries are making efforts to integrate the TB data collection and reporting with national health information systems (Centers for Disease Control and Prevention (CDC), 2012,). Through IDSR, data is collected on different diseases of public health importance including TB, and more recently MDR-TB in an integrated manner, using integrated data collection tools, and is analyzed at different levels of the health system, and transmitted to the national level monthly where it is stored in a national data bank (World Health Organisation, 2012a). Different programmes can then access relevant data from the data bank as necessary, analyze and use it for monitoring programme performance and to inform programme planning. Globally the case notification rate and treatment success rate are being used as key programme indicators, with targets for good performing programmes being 75% and 80% respectively. Whereas global estimates are at 67% for case notification rate and 85% treatment success rate, the achievements in most resource limited countries are much lower than this (World Health Organisation, 2012).

5.1   Health Information System Bottlenecks for TB Control

One critical bottleneck for the TB programmes in many resource limited settings is the inaccuracy and poor quality of the data used to compute the programme monitoring indicators. The denominator of most of the indicators is inaccurate due to lack of prevalence surveys (De Cock & Chaisson, 1999). As a result, most countries use WHO estimates of burden of disease to compute their indicators. There is however increased interest in TB prevalence surveys in many countries, with support from partners, although these are very resource intensive and their implementation challenging. Quality and completeness of data used to determine the numerators is also a bottleneck related to staff turnover, inadequate capacity, poor medical record keeping, and failure to collect data from the private sector (World Health Organisation, 2012a).Lack of or inadequate analysis and use of the data to inform programme management is another major challenge in resource limited settings. This is often due to lack of adequate skill in data analysis, lack of appreciation of its importance, and a weak culture of evidence-based planning (Orem *et al.*, 2012). More data is now needed on HIV related indicators among TB patients; the TB programme has to make adjustments to ensure availability of this data (De Cock & Chaisson, 1999). Vertical reporting on TB interventions implemented by some resource limited countries has also faced challenges of sustainability and hence results in some gaps in data especially due to attrition of the responsible health worker in a facility (Nsubuga, Brown, *et al.*, 2010; Nsubuga, Nwanyanwu, Nkengasong, Mukanga, & Trostle, 2010).

5.2   Health System Considerations

Integrated reporting systems: Strengthening integrated information systems such as IDSR should be prioritized as this would provide data not only on TB but also other related conditions *e.g.*, HIV. Moreover such systems are more sustainable than vertical reporting systems (World Health Organisation, 2012b). Increasing funding for TB control could be used to strengthen the integrated national health information systems that will benefit the whole health system. The tools and instruments should likewise be integrated to minimize duplications in data collection that strains data collectors (World Health Organisation, 2012a). Some countries *e.g.*, Russia still use vertical TB reporting systems, however most countries have now introduced TB variables and indicators in the integrated national health information systems with success; this has resulted in stronger and sustainable health information systems (Atun *et al.*, 2010). A set of agreed, simple and clear indicators should be used for monitoring progress (Nsubuga, Brown, *et al.*, 2010).

TB prevalence surveys: These are needed to generate more accurate data on the burden of disease (the denominator) (De Cock & Chaisson, 1999). There is increased interest in TB prevalence surveys in many countries, with support from partners, however these are very resource intensive and their implementation challenging (Atun *et al.*, 2010). Capacity building in this area is critically needed in the resource limited countries to enable accurate determination of the burden of disease.

Capacity building: Training of health workers at all levels on the use of integrated data collection tools, data collection, validation, compilation and reporting using paper-based and/or electronic tools is important (World Health Organisation, 2012a). For effective TB control, the training should target several staff in every facility, integration of data from the private sector, use of standardized registers and other medical records. In addition, capacity for data analysis and use should be developed at all points of collection; it's at this point that it can be useful to inform programme improvements (World Health Organisation, 2012b).

Data quality assessments: Data quality assessments (DQA) and audits that aim at continuous improvement of data quality within the national health information system should be conducted periodically and, gaps identified systematically addressed. The DQA should be integrated, using indicators from different programmes as the tracer indicators. DQA should include TB indicators among the tracking indicators.

Electronic reporting systems: Electronic reporting using computers and/or mobile phones could improve greatly the quality, accuracy, completeness and timeliness of integrated reports including TB and HIV data among others (World Health Organisation, 2012a). However, this requires hands-on training of the people collecting the data on how to conduct the electronic reporting. Electronic reporting can also enhance data analysis and utilization given that an electronic database is easily available (World Health Organisation, 2012a).

Key Bottlenecks	Health systems considerations
Inaccuracy and incompleteness of the data used to compute the TB programme monitoring indicators	*Conduct TB prevalence surveys* to get more accurate data for denominators *Training of health workers* at all levels of the health systems on use of integrated tools for data collection. *Introduction of electronic reporting systems* where feasible,
Poor quality data	
Lack of or inadequate analysis and use of the data to inform programme management	*Capacity and skills building* in data analysis and use
Need for HIV related data among TB patients	*Strengthening integrated information systems* such Integrated Disease Surveillance and Response that collect data on more than one disease/condition.
Non-sustainability of TB vertical reporting systems	*Invest more in integrated reporting systems* that are more sustainable.

Table 3: Bottlenecks and health systems considerations in the Health Information building block for TB control in resource limited settings.

6   Access to Essential Medicines, Vaccines, and Technologies

One of the pillars of effective TB control is early detection and effective treatment (World Health Organisation & Stop TB Partnership, 2006). To achieve this, access to good quality laboratory services and anti-TB medicines is critical (World Health Organisation & Stop TB Partnership, 2006). Access to good quality laboratory services requires trained laboratory workers with good diagnostics skills, availability of equipment and good quality reagents, materials and supplies for the laboratory testing, a system that ensures timely delivery of specimens to the laboratory, timely testing and appropriate feedback on the results (World Health Organisation & Stop TB Partnership, 2006). Microscopy has been the main stay of TB diagnosis for decades (World Health Organisation & Stop TB Partnership, 2006), however this is not very sensitive especially in patient co-infected with HIV and children, and misses out on detection of drug resistance (Parsons *et al.*, 2011; World Health Organisation & Stop TB Partnership, 2006). In addition, accurate microscopy requires skilled technicians (Parsons, *et al.*, 2011; World Health Organisation & Stop TB Partnership, 2006). Increasingly, culture and drug sensitivity testing facilities are becoming established in some resource limited settings. However, due to the costs involved in setting up and sustaining these, resource limited countries need to be very rational when making decisions on their deployment (World Health Organisation & Stop TB Partnership, 2006). There is increasing need for new, highly sensitive, point of care rapid tests to complement microcopy in diagnosis of TB; in addition the rapid tests should have capability for drug sensitivity testing so as to quickly detect MDR-TB cases (Parsons *et al.*, 2011; Quezada *et al.*, 2007; World Health Organisation & Stop TB Partnership, 2006).

Accurate quantification, timely procurement and distribution of good quality medicines to all health facilities where it is needed is requisite for effective TB treatment (World Health Organisation & Stop TB Partnership, 2006). Countries handle procurement and supply of the laboratory reagents, materials, and supplies as well as medicines differently; some procure vertically as the TB control programme whereas some use a centralized, integrated system of procurement; several countries procure anti-TB medicines through the Global Drug Facility (GDF), a facility that ensures competitive prices globally as well as high quality medicines whereas others procure directly from the manufacturers (Atun *et al.*, 2010). Vertical procurement and distribution of anti-TB drugs and laboratory supplies is often supported by donor-funded projects in most resource limited settings while integrated procurement is mostly undertaken by governments through the national procurement systems or national medical stores (Khan *et al.*, 2010).

6.1   Essential Medicines, Vaccines, and Technologies Bottlenecks for TB Control

Challenges faced in this area include inadequate numbers of good quality diagnostic centres due to lack of infrastructure, adequately trained laboratory technologists, and appropriate equipment in many health facilities, and irregular supply of reagents (Parsons *et al.*, 2011). This contributes to low case notification rates that are common in most resource limited settings. Microscopy that is the main TB diagnostic used is not very sensitive in HIV infected people and children, and does not detect drug resistance (Parsons *et al.*, 2011). In addition highly trained technicians are needed to run microscopy, yet these are not always available at health facilities, contributing to the limited numbers of inadequate diagnostic centres. Culture and drug sensitivity testing are resource intensive (Parsons *et al.*, 2011).

Periodic anti-TB medicine stock outs, common in resource limited settings, result in treatment interruptions and emergence of multi-drug resistant TB (Parsons *et al.*, 2011). On the other hand, over-stocking and mal-distribution of anti-TB medicines resulting in expiry of medicines is experienced in some areas alongside stock out of medicines in other areas are other challenges. Lack of consumption data and inaccurate quantifications contribute to the stock outs and mal-distribution of drugs (World Health Organisation & Stop TB Partnership, 2006). Whereas vertical procurement has resulted in timely distribution of medicines and supplies to health facilities in several countries, its sustainability remains an issue of concern. It often faces challenges when there are delays in release of funding from donors and when the projects come to an end (Atun *et al.*, 2010). On the other hand national integrated procurement and supply chain management systems though more sustainable, are weak in many resource limited settings and significant wastage has been documented (Harmonisation for Health in Africa, 2010).

6.2   Health Systems Considerations

Integrating procurement of anti-TB drugs into national procurement systems: In order to ensure availability of anti-TB medicines, procurement of anti-TB medicines and supplies should be integrated into national procurement systems for health products to ensure sustainability (Atun *et al.*, 2010). Where national procurement systems are still weak, concerted efforts by TB and other programmes should be put on supporting and strengthening the systems, with special focus on supply chain management to ensure accurate forecasting and; timely and accurate procurement, distribution and orders from the health facilities. This requires capacity building at different levels of the health system, which should be put into consideration when planning for TB and other disease control programmes, in collaboration with the national procurement entity, which in many countries is the National Medical Stores (Atun *et al.*, 2010). Integrated procurement systems have worked with success in Cambodia and India (Saw *et al.*, 2009). In Cambodia the National TB programme also supported capacity building at sub-national level to ensure accurate forecasting and ordering (Uchiyama *et al.*, 2006). Furthermore, to ensure high quality of medicines procured, the GDF should be used by countries without appropriate quality control mechanisms (World Health Organisation & Stop TB Partnership, 2006). Several countries including Tanzania and Uganda have been procuring anti-TB medicines through the GDF and have not reported quality issues (Atun *et al.*, 2010).

Bundling of medicines and diagnostic supplies: To ensure that diagnostic reagents, supplies and anti-TB medicines are readily available at the health facilities, orders from health facilities should include well quantified needs, and bundling of medicines and laboratory supplies during distribution should be considered.

Increasing funding for Medicines, vaccines and technologies: National governments should work towards funding all procurement of first line anti-TB medicines, second line medicines, and laboratory reagents and supplies requirements to minimize the stock out challenges created by projectized donor-funded vertical procurements (Atun *et al.*, 2010). India has taken positive action in this aspect whereby the government procurement system procures anti-TB drugs with government funds but has a back-up emergency procurement system financed donors to bridge gaps in case of any delays in government procurements (Atun *et al.*, 2010).

Monitoring drug consumption and stocks: Mechanisms for monitoring medicine consumption rates and innovative methods of tracking stocks of medicines should be established in all countries to ensure adequate amounts of medicines are available in health facilities at all times. In Uganda, a mobile phone rapid SMS based system has been established to monitor and report on medicine stocks weekly. This ensures quick identification of facilities that have minimum stocks of medicines and informs distribution plans within in the district where there is overstocking in some facilities, or from central to district levels when this is needed. In order to curb the increasing prevalence of MDR-TB, and the increasing expenditures on second line medicines, countries should have zero tolerance for anti-TB drug stock outs.

Integrated training of laboratory workers: Integrated training of laboratory workers should be done to enhance accuracy of diagnosis of TB as well as other common diseases in the locality instead of training them on only TB diagnosis as has been done in some countries. An example is Uganda where TB microscopists have been trained (Awofeso *et al.*, 2008; World Health Organisation & Stop TB Partnership, 2006). This ensures that the laboratory workers keep busy when there are no TB specimens and thus do not lose skills.

Develop point of care rapid tests to complement microcopy in diagnosis of TB: Such tests should be highly sensitive and fairly easy to use. In addition the rapid tests should have capability for drug sensitivity testing so as to quickly detect MDR-TB cases (Parsons *et al.*, 2011; Quezada *et al.*, 2007; World Health Organisation & Stop TB Partnership, 2006).

Innovative specimen referral mechanisms: Where building of TB diagnostic capacity is not possible within a short distance (<5km), innovative specimen referral systems should be established. For example, only a few, or none of the laboratories in resource limited settings may be able to confirm MDR or XDR-TB (World Health Organisation & Stop TB Partnership, 2006); but with effective specimen referral mechanisms specimens could be referred for testing at the one laboratory in the country or in a neighboring country with the diagnostic capacity as is happening in some African countries. Uganda has one national reference laboratory for TB that provides diagnostic facilities for MDR-TB. A specimen referral mechanism has been established country-wide that ensures that specimens referred for testing to this laboratory reach it within 1 – 2 days. The laboratory also provides diagnostic services for some of the countries within the African region.

Integrating routine immunization services into maternity services: BCG vaccines have been integrated into the routine immunization system in all countries. Considerations should be on supporting and strengthening the immunization systems to ensure very high coverage of vaccines, including BCG vaccine soon after birth. To ensure this, vaccination services should be available at all maternity centers either as static or outreach sites; this will minimize missed opportunities for vaccination. Quality of vaccines should be ensured and national systems for monitoring severe adverse reactions, which in most countries are managed by the national medicines regulatory authorities, be strengthened to monitor adverse reactions following immunization.

Bottlenecks	Health Systems Considerations
Inadequate numbers of diagnostic centres due to lack of infrastructure, adequately trained laboratory technologists, appropriate equipment, and irregular supply of reagents in many health facilities	*Integrated training* of laboratory workers *Bundling laboratory supplies and reagents with anti-TB drugs* Development and introduction of easy to use *point of care TB rapid diagnostic tests*
Microscopy not very sensitive in HIV infected people and children, and does not detect drug resistance	*Establishment of culture and drug sensitivity testing facilities* *Innovative specimen referral mechanisms* to the few facilities established
Lack of consumption data and inaccurate quantifications of drug needs resulting into stock outs and mal-distribution	*Innovative drug consumption and stock monitoring mechanisms*
Non-sustainability of vertical procurement systems that are mainly donor-driven	*Integrating procurement of anti-TB drugs into national procurement systems* *Increasing government funding* for Medicines, vaccines and technologies

Table 4: Bottlenecks and health systems considerations in medicines, vaccines, and technologies building block for TB control in resource limited settings.

7   Health Financing

Financing for health services in sub-Saharan Africa falls below recommended investments and as a result, majority of countries cannot ensure access to health services for the whole population. For example, by 2010, over a third of African Union countries had not reached the recommended level of health expenditure per capita to fund a minimum package of health services estimated at US$ 44, while only five countries were allocating 15% of their national budget to health a target set in the Abuja declaration (Musango, Orem, Elovainio, & Kirigia, 2012).

Global efforts have tried to cover funding shortages in low income countries and among these is the Global Fund, UNITAID, bilateral agencies and philanthropic sources. Funding from these sources for the 22 TB high-burden countries increased from approximately $1.84 billion in 2006 to almost $2.64 billion in 2010 (Atun *et al.*, 2010). The Global fund alone provides around 63% of all international financing for tuberculosis control globally (Lal *et al.*, 2011). Returns on these investments have been realized to varying levels due to a number of challenges among which is weak financial management, weak accountability, low absorption capacity and weak procurement mechanisms (Kapiriri & Martin, 2006).

In an effort to improve access to health services, several countries provide health services free at the point of use. Financial barriers to patients' access to tuberculosis health services are still eminent despite tuberculosis services having been included in the free basic health package. This is due to gaps in service delivery partly as a result of under-investment in health (Atun *et al.*, 2010; World Health Organisation, 2012). Current estimate show that, in the case of WHO Africa Region member states, available funding for TB control is only 55% and 47% of estimated requirement in 2012 and 2013 respectively and, over 50% is being funded by the Global fund (World Health Organisation, 2012). A call for increasing domestic funding for health has been made in the several health financing panels held between ministers of health and finance but progress remains slow (Musango *et al.*, 2012). Effective TB control calls for increased investment in health alongside improving effectiveness of donor aid.

7.1 Bottlenecks in Health Financing for TB Control

Overall under-investment in health has implications on implementation of TB control strategies as evidenced by suboptimal coverage of TB interventions, and poor quality of TB services in several resource limited settings (World Health Organisation, 2012). Although investments in TB falls short of estimated requirements on the one hand, in 2005, expenditures were less than available funding in two WHO regions, particularly Africa and the Eastern Mediterranean, pointing to low absorption capacity issues (Floyd, Pantoja, & Dye, 2007).

As a results of inadequate investment and suboptimal coverage with TB control interventions, case detection rate in the WHO African Regions stands at 61% while TB success treatment rate stands at 82% falling short of targets set at 70% and 85% respectively (World Health Organisation, 2012). Public sector expenditure on medicines for countries in the WHO Africa Region is far inadequate below US$2 percapita in several countries (WHO Africa Regional Office, 2013). As a result, some countries are experiencing emergence of MDR and XDR alongside a worsening TB epidemic with implications of higher cost of service delivery (World Health Organisation, 2012). The significant reliance of donor funding to finance TB programme poses several challenges. In the recent past, the economic crisis affecting several of the developed economies, who make significant investments in health, has had negative implications on funding for health services in low income countries (Kirigia, Nganda, Mwikisa, & Cardoso, 2011). This has raised concerns on suitability of funding for programme implementation and sustaining achievements made. This is further compounded by the rising costs of providing TB services largely driven by MDR TB and XR TB emergence (World Health Organization, 2012). Furthermore, aligning donor funding to government priorities and ensuring predictability are long standing challenges (Nabyonga-Orem, Ssengooba, & Okuonzi, 2009).

Inefficient use of available resources has also been highlighted. A study in Rwanda documented a significant cost saving by changing the service delivery model from General Practitioner clinics to the public sector (Kirigia *et al.*, 2011). A loss of close to US$ 12 million in the health sector was estimated in health worker absenteeism in Uganda (World Bank, 2009). The WHO, World health report estimated that 20% - 40% of health resources are wasted mainly in drug procurement (World Health Organisation, 2010a). Although this is a global estimate, the picture in African countries is close given the fact that African governments pay 2.5 to 6.5 times higher than international reference prices (United Nations (UN), 2012)).

7.2   Health Systems Considerations

Financing for TB programs: Augments have been made for countries in SSA to wean themselves off donor funding and among the strategies suggested is; reduction in economic inefficiencies; reprioritizing public expenditures; raising additional tax revenues; increased private sector involvement in health development; and fighting corruption (Kirigia & Diarra-Nama, 2008). The call to increasing domestic funding by low income countries has been made repeatedly which needs to be implemented (Hafidz, & Rostina, 2013; Musango *et al.*, 2012). Some countries have taken bold steps to raise more funding for health through collecting earmarked taxes for health for example, a 2.5% of VAT in the case of Ghana. Earmarked taxes for health have been imposed on tobacco and alcohol in the case of Benin and Mobile companies and Money gram in the case of Gabon (WHO Africa Regional Office, 2013). These innovative mechanisms provide opportunities to raise more funding for health.

Improved alignment of donor funding: Donor funding provides an opportunity to strengthen the health system but efforts have to be made to address identified challenges. The poor alignment could be reduced through ensuring strong government leadership and governance, comprehensive and participatory planning processes and, monitoring. The principles of the International Health Partnerships (iHP+) which emphasize increased alignment behind one plan, joint approaches, greater use of country systems especially financial management and one platform for monitoring and accountability for results offer enormous opportunities for improving effectiveness of donor aid (International Health Partnerships, n.d.).

Improving efficiency in resource allocation and use: Strengthening medicines procurement mechanisms will minimize losses and subsequently reduce medicines stock outs. Regionally based procurement arrangements named "voluntary pooled procurement"; where a number of countries negotiate with a given supplier as a block, offer stringent quality standards and better negotiation opportunities and these need to be further explored (i+Solutions, n.d.). Financial management mechanisms need to be strengthened and among the suggested options is training MoH staff in accountability processes (Musango, *et al.*, 2012). Other measures include linking money to results under result/performance based financing mechanisms that have shown good results in several countries. They offer opportunities for system wide improvements depending on how they are implemented (Meessen, Soucat, & Sekabaraga, 2011)

Key Bottlenecks	Health systems considerations
Inadequate financing for TB control	*Increase domestic funding for TB control* through allocating more funds from available government budget and reprioritizing public expenditures. *Raise more funding* from innovative financing mechanisms to finance TB programmes.
Alignment of donor aid to government plans	*Improved alignment of donor funding by* ensuring strong government leadership and governance, comprehensive and participatory planning processes and, monitoring. Greater use of country systems especially financial management.
Inefficiency in the use of resources	*Improving efficiency in resource allocation and use through* strengthening medicines procurement mechanisms and financial management systems. Explore mechanisms that link funding to results.

Table 6: Bottlenecks and health systems considerations in the financing building block for TB control in resource limited settings.

8   Leadership and Governance

The importance of good leadership and management, for effective health program implementation is already documented (Keugoung, Macq, Buve, Meli, & Criel, 2013). Decentralization of governance and financing for service delivery occurred in many low and middle income countries in the 1990s aimed at improving access, equity and efficiency in the health sector among others. However, inadequate financing, low planning capacity and political conflicts weakened these reforms and hindered fulfillment of their mandates (Atun *et al.*, 2010). In some instances decentralization of governance and financing led to reduced programmatic financing, poor monitoring of programme performance, interrupted drug supplies as a result of disrupted supply chain systems, impaired case reporting further compromising effective service delivery (Atun *et al.*, 2010).

8.1   Leadership and Governance Bottlenecks for TB Control

Weak management of HRH at the decentralized level has led to low retention, reduced morale of health workers and further compromising quality of health services (Figueroa-Munoz *et al.*, 2005). In an effort to respond to the several managerial challenges at decentralized levels, vertical programmes have attempted to designate focal points for specific diseases at the decentralized level. This has not been successful in several cases where the designated person lacks clout to engage within the overall decentralized leadership set up. In addition, due to staffing constraints, designated officers also do have other responsibilities, which limit the amount of time they can commit to a given disease. On the other hand however, incentive mechanisms accompanying such designations have led to reduced attention being paid to other programmes. The ability to improve quality of tuberculosis services depends crucially on the good practice of the managers at the level of the basic management unit. Decentralization of treatment to peripheral health centers and the community has been undertaken but this requires strong managerial capacity to ensure the logistics for DOTS, drug security, supervision, monitoring and recording in the community are in place. These are however not in place in majority of countries (Maher, Harries, & Getahun, 2005).

8.2   Health System Considerations

Strengthening leadership and management especially at the decentralized and service delivery level is essential. This could be through provision of management short courses as part of in-service training and, undertaking supervision visits to offer mentorship and problem solving. Pre-service curriculum for schools of public health should also be strengthened on management aspects as a medium to long term measure. The environment within which managers work must be supportive for them to be effective, the institutional set up must be strengthened, policies and guidelines put in place and roles and responsibilities spelt out.

Managerial constraints in tuberculosis control at decentralized levels cannot be resolved by NTPs in isolation and it is therefore essential strengthen overall management for health services at the decentralized level (Figueroa-Munoz *et al.*, 2005).

Key Bottlenecks	Health systems considerations
Weak leadership and management capacities especially at the decentralized and service delivery levels	*Strengthening leadership and management* through provision of management short courses as part of in-service training. *Supportive supervision visits* to offer mentorship and problem solving. *Pre service curriculum for schools of public health should also be strengthened* on management aspects as a medium to long term measure. *Put in place a supportive environment*, polices and guidelines including spelling out roles and responsibilities. *Leadership and managerial skills should be strengthened as part of the overall management for health services at the decentralized level.*

Table 6: Bottlenecks and health systems considerations in the financing building block for TB control in resource limited settings.

9   Conclusion

Efforts to control TB require strengthened HSS able to deliver needed intervention to the whole population in a timely manner. The HSS functions as a whole and efforts to strengthen it should undertake evidence based prioritized actions in each of the six building blocks. This will involve undertaking an assessment of the current status of a given HSS following which prioritized strategies will be identified. Improving coverage of interventions for a given diseases has implication on all the six HSS building blocks and this should be factored in the planning, implementation and evaluation of any disease programme. We do not attempt to suggest which building block is more important or where does one lay more emphasis; instead we emphasize a country specific approach based on evidence.

We also emphasize a holistic approach to HSS strengthening underpinned by robust national health policies and sector strategic plans developed a participatory and inclusive manner, bringing together all relevant stakeholders. The stewardship role of government needs to be strengthened at the national and decentralized levels to be able to harness the contribution of all actors, align all available resources to agreed priorities, regulate the private sector and oversee implementation of agreed strategies. Where vertical governance, funding and service delivery systems exist, integration will be difficult and changes must be underpinned by legal and regulatory adjustments aimed at linking the governance, organization and funding of vertical programmes with mainstream health systems.

References

Adatu, F., Odeke, R., Mugenyi, M., Gargioni, G., McCray, E., Schneider, E., Maher, D. (2003). *Implementation of the DOTS strategy for tuberculosis control in rural Kiboga District, Uganda, offering patients the option of treatment supervision in the community, 1998-1999. International Journal of Tuberculosis and Lung Diseases, 7(9 Suppl 1), S63-71.*

Atun, R. A., Bennett, S., Duran, A. (2008). *When do vertical (stand-alone) programmes have a place in health systems? Geneva, Switzerland: World Health Organization.*

Atun, R., Weil, D. E., Eang, M. T., Mwakyusa D. (2010). *Health-system strengthening and tuberculosis control. Lancet, 375(9732), 2169-2178.*

Awofeso, N., Schelokova, I., Dalhatu, A. (2008). Training of front-line health workers for tuberculosis control: Lessons from Nigeria and Kyrgyzstan. Human Resources for Health, 6,20.

Centers for Disease Control and Prevention (CDC). (2012). Current status of integrated disease surveillance and response (IDSR) in countries. Availableat http://www.cdc.gov/globalhealth/dphswd/idsr/progress/status.html.

Collins, D., Hafidz, F., Rostina, J. (2013). International workshop on sustainable financing for TB programs, including experiences from HIV/AIDS and malaria programs. Submitted to USAID by the TB CARE I Program. In. Edited by Management Sciences for Health TCII. Indonesia: Management Sciences for Health.

Corbett, E. L., Marston, B., Churchyard, G. J., De Cock, K. M. (2006). Tuberculosis in sub-Saharan Africa: Opportunities, challenges, and change in the era of antiretroviral treatment. Lancet, 367(9514), 926-937.

De Cock, K. M., Chaisson, R. E. (1999). Will DOTS do it? A reappraisal of tuberculosis control in countries with high rates of HIV infection. International Journal of Tuberculosis and Lung Diseases, 3(6), 457-465.

Figueroa-Munoz, J., Palmer, K., Poz, M. R., Blanc, L., Bergstrom, K., Raviglione, M. (2005). The health workforce crisis in TB control: A report from high-burden countries. Human Resources for Health, 3(1), 2.

Floyd, K., Pantoja, A., Dye, C. (2007). Financing tuberculosis control: The role of a global financial monitoring system. Bulletin of the World Health Organization, 85(5):334-340.

Gabriel, A. P., Mercado, C. P. (2011). Evaluation of task shifting in community-based DOTS program as an effective control strategy for tuberculosis. Scientific World Journal, 11,2178-2186.

Harmonisation for Health in Africa (HHA). (2010). Investing in Health for Africa: The Case for Strengthening Systems for Better Health Outcomes. Available at http://www.hha-online.org/hso/system/files/AIC_en_Summary.pdf

Harries, A. D., Hargreaves, N. J., Chimzizi, R., Salaniponi, F. M. (2002). Highly active antiretroviral therapy and tuberculosis control in Africa: Synergies and potential. Bulletin of the World Health Organization, 80(6), 464-469.

Harries, A. D., Zachariah, R., Corbett, E. L., Lawn, S. D., Santos-Filho, E. T., Chimzizi, R., ... De Cock, K. M. (2010). The HIV-associated tuberculosis epidemic--when will we act? Lancet, 375(9729), 1906-1919.

He, G. X., Wang, H. Y., Borgdorff, M. W., van Soolingen, D., van der Werf, M. J., Liu, Z. M., ... van den Hof, S. (2011). Multidrug-resistant tuberculosis, People's Republic of China, 2007-2009. Emerging Infectious Diseases, 17(10), 1831-1838.

International Health Partnerships (ihp+) (n.d.) Aligning for better results. Accessed on 19th September 2013 at http://www.internationalhealthpartnership.net/en/,

i+ Solutions (n.d.) Voluntary pooled procurement. Available at http://www.iplussolutions.org/en/content/voluntary-pooled-procurement

Kapiriri, L., Martin, D. K. (2006). The Global Fund Secretariat's suspension of funding to Uganda: How could this have been avoided? Bulletin of the World Health Organization, 84(7), 576-580..

Keugoung, B., Macq, J., Buve, A., Meli, J., Criel, B. (2013). The interface between the national tuberculosis control programme and district hospitals in Cameroon: Missed opportunities for strengthening the local health system - a multiple case study. BioMed Central Public Health, 13, 265.

Khan, F. A., Minion, J., Pai, M., Royce, S., Burman, W., Harries, A. D., Menzies, D. (2010). Treatment of active tuberculosis in HIV-coinfected patients: A systematic review and meta-analysis. Clinical Infectious Diseases, 50(9), 1288-1299.

Kirigia, J. M., Diarra-Nama, A. J. (2008). Can countries of the WHO African Region wean themselves off the donor funding for health? Bulletin of the World Health Organization, 86(11):889-892.

Kirigia, J. M., Nganda, B. M., Mwikisa, C. N., Cardoso, B. (2011). Effects of global financial crisis on funding for health development in nineteen countries of the WHO African Region. BioMed Central International Health Human Rights, 11, 4.

Lal, S. S., Uplekar, M., Katz, I., Lonnroth, K., Komatsu, R., Yesudian, D. H. M., Atun, R. (2011). Global Fund financing of public-private mix approaches for delivery of tuberculosis care. Tropical Medicine and International Health, 16(6), 685-692..

Mafigiri, D. K., McGrath, J. W., Whalen, C. C. (2012). Task shifting for tuberculosis control: A qualitative study of community-based directly observed therapy in urban Uganda. Global Public Health, 7(3), 270-284.

Maher, D., Harries, A., Getahun, H. (2005). Tuberculosis and HIV interaction in sub-Saharan Africa: Impact on patients and programmes; implications for policies. Tropical Medicine and International Health, 10(8), 734-742.

Malmborg, R., Mann, G., Thomson, R., Squire, S. B. (2006). Can public-private collaboration promote tuberculosis case detection among the poor and vulnerable? Bulletin of the World Health Organization, 84(9),752-758.

Meessen, B., Soucat, A., Sekabaraga, C. (2011). Performance-based financing: Just a donor fad or a catalyst towards comprehensive health-care reform? Bulletin of the World Health Organization, 89(2), 153-156.

Musango, L., Orem, J. N., Elovainio, R., Kirigia, J. (2012). Moving from ideas to action - developing health financing systems towards universal coverage in Africa. BioMed Central International Health and Human Rights, 12, 30.

Nabyonga, Orem. J., Mugisha, F., Kirunga, C., Macq, J., Criel, B. (2011). Abolition of user fees: The Uganda paradox. Health Policy and Planning, 26(Suppl 2), i41-51.

Nabyonga, O. J., Ssengooba, F., Okuonzi, S. (2009). Can donor aid for health be effective in a poor country? Assessment of prerequisites for aid effectiveness in Uganda. Pan African Medical Journal, 3(1).

Nsubuga, P., Brown, W. G., Groseclose, S. L., Ahadzie, L., Talisuna, A. O., Mmbuji, P., ... White, M. (2010). Implementing integrated disease surveillance and response: Four African countries' experience, 1998-2005. Global Public Health, 5(4), 364-380.

Nsubuga, P., Nwanyanwu, O., Nkengasong, J. N., Mukanga, D., Trostle, M. (2010). Strengthening public health surveillance and response using the health systems strengthening agenda in developing countries. BioMed Central Public Health, 10 (Suppl 1), S5.

Nunn, P., Harries, A., Godfrey-Faussett, P., Gupta, R., Maher, D., Raviglione, M. (2002). The research agenda for improving health policy, systems performance, and service delivery for tuberculosis control: A WHO perspective. Bulletin of the World Health Organization,80(6), 471-476.

Orem, J. N., Mafigiri, D. K., Marchal, B., Ssengooba, F., Macq, J., Criel, B. (2012): Research, evidence and policymaking: The perspectives of policy actors on improving uptake of evidence in health policy development and implementation in Uganda. BioMed Central Public Health, 12,109

Oxman, A. D., Fretheim, A. (2009). Can paying for results help to achieve the Millennium Development Goals? A critical review of selected evaluations of results-based financing. Journal of Evidence Based Medicine, 2(3), 184-195.

Parsons, L. M., Somoskovi, A., Gutierrez, C., Lee, E., Paramasivan, C. N., Abimiku, A., ... Nkengasong, J. (2011). Laboratory diagnosis of tuberculosis in resource-poor countries: Challenges and opportunities. Clinical Microbiology Review, 24(2), 314-350.

Perry, H. N., McDonnell, S. M., Alemu, W., Nsubuga, P., Chungong, S., Otten, M. W. Jr., ... Thacker, S. B. (2007). Planning an integrated disease surveillance and response system: A matrix of skills and activities. BioMed Central Medicine, 5:24.

Quezada, C. M., Kamanzi, E., Mukamutara, J., De Rijk, P., Rigouts, L., Portaels, F., Amor, B. Y. (2007). Implementation validation performed in Rwanda to determine whether the INNO-LiPA Rif.TB line probe assay can be used for detection of multidrug-resistant Mycobacterium tuberculosis in low-resource countries. Journal of Clinical Microbiology, 45(9), 3111-3114..

Rangan, S. G., Juvekar, S. K., Rasalpurkar, S. B., Morankar, S. N., Joshi, A. N., Porter, J. D. (2004). Tuberculosis control in rural India: Lessons from public-private collaboration. International Journal of Tuberculosis and Lung Diseases, 8(5), 552-559.

Rifat A. Atun, Sara Bennett, & Antonio Duran. (2008). When do vertical (stand-alone) programmes have a place in health systems? Geneva, Switzerland: World Health Organization

Rutebemberwa, E., Pariyo, G., Peterson, S., Tomson, G., Kallander, K. (2009). Utilization of public or private health care providers by febrile children after user fee removal in Uganda. Malaria Journal, 8,45.

Saw, S., Manderson, L., Bandyopadhyay, M., Sein, T. T., Mon, M. M., Maung, W. (2009). Public and/or private health care: Tuberculosis patients' perspectives in Myanmar. Health Research Policy and Systems, 7, 19.

Shargie, E. B., Lindtjorn, B. (2005). DOTS improves treatment outcomes and service coverage for tuberculosis in South Ethiopia: A retrospective trend analysis. BioMed Central Public Health, 5, 62.

Ssengooba, F., Cruz, V. O., Yates, R., Murindwa, G., & McPake, B. (2006). Health systems reforms in Uganda: processes and outputs. London, United Kingdom: London school of hygiene and tropical medicine. Health systems development programme (HSD).

Travis, P., Bennett, S., Haines, A., Pang, T., Bhutta, Z., Hyder, A. A., ... Evans, T. (2004). Overcoming health-systems constraints to achieve the Millennium Development Goals. Lancet, 364(9437), 900-906.

Uchiyama, Y., Mao, T. E., Okada, K., Chay, S., Kou Soum, M., Leng, C. (2006). An assessment survey of anti-tuberculosis drug management in Cambodia. International Journal of Tuberculosis and Lung Disease, 10(2), 153-159..

United Nations (UN). (2012). UN-MDG Gap task force report. Retrieved on 6th Sepetmber, 2013from http://www.who.int/medicines/mdg/mdg8report2012_en.pdf.

WHO Africa Regional Office. (2013). Medines Pricing and Financing. Retrieved on 9th September 2013 from http://www.afro.who.int/en/cluster-a-programmes/hss/essential-medicines/programme-components/medicines-pricing-and-financing.htlm.

WHO Africa Regional Office. (2013). State of health financing in the African region. Brazzaville, Congo: World Health Organization.

Wilkinson, D., Floyd, K., Gilks, C. F. (1997). Costs and cost-effectiveness of alternative tuberculosis management strategies in South Africa--implications for policy. South African Medical Journal,87(4), 451-455.

Willis-Shattuck, M., Bidwell, P., Thomas, S., Wyness, L., Blaauw, D., Ditlopo, P. (2008). Motivation and retention of health workers in developing countries: A systematic review. BioMed Central Health Services Research, 8, 247.

World Bank. (2009). Fiscal space for health. Kampala, Uganda: World Bank.

World Bank. (2013). How we classfy countries. Accessed September 2013 from http://data.worldbank.org/about/country-classifications

World Health Organization (WHO). (1994). TB: A global emergency. WHO report on the TB epidemic. WHO/TB/94.177. Geneva, Switzerland: World Health Organisation.

World Health Organisation (WHO). (2000). Health Systems: Improving Performance. World Health Report. Geneva, Switzerland: World Health Organisation.

World Health Organizion (WHO). (2003). Adherence to long-term therapies: Evidence for action. Geneva, Switzerland: World Health Organization.

World Health Organisation (WHO) & Stop TB Partnership. (2006). The Stop TB Strategy: Building on and enhancing DOTS to meet the TB-related Millennium Development Goals. Geneva, Switzerland: World Health Organization.

World Health Organisation (WHO). (2007). Everybody's business - strengthening health systems to improve health outcomes: WHO's framework for action. Geneva, Switzerland: World Health Organisation

World Health Organisation (WHO). (2012). Global tuberclosis report. Geneva, Switzerland: World Health Organization.

World Health Organisation (WHO). (2010). The Stop TB strategy. Geneva, Switzerland: World Health Organization.

World Health Organisation (WHO). (2010a). The World Health Report: Health Systems Financing—the Path to Universal Coverage. Geneva, Switzerland: World Health Organization.

World Health Organisation (WHO). (2012a). Electronic recording and reporting for tuberculosis care and control. Geneva, Switzerland: World Health Organization. Available at http://whqlibdoc.who.int/publications/2012/9789241564465_eng.pdf.

World Health Organisation. (2012b).Integrated Disease Surveillance: Technical Guidelines for Integrated Disease Surveillance and Response in the African Region. Available at http://www.afro.who.int/en/clusters-a-programmes/dpc/integrated-disease-surveillance/features/2775-technical-guidelines-for-integrated-disease-surveillance-and-response-in-the-african-region.html,

World Health Organisation (WHO). (2013). The human resources for health action framework and human resources development for implementation of the Stop TB Strategy. Available at http://www.who.int/tb/health_systems/human_resources/hrh_action_framework/en/index2.html

World Health Organisation (WHO). (2013a). Multi Drug resistant Tuberclosis (TB). Available at http://www.who.int/tb/challenges/mdr/en/

Directly Observed Treatment: Implementation and Validation of an Original Model

Beatriz Mejuto
Pharmacy Department
Hospital da Costa, Burela, Spain

Victoria Tuñez
Tuberculosis Unit, Preventive Medicine Department
Complexo Hospitalario Universitario de Santiago, Santiago de Compostela, Spain

María Luisa Pérez del Molino
Microbiology Department
Complexo Hospitalario Universitario de Santiago, Santiago de Compostela, Spain

Rosario García-Ramos
Pharmacy Department
Complexo Hospitalario Universitario de Santiago, Santiago de Compostela, Spain

1 Introduction

The Tuberculosis (TB) is, in most instances, a curable disease. History has shown that improved social and economic conditions can greatly facilitate TB control, while economic crises can rapidly worsen the situation (Global Plan to Stop TB 2011-2015). The clear link between HIV trends and TB trends demonstrates the importance of direct TB risk factors for TB control. Epidemics of smoking, diabetes and substance abuse could have similar effects. The Global Plan to Stop TB acknowledges the importance of such preventive actions for effective future TB control. However, it is important to highlight that the plan focuses on the actions that should be pursued by National TB Control programs (NTPs). These include co-ordinated diagnosis and management of TB risk factors and co-morbidities and joint advocacy for social mobilization and development (Global Plan to Stop TB 2011-2015).

Recognizing the scale of the problem, global targets for reductions in the burden of TB disease (measured as incidence, prevalence and mortality) have been set within the context of the Millennium Development Goals (MDGs) and by the Stop TB Partnership. The target set within the MDGs is to halt and reverse the incidence of TB by 2015. In addition, the MDGs include three other indicators for measurement of progress in TB control: prevalence and death rates, and the proportion of cases that are detected and cured in DOTS programmes (Global Plan to Stop TB 2011-2015).

The incidence rate, estimated by WHO, in Spain in 2011 was 15 cases (14-17) / 100.00 inhabitants, while in Europe was 42 cases/100.000 inhabitants (http://apps.who.int/ghodata/). In Galicia, northwest region of Spain, with 2.762.198 inhabitants, the development, in 1995, of the Galician Program for Prevention and Control of Tuberculosis (PGPCTB) (PGPCTB, 1995; report PGPCTB, 2003), has allowed us to know our epidemiological reality. Despite the number of cases decreased by about 50%, the incidence still remains figures do not agree with our level of economic and health development. In 1996, the incidence of TB in Galicia was found to be about 72.3 cases/100.000 inhabitants and in 2011 about 24.6 cases/100.000 inhabitants, which indicates 7% annual decrease (report PGPCTB 2012; www.sergas.es).

Several studies worldwide identified the following factors as the most important cause of the lack control of the disease (report PGPCTB 2003): diagnostic delay, that determines an increase in the risk of transmission of the disease (Altet, 2006); patients who have interrupted their treatment; and poor management of the disease, due to incorrect handling of the established drug regimens.

Coordinated strategies are necessary to control TB: early diagnosis and treatment, *M. tuberculosis* susceptibility analysis to specific drugs, contacts study and treatment. Moreover, is it necessary to intensify the treatment adherence?

A new strategy to control this disease called Stop TB was launched by the World Health Organization (WHO) in 2006. The first component of the Stop TB strategy, directly observed therapy, short course (DOTS) expansion and enhancement, is the cornerstone, proposed by the WHO in 1994 (WHO Stop TB Strategy, 2006). DOTS is a method of treatment administration that ensures adherence to it and which requires that a health worker or another person designated for this purpose, witness medication intake by the patient (ATS / CDC / IDSA, 2003; WHO Stop TB Strategy, 2006).

The basic components of the DOTS strategy are: political commitment with adequate and sustained financing; early case detection and diagnosis through quality-assured bacteriology; standardized treatment with supervision and patient support; effective drug supply and management; monitoring and evaluation of performance and impact (WHO Stop TB Strategy, 2006).

The Global Plan to Stop TB 2011-2015 includes the importance of the DOTS including as an indicator (6.10): "proportion of TB cases detected and cured under DOTS".

The PGPCTB, promotes the establishment of DOT, at least in certain groups of patients for their clinical and/or social characteristics, considering the progressive establishment in the following cases:

- All retreatments: including treatment failures, relapses, previously treated cases for over a month and all recovered dropouts.

- Patients with associated factors to suspect an increased risk of treatment dropout. It recommends the establishment of DOT to patients with:

  o Addiction habits (drug users and alcohol users).

  o HIV positive.

  o Without fixed residence.

  o Social distocia (people with social and/or economic problems).

  o Mental illness.

  o Immigrants.

  o Malignancies.

  o Silicosis, sailor, gastrectomy, chronic renal failure, chronic disease and low birth weight.

- All patients with resistance to at least isoniazid (H) and rifampicin (R).

- All patients with intermittent treatment.

- All patients with self-administered treatment, which have not gone to the follow-up and treatment adherence control visit.

The application of this treatment regimen in the health area of Santiago de Compostela began with the development of a structured program of health care provision in which collaborated Tuberculosis Unit (UTB) and the Pharmacy Service (PhS) of the University Hospital of Santiago de Compostela (CHUS), a program implemented in 1996 and currently in force. With this program, hereinafter "Compostela DOT", both dispensing and pharmaceutical care were conducted from the hospital.

2   Description of the "Compostela DOT"

In the diagram below lists the operating flow and resources used in TB DOT in the area of Santiago de Compostela. There is an individualized pharmaceutical provision by patient. This one has the same unit dose methodology distribution of drugs than the one used for the patients admitted in the hospital. However, the pharmaceutical provision differs in some points. The UTB doctor sends the medical order to the PhS, which validates treatment and expected duration. Once in the PhS, the information system is fulfilled with patient and treatment data. If it is possible the complete treatment is programmed. Medication is prepared in individual pillboxes with 21 holes labeled with the days of the week, 21 daily doses. The pillboxes (two per patient) are conditioned weekly and divide in three large geographic areas that provide transport and monitoring patients. Programming leads to assign the supervision area, prepare the planning treatment, compliance sheets and pillboxes. Weekly is printed a list with the drugs needed for each pillbox. The common sanitary transport systems are used for their distribution. Monitoring treatment decision is made by different professionals who are assigned by the UTB by type of TB and reason for monitoring.

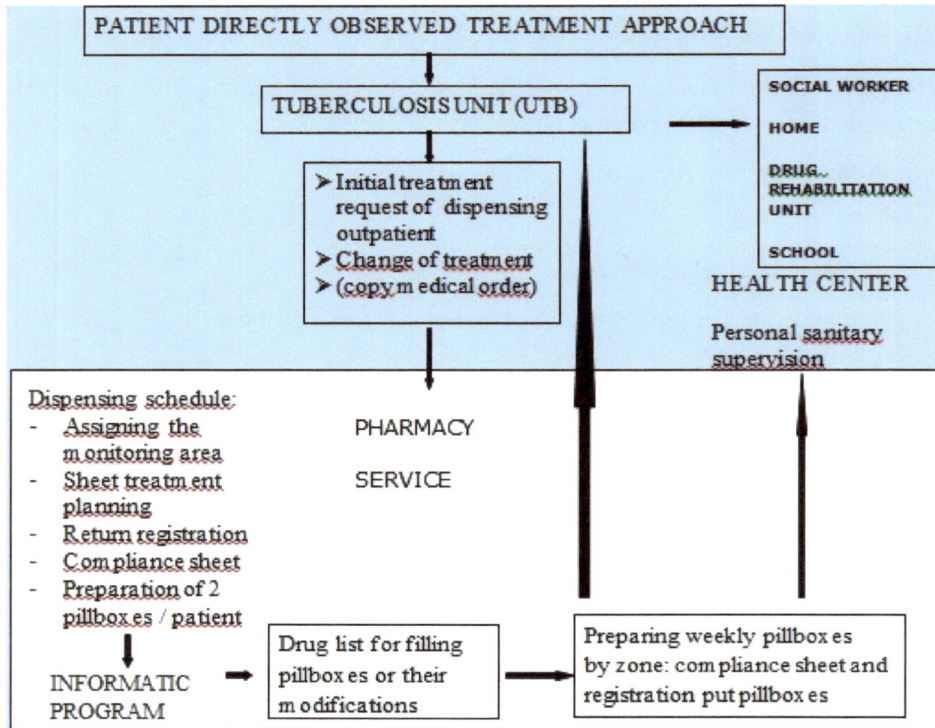

Figure 1: Operation flow diagram of the DOT

3   Results and analysis of the "Compostela DOT"

The implementation of the PGPCTB in 1996 with the creation of a register of the cases, has shown the epidemiological situation of the disease and its evolution over time, during the eleven years of the study period (1996-2006) were diagnosed in the area of Santiago de Compostela a total of 2.455 cases.

The TB rate in our health area was 19.5 cases/100,000 inhabitants in 2011. Despite this reduction, the rates are higher than expected if we consider the social and economic status of our area, and, more alarmingly, too high when compared to the rates in other Western European countries such as Germany (6.5 cases/100,000 inhabitants) or the United Kingdom (14 cases/100,000 inhabitants). Fortunately the figures are lower than the ones in Eastern European countries such as Russia (106.3 cases/100,000 inhabitants) or Georgia (143.1 cases/100,000 inhabitants) (Global Tuberculosis report 2012).

The distribution of total cases under DOT by type of TB, defined by WHO (Global Tuberculosis report 2012) over two time periods (1996–2000 and 2001–2006), is shown in Table 1.

Period	New Tuberculosis cases	Treatment after default	Relapsed	Chronic	Total
1996-2000	1263	28	98	4	1393
2001-2006	997	7	58	0	1062
Total	2260	35	156	4	2455

Table 1: Distribution of TB cases in Santiago de Compostela by period and type of tuberculosis

In the UTB of Santiago de Compostela, during the years under study, we have established 255 DOT, the 10.4% of cases of TB diagnosed and recorded in our area. This proportion is similar to other Spanish regions (Caylà *et al.*, 2009) and lowers other countries such as Canada, that with a rate of 7.5/100.000, supervise in DOT 49% of cases (Kim *et al.*, 2008). Following the guidelines of PGPCTB were monitored 100% of the cases diagnosed as chronic, 85.7% of treatment after default, 28.8% of relapsed, 7.8% of initial cases and 100% of MDRTB cases. The low rate of DOT in relapses is due to many cases have an old tuberculosis episode. Therefore, we haven´t found documented data from previous episodes when the treatment was not as effective.

The number of DOT per year over the total recorded cases depicted in Figure 2.

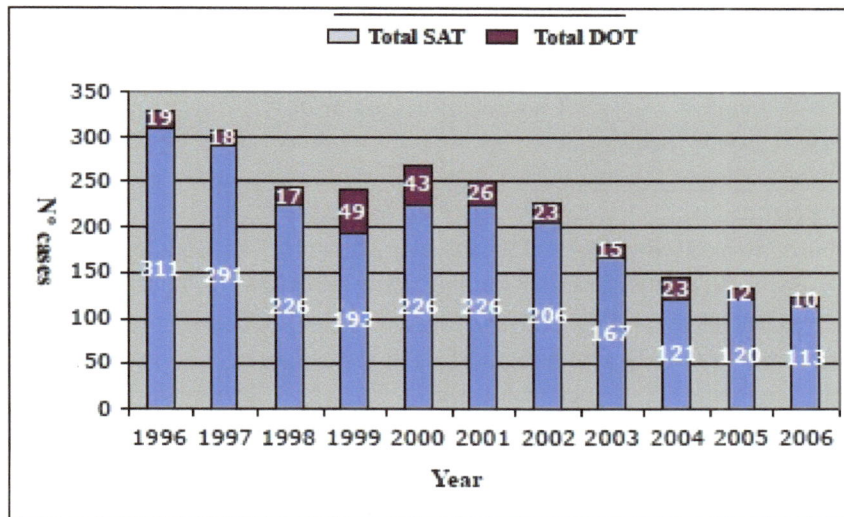

SAT: self-administered treatment; DOT: direct observed treatment

Figure 2: Evolution DOT TB cases between 1996-2006

Epidemiological characteristics of patients under DOT: The mean age of the patients was 39.67 ± 17.0 years (range: 0-83). Age groups distribution: 18 cases < 17 years, 174 between 18-50 years and 63 > 51 years. There were 23.9% women and 76.1% men under DOT. The demographic profile of the patient who was started DOT is not different to the rest of the patients diagnosed with TB in our area (Galicia TB Report, 2010). The patient profile described in the WHO report is very similar to the one shown in our patients where most were male and the average age was 39.9 years. This is consistent with the classical studies performed on populations in high TB incidence areas, which show men are in the majority and that there is a bimodal curve with a first high peak for young patients (Bayer, 1995).

Monitoring criteria: The risk of give up the treatment was the primary, 59.1% of cases; followed by retreatment cases, 31.8%, which include treatment after default, relapse and chronic cases.

Clinical characteristics: With regards to TB type, 176 (69.0%) of these patients were newly diagnosed cases and 79 (31%) were being retreated for TB. Among the latter, 30 were classified as treatments, after default, 45 were relapse cases and 4 had chronic illness.

The distribution by type of TB DOT throughout the period studied is shown in Table 2.

Period	New TB cases	Treatment after default	Relapsed	Chronic	Total
1996-2000	93	25	24	4	146
2001-2006	83	5	21	0	109
Total	**176** (69%)	**30** (11,8%)	**45**(17,6%)	**4** (1,6%)	**255** (100%)

DOT: direct observed treatment; TB: tuberculosis

Table 2: Distribution of DOT TB cases in Santiago de Compostela by period and type of tuberculosis

It is essential to know the quality of a DOT program. For this it is necessary to establish the decrease in the treatment after default rate and chronic cases of TB in the area where DOT has been implemented (Snyder & Chin, 1999). The analysis of the results shows a statistically significant decrease in the number of treatments after default and the elimination of chronic cases in the last six years of the studied period ($p < 0,05$). We believe this is an effect of treatment thorough monitoring of all cases in our area, which has not allowed the emergence of new chronic cases and has managed the reuptake of the treatment after default.

Risk factors associated with DOTS patients: The most frequently associated has been addiction habits (47.8%), factor that determines social and family problems, which in turn result in poorly performed treatments. Social dystocia, 18.4%, is the second major factor, which in our enviroment make conditional a significant percentage of poor therapeutic compliance. The analysis of risk factors - grouped into three categories: none, a risk factor and two or more risk factors- shows that were associated to a single risk factor 51.8% of cases. In the initial TB, 61.4% are associated with a single risk factor and in treatments after default 40.0%. In 53.3% of relapsed was not documented any risk factors. The HIV-infected patients in the study occupy third place, only one of them had a MDR. A recently published study evaluated the effects of a supportive intervention in patients co-infected HIV-TB, obtaining in the intervention patients better clinical outcomes and lower utilization of the health system. Moreover, in the two years of monitoring, it was determined a reduction in the use of clinical resources significantly offset the costs of the intervention (Cerda *et al.*, 2011). HIV infection has a high impact on TB epidemiology in many countries, including Spain, one of the European countries with higher AIDS and tuberculosis coinfection (Surveillance of tuberculosis in Europe -Euro TB, 2008, Global tuberculosis report 2012). However, in Galicia, from the very beginning of the PGPCTB, it has been demonstrated that TB continues to show a classical epidemiologic distribution, without the influence of HIV. The statistics reveal a coinfection rate of about 4.3% in 1996 and 3.3% in 2006. In none of the years of the study was this coinfection rate higher than 10% (Cruz & Fernandez Nogueira, 2007).

Mortality among HIV patients was 13.8%, not being the cause in any case the TB. The abandonment of these patients accounted for 10.3%, data higher than that found in a similar study in which 3.3% was observed and in which the percentage of patients with this disease is also lower than the present study (4.4% vs 10.4%) (Cayla *et al*, 2009).

TB location was pulmonary in 87,6%, 9.7% also had extrapulmonary. Primary TB represented 2,4% of the instances. The location was only extrapulmonary in 7.8% cases: pleural (35%), lymph node (30%), osteo-articular (15%) and meningitis (5%). Cases of pulmonary TB probably take priority when a TB control program is conducted because of their potential to infect others if left untreated (Murray *et al.*, 1990).

In our study, almost half of pulmonary TB evidenced cavitated forms in chest radiology; three quarters of patients had positive AFB smears. Positive AFB TB incidence is still important even though it has declined significantly during eleven years (27.1 cases/100.000 inhabitants in 1996 *vs* 9.2 cases/100.000 inhabitants in 2006). The incidence of TB pulmonar in our health area was 44.6 cases/100.000 inhabitants in 1996 and 15.8 cases/100.000 inhabitants in 2006. In our area, epidemiological data of positive AFB smear in pulmonary TB (58%) are similar to global data (56%) and a bit higher than Spanish data (43%) (Global Tuberculosis report 2012; Centro Nacional de Epidemiología, 2010). The high number of positive AFB smears in our DOT study is probably related to patient selection.

The high percentage of cavitated pulmonary tuberculosis, the incidence of positive AFB smears and the high incidence of TB in children under four years, suggest that there may be a diagnostic delay, which is making it difficult to control the disease in our environment.

Diagnostic delay, time interval since the patient feels the first symptoms of his illness until initiates an appropriate chemotherapy is an indicator for evaluating TB programs (Altet *et al.*, 2003; Altet, 2006). Until 2009, in Galicia only diagnostic delay estimates based on indirect data were possible. In 2010 a software to assess the diagnostic delay was performed. Nowadays a prospective study is ongoing.

Microbiological studies: Microscopy and culture: There was bacteriological confirmation in 197 patients (77.3%), of which 188 corresponded to pulmonary TB (83.2%), with only one bacteriological confirmation on the primary TB (16.7%) and 30.0% extrapulmonary TB.

One of the main strategies of PGPCTB is controlling the resistance of strains of *M. tuberculosis* in Galicia and consequently, the health area of Santiago de Compostela performed, in collaboration with WHO, studies of drug resistance of 1st line since 1998. From the year 2004, and by order of the Ministry of Health, antibiogram is performed on all isolates in our region. All these activities have allowed us to verify that our resistance is low (WHO / IUATLD, 2004; Pérez del Molino *et al.*, 2006; WHO / IUATLD, 2008).

Showed resistance to at least H, 8.2% and 3.9% MDR and in one case on the basis of epidemiological criteria (contact MDR), was treated as such. Three MDR strains were not viable. Although we can not post as DOT, in 2006 was MDR diagnosed post-mortem, which is included in the microbiological studies described below, by its epidemiological interest drug sensitivity studies (proportion method MIGIT 960.BD ®) and resistance genes to H and R (GenoType MTBDRplus ®) are shown in Table 3.

A novel data management system, which standardizes and improves strains study with erratic or kinetic complex, has been used in the phenotypic characterization of these resistant strains (Springer *et al*, 2009).

| N° | Year | Isoniazid | | | | Rifampicin | | S* | E | Z | ETH | OFLO 1-4* | LZ 0,5-2* | A 0,5-2* |
		H 0,1	H 0,4	*katG*	*inhA*	R	*rpoB*							
1	1996	R	R	S315T1	N	R	WT8/MUT3	S	S	S	S	≤1	1	≤0,5
2	1997	R	R	N	N	R	WT7	R	R	S	S	≤1	1	≤0,5
3	1998	R	R	S315T1	N	R	WT7/H526Y	S	S	S	S	≤1	≤0,5	≤0,5
4	1998	R	S	N	N	S	N	S	S	S	S	≤1	≤0,5	≤0,5
5	1999	R	S	N	C15T	S	N	R	S	S	S	≤1	1	≤0,5
6	2000	R	R	D	N	S	N	S	S	S	S	4	≤0,5	≤0,5
7	2000	R	R	S315T1	N	R	WT8	S	S	S	S	≤1	≤0,5	≤0,5
8	2000	R	S	N	C15T	S	N	S	S	S	S	≤1	≤0,5	≤0,5
9	2000	R	R	N	N	S	N	S	S	S	S	≤1	≤0,5	≤0,5
10	2002	R	R	N	N	S	N	S	S	S	S	≤1	≤0,5	≤0,5
11	2002	R	R	N	N	S	N	S	S	S	S	≤1	≤0,5	≤0,5
12	2003	R	R	S315T1	N	R	WT7	R	R	S	S	≤1	≤0,5	≤0,5
13	2004	R	R	S315T1	N	R	WT8	S	S	S	S	≤1	≤0,5	≤0,5
14	2005	R	R	N	N	S	N	R	S	S	S	≤1	1	≤0,5
15	2006	R	S	N	N	S	N	S	S	S	S	≤1	≤0,5	≤0,5
16	2006	R	R	S315T1	N	R	WT8	S	S	S	S	≤1	≤0,5	≤0,5
17	2006	R	R	S315T1	N	R	WT8	S	S	S	S	≤1	≤0,5	≤0,5
18	2006	R	R	S315T1	N	S	N	R	S	S	S	≤1	≤0,5	≤0,5

H: isoniazid; R: rifampicin; S*: estreptomicina; E: ethambutol; Z: pyrazinamide; ETH: ethionamide; OFLO: ofloxacin; LZ: linezolid; A: amikacin; R: resistent; S: sensible; D: no hybridization WT; WT7: codon 526-529; WT8: codon 530-533.* Concentration (ug/ml)

Table 3: Drug susceptibility study on strains resistant to isoniazide

Of the strains studied, 77.8% had high-level resistance to H, of these, 64.3% had mutations in the *kat*G gene. In 61.1% were detected changes in the genes studied: 11.1% had C15T mutation in *inh*A promoter and 50% had mutations in *kat* G (4% S315T1). 38.9% (1 MDR) did not show any changes. All MDR strains (No. 1, 2, 3, 7, 12, 13, 16, 17) exhibit variations in *rpo*B, being 22.2% identical strains which presents absence of WT8 (codon 530-533) and mutation S315T1 in *kat*G.

Regarding the 2nd line drugs, generally, only performed their susceptibility to clinical indication for MDR-TB strains. In this paper not found any XDR-TB strain, resistant strains studied maintaining high sensitivity to 2nd line drugs and linezolid. Recently, it has published a classification of tuberculosis drugs with highly practical interest for the treatment of MDR-TB (Caminero *et al.*, 2010;GPTC, 2010), which considers the fluoroquinolones (FQ) as group two, and assumes that it is one of the four groups of drugs more active for the treatment of MDR-TB (WHO Report, 2008). Between the resistant strains studied, we found a single ofloxacin resistant strain also showed resistance to isoniazid. Currently, FQs are used to treat TB with resistance and / or complications due to side effects of 1st line drugs, the increase in resistance increases the risk of treatment failure in MDR-TB (Migliori *et al.*, 2008). Recent publications include a frequency of FQ resistance of 0.5 to 1.8% (El Sahly *et al.*, 2011; Jeon *et al.*, 2011).

Quinolone use in the treatment of tuberculosis is a subject currently discussed. In our serie were used in just over a tenth of treatments and in all cases of MDR-TB; until 2000 ciprofloxacin was used, and in recent years, levofloxacin, fourth generation quinolone, which together with the moxifloxacin and gatifloxacin, are the FQs with more activity against *M. tuberculosis*. Data from published multicentre studies do not show superiority in the use of the FQs with respect to treatment regimens that include isoniazid. At present, its use for the treatment of uncomplicated TB is not approved (Ziganshina & Squire, 2008; Sanchez *et al.*, 2011).This group of antibiotics is widely used in other infections, unlike the first-line drugs for treatment of tuberculosis, particularly suitable in community-acquired pneumonia, having described a clear association of it use with the delay in the diagnosis of TB, as well as a higher risk of resistance development (Chen *et al.*, 2011).

Available data in the process of researching new drugs have found different properties of these that create expectations about future indications. Therapeutic models including high dose rifamycins and patterns which associated rifapentine with moxifloxacin or gatifloxacin might shorten the treatment of TB (Ginsberg, 2010; Sanchez *et al.*, 2011). If research and development in new TB treatments is significantly enhanced and amplified according to the strategic framework on Global Plan to Stop TB 2011-2015, the following achievements are expected by 2015: a new four-month TB treatment regimen – including one new or repurposed drug approved by regulatory authorities for drug- sensitive TB – will be recommended by WHO and available for use; two new drugs will be approved by regulatory authorities for drug-sensitive TB; at least one new drug for the treatment of drugresistant TB will be introduced into the market (Global Plan to Stop TB 2011-2015). Rapid diagnosis of TB and MDR-TB is one of the cornerstones in the control of this disease, because it allows an epidemiological and early therapeutic action. In recent years there has been significant progress in the development of new diagnostic tools, particularly molecular, for the direct diagnosis of clinical samples. These methods rely on the amplification of different nucleic acid targets for the identification of the *M. tuberculosis* and detection of chromosomal mutations most frequently associated with phenotypic resistance to various drugs. Currently, there are three commercial methods for use in clinical laboratories, two of them only detect rifampicin resistance (Ling *et al.*, 2008) and the third also detected resistance genes for the H (GenoType MTBDRplus®). The total strains tested are carriers of mutations in *rpo*B, so the technique detected 100% of strains resistant to rifampicin. This high sensitivity is consistent with data from a recently published meta-analysis, 94-100% (Ling *et al.*, 2008). Sensitivity for the detection of MDR-TB is 88.9%, however other publications detected between 73% - 89% (Hillemann *et al.*, 2005; Miotto *et al.*, 2008).

All quick techniques detected with great specificity the rifampicin resistance, so they are especially useful in areas with high rates of MDR-TB or special situations, cases of immigrant patients from areas with high resistance to this drug (Boehme *et al.*, 2010; Alcaide & Coll., 2011). By the above, it is obvious that we must always make additional confirmation of the phenotype. Although aspects such as cost-effectiveness and indications for the proper implementation of these techniques are not entirely well-established, organizations such as the WHO firmly support of the application and universal use of these new molecular methods, especially in countries with high incidence of MDR and TBXDR, and in particular, due to its characteristics, the Xpert MTB / RIF® technique (Global Plan to Stop TB 2011-2015).

Molecular typing: We carried out molecular analysis of strains by rep-PCR technique automated (DiversiLab System ®). 13 different patterns were found (72.2%); 6 strains (33.3%) had a similar pattern. The four MDR strains that showed equal resistance genes belong to this cluster. These strains had previously been confirmed to be identical by RFLP technique-6110 and belong to a cluster of Spanish distribution and previously published (Vázquez-Gallardo *et al*, 2007; Gavín *et al* 2012).

Pharmacotherapeutic characteristics: The initial treatment by type of TB are summarized in Table 4:

	New TB cases	Treatment after default	Relapsed	Chronic	Total
2HRZ+4HR	102 (85,0%)	12 (10,0%)	6 (5,0%)	0	120 (47,1%)
2HRE+7HR	10 (71,4%)	2 (14,3%)	2 (14,3%)	0	14 (5,5%)
2HRZS+4HR	0	0	1(100)	0	1 (0,4%)
2HRZE+4HR	45 (58,4%)	15 (19,5%)	17 (22,1%)	0	77 (30,2%)
OMS (2HRZES/1HRZE/5HRE)	5 (31,3%)	0	11 (68,8%)	0	16 (6,3%)
OTRO	14 (51,9%)	1 (3,7%)	8 (29,6%)	4 (14,8%)	27 (10,6%)
Total	176	30	45	4	255 (100%)

H: isoniazid; R: rifampicin; S: estreptomicin; E: ethambutol; Z: pyrazinamide

Table 4: Initial treatment patterns by type of TB (n=255).

In our series of DOT, the pattern 2RHZ + 4HR was originally instituted in more than half of the initial cases due to WHO endorses this regimen in areas where primary resistance to isoniazid is lower than 4%. In our province, resistance prevalence to H in new cases was 3,5 % (WHO/IUATLD, 2008). In a quarter of them, the initial regimen used included ethambutol also accepted by the international organizations (WHO, UICITER, ATS) whose effectiveness is well proven even in countries where drug resistance are higher than those quoted. Other standard guidelines were implemented in less than one tenth of the initial cases and in a similar percentage of cases was necessary to use second-line drugs, for reasons of resistance and / or intolerance. In these cases the patient management in DOT regime is essential due to its toxicity and route of administration.

According to WHO, appropriate first-line treatment for sensitive cases is the best way to prevent the acquisition of drug resistance. Primary transmission may be stopped with the identification in time of resistant cases and the use of appropriate treatment regimes. DOT implementation strategies for the treatment of resistant cases would act in a synergistic manner to eliminate most of the potential sources of transmission of drug-resistant tuberculosis (GPCT 2010; WHO report, 2006).

In the treatment after default cases, standard guidelines were initially used in most cases, being somewhat lower percentage in the case of relapses. Highlight that more than a half of the OMS patterns have been set up in recidive patients. In chronic cases, proper guidelines were designed to the results of susceptibility and previous history of drug use, as three of them were MDR.

The average duration of treatment for all cases was 8.0 months (SD = 4.4) with a range of 1-33 months. For chronic average duration was 23.0 months (SD: 7.0, range: 18-33).

The initial regimen remains 2HRZ +4HR majority also as final pattern, 89 (34.9%). The initial pattern 2HRZE + 4HR is established unchanged in 50 cases (19.6%). In more than one third of cases of DOT treatment modifications were made. 29.3% prolonged treatment and in a fourth of these cases, the change of treatment was due to treatment after default. Note that in the final guidelines in 23 (9%) of the pattern of "other drugs" was introduced levofloxacin.

Only 2.3% of patients were treated in an intermittent drug administration schedule. Intermittent regimens have shown to be as effective as the ones based on once-daily administration and are, as well, the less costly option (Mwandumba & Squire, 2001). Therefore, in our case, the increased use of intermittent treatments have cheapened the cost of DOT, but not have the resources for comprehensive monitoring, that is required to ensure the appropriate treatment. Studies have also shown that intermittent regimens do not increase the rate of TB drug resistance (Alvarez *et al.*, 2009). Now that some of these infrastructure problems have been solved, it would be very interesting to implement this kind of regimen (Mejuto *et al.*, 2010).

Adverse reactions have been reported in 9.0% of the series, being majority hepatotoxicity, forcing, in 57.1% of cases to change treatment because of intolerance, in line with data published by Tostmann et al (2008). In general, the treatments were well tolerated.

Hospital admissions: 43% of DOT cases resulted in hospitalization, corresponding to the first five years of the study, 65.2% There was a statistically significant reduction in hospital admissions in the second period of the study (p <0,05).

The **recurrence** in the study period was 1.5%. This parameter is a useful indicator of treatment efficacy under the DOT strategy. Few studies carried out under routine program conditions have reported disease recurrence. Published values range from 0% to 14% (Cox *et al.*, 2008). In our series, the recurrence is low, indicating the efficacy of the program. Given the high difficulty to achieve adherence to treatment in this group of patients, even in two cases, a court order was necessary to ensure therapeutic compliance, we believe that our results are good.

Places of treatment supervision: In the UTB were monitored 36.5% of the DOT and in primary care centers, 28.2%. A case of TB relapse was monitored in hospital admission by court order.

UTB both as primary health care centers the percentage of cases with two or more risk factors was higher than in the rest of the monitoring locations. Notably, 40.6% of patients without any risk factors in the monitoring carried out by a family member. If we regroup the monitoring sites: drug unit, school and hospital as a new variable "*others*", we obtain statistically significant differences (p = 0.006). In ideal conditions, treatment monitoring should be performed by health personnel but not always is possible due to multiple factors, including the enormous dispersion of the population. UTB team is the one that decides the appropriateness of monitoring place. Successful cases have been similar in the health center, social services and the family follow-up. Similar data were obtained by other authors (Wandwalo *et al.*, 2004; Lwilla *et al.*, 2003; Wright *et al.*, 2004; Newell *et al.*, 2006). However, the percentage is somewhat lower in the case of UTB, possibly due to the difficulty of cases monitored by it.

Final status of the treatment and the case: There were 88.6% of cases with completed treatment, of whom 36.1% had a treatment modification. 70.7% were treatment changes (16.9% was due medication intolerance and 7.7% drug resistance) and 29.3% treatment prolongation. Treatment discontinuation was documented in 11.4%, being the major causes, mortality from other causes (3.5%) and the transfer of area 8 (3.1%).

The highest percentage of cases with interruption of the treatment was observed in the relapses (22.2%), while the highest percentage completed treatment was found in the treatment after default (66.7%).

Within the monitoring criteria, interruption of the treatment was found in retreatment cases and risk of abandonment (16% vs 10.6% respectively). The highest percentage of completed treatment was observed in the risk of abandonment group (58.9%). Modification of treatment was done in the total of cases of non-compliance of self-administered treatment (SAT), also performed in 90% of cases of resistance to H and R. Statistically significant differences were observed in relation to the final status of the case between the two main reasons for monitoring: retreat and risk of abandonment (p = 0.027).

DOT cases with 2 or more risk factors interrupted their treatment by 26.1% compared to 7.7% observed among those with one or no risk factors. The highest percentage of cases who completed treatment was found among those with one risk factor, 61.4% (p = 0.001). The percentage of cases with satisfactory resolution was lower in those with two or more risk factors (71.7% vs 90.3%), and this group also increased mortality (13.0%) and potentially unsatisfactory cases (15.2%) (p = 0.011).

	Final status of the treatment				
	Completed treatment	Treatment modification	Treatment interruption	Total	p value
Type of TB					
Initial	92 (52,3%)	68 (38,6%)	16 (9,1%)	176	0,066(*)
Treatment after default	20 (66,7%)	7 (23,3%)	3 (10,0%)	30	
Relapsed	21 (46,7%)	14 (31,1%)	10 (22,2%)	45	
Chronic	1 (25%)	3 (75%)	0	4	
Total	134 (52,5%)	92 (36,1%)	29 (11,4%)	255 (100%)	
Monitoring criteria					
Retreatment	43 (53,1%)	25 (30,9%)	13 (16,0%)	81	
Risk of give-up	89 (58,9%)	46 (30,5%)	16 (10,6%)	151	
Resistance H and/or R	1 (10%)	9 (90%)	0	10	
Non-compliance of self-administered treatment (SAT)	0	6 (100%)	0	6	
Medical motive	1 (14,3%)	6 (85,7%)	0	7	
Total	134 (52,5%)	92 (36,1%)	29 (11,4%)	255(100%)	
N° risk factors					
None	33 (42,9%)	37 (48,1%)	7 (0,1%)	77	0,001
1	81 (61,4%)	41 (31,1%)	10 (7,6%)	132	
≥ 2	20 (43,5%)	14 (30,4%)	12 (26,1%)	46	
Total	134 (52,5%)	92 (36,1%)	29 (11,4%)	255(100%)	

TB: tuberculosis; H: isoniazid; R: rifampicin.

p (*) Analysis excluding the 4 chronic cases.

Table 5: DOT final status of the treatment related with clinical endpoints.

HIV-positive patients had a higher percentage of treatment interruptions (31.0% vs 8.8%) and a lower percentage of completed treatment (27.6% vs 55.8%) compared to the uninfected. These differences were statistically significant (p = 0.0001). Also, a higher percentage of unsatisfactory cases (20.7% vs 5.3%) and higher mortality compared to non-infected (13.8% vs 4.9%) (p = 0.001).

Final status of the case was satisfactory in 87.1% (157 of initial TB cases, 35 relapse, 26 treatment after default, 4 chronic), with 4.7% bacteriological cure. Potentially unsatisfactory cases (7.1%) corresponded to a transfer of area 44.4%, so we do not know the final outcome. Final status of the case presents statistically significant differences between the initial cases, treatment after default and relapses (p = 0.007). In the seven cases of abandonment (2.8%) should be noted that three cases were infected with HIV and three were drug users, each with multiple social factors that conditioned a high risk of default. WHO estimates the abandonment of TB treatment between 1-20%, but these figures vary greatly in selected populations (Alvarenga & Veleres, 2008). In our work, the abandonment rate observed is lower than in other studies (2.8% vs 7.1%) (Caylà *et al.*, 2009), taking into account, in addition, that the above study excluded patients with known resistances. Potentially unsatisfactory results by type of TB have been higher in cases of treatment after default, being these statistically significant results.

Overall mortality was 5.9%, representing the greater part of the cases, patients with two or more risk factors and relapses, among the latter are the totality of deaths due to TB (1.2%), one MDR. Of the

12 with no mortality associated with TB, 5 of them were immunocompromised patients (4 HIV-infected and 1 neoplasm), all aged 25-40 years; another 4 cases (33.3%) correspond to patients with more than 65 years and comorbidities.

In 90.5% of tuberculosis resistant to at least H was obtained a satisfactory result, with the mortality rate of 9.5% (as only one death from TB). Within the subgroup of patients with MDR in 80.0% was obtained a satisfactory result, with 20% mortality. Published data show higher mortality for this group of patients, the figures are closer to 30% (Cox *et al.*, 2006).

	Final status of the case				
	Satisfactory	**Death**	**Potentially unsatisfactory**	**Total**	**p valor**
Type of TB					
Initial	157 (89,2%)	6 (3,4%)	13 (7,4%)	176	
Treatment after default	26 (86,7%)	1 (3,3%)	3 (10,0%)	30	0,007 (*)
Relapsed	35 (77,8%)	8 (17,8%)	2 (4,4%)	45	
Chronic	4 (100%)	0	0	4	
Total	222 (87,1%)	15 (5,9%)	18 (7,1%)	255 (100%)	
Monitoring criteria					
Retreatment	67 (82,7%)	9 (11,1%)	5 (6,2%)	81	
Risk of give-up	135 (89,4%)	4 (2,6%)	12 (7,9%)	151	
Resistance H and/or R	10 (100%)	0	0	10	0,027 (**)
Non-compliance of self-administered treatment (SAT)	5 (83,3%)	1 (16,1)	0	6	
Medical motive	5 (71,4%)	1 (14,3%)	1 (14,3%)	7	
Total	222 (87,1%)	15 (5,9%)	18 (7,1%)	255 (100%)	
N° risk factors					
None	69 (89,6%)	5 (6,5%)	3 (3,9%)	77	
1	120 (90,9%)	4 (3,0%)	8 (6,1%)	132	0,011
≥2	33 (71,7%)	6 (13%)	7 (15,2%)	46	
Total	222 (87,1%)	15 (5,9%)	18 (7,1%)	255 (100%)	
HIV					
Yes	19 (65,5%)	4 (13,8%)	6 (20,7%)	29	
No	203 (89,8%)	11 (4,9%)	12 (5,3%)	226	0,001
Total	222 (87,1%)	15 (5,9%)	18 (7,1%)	255 (100%)	

TB: tuberculosis; H: isoniazid; R: rifampicin;
p (*) Analysis excluding the 4 chronic cases.
p (**) Analysis between the 2 major monitoring criteria (retreatment and risk of give-up)

Table 6: DOT final status of the case related with clinical endpoints.

4   Conclusions

The foremost strategy of the WHO to achieve TB control is to apply DOTS to every single TB patient (Bayer, 1995). As this recommendation addresses mainly the poorest countries of the world, every country needs to adapt this WHO proposal to its own social, epidemiologic, and economic situation (Mejuto *et al.*, 2010). All experts in TB management agree that there are great difficulties in distinguishing patients "reliable" of the "non-reliable" because of the many factors of individual, family, social, cultural or even healthcare may be involved in the complex issue of therapeutic compliance. The duration of treatment and the number of drugs administered are also factors that affect compliance. Although DOTS is not used in all cases of the disease, it is important to determine the groups which it is necessary to establish this treatment regimen (WHO Resolution WHA53.1, 2000; WHO Stop TB Strategy, 2006).

The WHO report 2008 shows that DOTS has a very different distribution throughout Europe, ranging from 0% to 100% (67% average). The statistics in this report emphasize that Western European countries, with low TB incidence, do not use the DOTS strategy (WHO report, 2008).

The provision of diagnosis and treatment according to the DOTS/Stop TB Strategy has resulted in major achievements in TB care and control. Between 1995 and 2011, 51 million people were successfully treated for TB in countries that had adopted the DOTS/ Stop TB Strategy, saving 20 million lives (Global Tuberculosis report 2012). "Compostela DOT" allows optimize health care resources. The preparation of medication is centralized in the Hospital Pharmacy Service, with a distribution in unit dose system, according to a schedule adapted to the geographical dispersion of the area, reducing the resources required for outpatient management as well as the global cost of the monitoring.

The introduction of the DOT strategy, together with strict control and follow-up of all TB diagnoses in our health area, has combined to reduce the illness incidence rate of TB, which ranged from 72.7 cases/100.000 inhabitants in 1996 to 27.1 cases/100.000 inhabitants in 2006. Even so, we are far from achieving total TB control. The TB needs from the perspective of the time to be able to analyze results and trends. The epidemiological results of these eleven years, demonstrate that possibly the selected groups were the suitable ones. On the other hand a recent publication realized by a group of pneumogists of the SEPAR, pleads for restoring DOT in the same groups of patient who decided the PGPCTB in 1995 (Cayla *et al.*, 2009). "Compostela DOT", given the good results obtained, it remains, with identical characteristics, effective today.

References

Alcaide F , Coll P. (2011). *Advances in rapid diagnosis of tuberculosis disease and anti-tuberculous drug resistance. Enferm Infecc Microbiol Clin, 29(Supl 1): 54-60.*

Altet Gómez MN, Alcalde Megías J, Canela Soler J, Milá Augé MA, Jiménez Fuentes ML, de Souza Galvao ML, Solsona Pereiró J. (2003). *Estudio del retraso diagnóstico de la tuberculosis pulmonar sintomática. Arch Bronconeumol.: 39: 146–152.*

Altet N. (2006). *Retraso diagnóstico en tuberculosis. Enf Emerg., 8: 163–168.*

Alvarez TA, Rodrigues MP, Viegas CA. (2009). *Prevalence of drug-resistant Mycobacterium tuberculosis in patients under intermittent or daily treatment. J Bras Pneumol., 35: 555–560.*

Alvarenga PE, Veleres J. (2008). *Meta-analysis of factors related to health services that predict treatment default by tuberculosis patients. Cad.Saúde Pública Río de Janeiro., 24 Sup 4: S485-S502.*

Bayer DW. (1995). Directly observed therapy for tuberculosis: history of an idea. Lancet, 345: 1545-1548.

Boehme C, Nabeta P, Hillemann D, Nicol MP, Shenai S, Krapp F,Allen J, Tahirli R, Blakemore R, Rustomjee R, Milovic A et al (2010). Rapid molecular detection of tuberculosis and rifanpin resistance. N Engl J Med, 363: 1005-15.

Caminero JA, Sotgiu G, Zumla A, Migliori GB. (2010). Best drug treatment for multidrug-resistant and extensively drug-resistant tuberculosis. Lancet Infect Dis, 10: 621–29.

Caylà JA, Rodrigo T, Ruiz-Manzano J, Caminero JA, Vidal R, García JM, Blanquer R, Casals M. (2009). Working Group on Completion of Tuberculosis Treatment in Spain (Study ECUTTE). Tuberculosis treatment adherence and fatality in Spain. Respir Res Dec 1; 10:12.

Centro Nacional de Epidemiología. (2010). Situación de la tuberculosis en España. Casos de tuberculosis declarados a la Red Nacional de Vigilancia Epidemiológica en 2009. Boletín epidemiológico. Vol. 18 n° 22/213-220 ISSN: 1135 – 6286.

Cerda R, Muñoz M, Zeladita J, Wong M, Sebastian JL, Bonilla C, Bayona J, Sanchez E, Arevalo J, Caldas A, Shin S. (2011). Health care utilization and costs of a support program for patients living with the human immunodeficiency virus and tuberculosis in Peru. Int J Tuberc Lung Dis, 15(3):363-368.

Chen TC, Lu PL, Lin CY, Lin WR, Chen YH. (2011). Fluoroquinolones are associated with delayed treatment and resistance in tuberculosis: a systematic review and meta-analysis. Int J Infect Dis, 15 (3), 211-216.

Cruz E, Fernández-Nogueira E. (2007). Epidemiology of tuberculosis in Galicia, Spain, 1996–2005. Int J Tuberc Lung Dis, 11: 1073–1079.

Gavín P, Iglesias MJ, Jiménez MS, Rodríguez-Valín E, Ibarz D, Lezcano MA, Revillo MJ, Martín C, Samper S; Spanish Working Group on MDR-TB. (2012). Long-term molecular surveillance of multidrug-resistant tuberculosis in Spain.Infect Genet Evol., 12(4):701-10.

Ginsberg AM. Drugs in development for tuberculosis. (2010). Drugs, 70 (17):2201-14.

Grupo de trabajo de la Guía de Práctica Clínica sobre el Diagnóstico, el Tratamiento y la Prevención de la Tuberculosis (GPTC). (2010). Centro Cochrane Iberoamericano, coordinador. Guía de Práctica Clínica sobre el Diagnóstico, el Tratamiento y la Prevención de la Tuberculosis. DL: B-3745-2010.

El Sahly H, Teeter LD, Jost KC Jr, Dunbar D, Lew J, Graviss EA. (2011). Incidence of Moxifloxacin Resistance in Clinical Mycobacterium tuberculosis Isolates in Houston. J Clin. Microbio, Jun. JCM.00231-11.

Hillemann D, Weizenegger M, Kubica T, Richter E, Niemann S. (2005). Use of the genotype MTBDR assay for rapid detection of rifampin and isoniazid resistance in Mycobacterium tuberculosis complex isolate Mycobacterium tuberculosis complex isolates. J Clin Microbiol, 43: 3699–3703.

Informe de tuberculose en Galicia. (Galicia TB report). (2010). Características dos casos de tuberculose de Galicia dos anos 2007 e 2008. Evolución no período 1996-2008. Ed. Xunta de Galicia, Consellería de Sanidade, Dirección Xeral de Saúde Pública e Planificación. DL: C8-2010.

Informe do programa galego de prevención e control da tuberculose (report PGPCTB). (2012). Evolución no período 1996-2011. Ed. Xunta de Galicia, Consellería de Sanidade, Dirección Xeral de Saúde Pública e Planificación.

Informe do programa galego de prevención e control da tuberculose (report PGPCTB). (2003). Documentos Técnicos de Saúde Pública. Ed. Xunta de Galicia. Consellería de Sanidade. Dirección Xeral de Saúde Pública. Santiago de Compostela, 2003. ISBN: 84-453-3763-X.

Jeon CY, Calver AD, Victor TC, Warren RM, Shin SS, Murray MB. (2011). Use of fluoroquinolone antibiotics leads to tuberculosis treatment delay in a South African gold mining community. Int J Tuberc Lung Dis, 15(1): 77-83.

Kim J, Langevin M, Wylie EL, McCarthy AE. (2008). The epidemiology of tuberculosis in Ottawa, Canada, 1995-2004. Int J Tuberc Lung Dis, 12(10):1128-33.

Ling DI, Zwerling AA, Pai M. (2008). GenoType MTBDR for the diagnosis of multidrug-resistant tuberculosis: a meta-analysis. Eur Respir J, 32: 1165-1174.

Lwilla F, Schellenberg D, Masanja H, Acosta C, Galindo C, Aponte J. (2003). Evaluation of efficacy of community-based vs. institutional-based direct observed short-course treatment for the control of tuberculosis in Kilombero district, Tanzania. Tropical Medicine and International Health, 8(3): 204-10.

Mejuto B, Tuñez V, Pérez del Molino ML, García R. (2010). Characterization and evaluation of the directly observed treatment for tuberculosis in Santiago de Compostela (1996-2006). Risk Manag Health Policy, 3:21-6. doi: 10.2147/RMHP.S8921. Epub 2010 Jun 22.

Migliori GB, Lange C, Girardi E, Centis R, Besozzi G, Kliiman K, Codecasa LR, Spanevello A, Cirillo DM; SMI-RA/TBNET Study Group. (2008). Fluoroquinolones: are they essential to treat multidrug-resistant tuberculosis? Eur Respir J, 31: 904–10.

Miotto P, Piana F, Cirillo DM, Migliori GB. (2008). Genotype MTBDRplus: a further step toward rapid identification of drug-resistant Mycobacterium tuberculosis. J Clin Microbiol, 46: 393–394.

Mwandumba HC, Squire SB. (2001). Fully intermittent dosing with drugs for treating tuberculosis in adults. Cochrane Database Syst Rev. (4): CD000970.

Newell JN, Baral SC, Pande SB, Bam DS, Malla P. (2006). Family-member el TODS and community el TODS for tuberculosis control in Nepal: cluster-randomised controlled trial. Lancet, 367(9514): 903-9.

Pérez del Molino ML, Túnez V, Pardo F, Cortizo S, Romero PA. (2006). Drugs resistance of Mycobacterium tuberculosis in Santiago de Compostela, Spain (2002-2005). 25th ICCS/17th ECCMID.Munich/Germany 31 March-3 April.

Programa galego de prevencion e control da tuberculose (PGPCTB). (1995). Documentos Tecnicos de Saúde Pública. Xunta de Galicia. Consellería de Sanidade e Servicios Sociais. Direccion Xeral de Saude Publica. Santiago de Compostela. ISBN: 84-453-1379-7.

Sanchez F, López Colomés JL, Villarino E, Grosset J. (2011). New drugs for tuberculosis treatment. Enf Infecc Microbiol Clin, 29(Supl 1):47-56.

Servicio Galego de Saúde. SERGAS. www.sergas.es

Snyder D, Chin D. (1999). Cost-effectiveness analysis of Directly Observed Therapy for patients with tuberculosis at low risk for treatment default. Am J Respir Care Med, 160: 582-6.

Springer, B., K. Lucke, R. Calligaris-Maibach, C. Ritter, and E. C. Böttger. (2009). Quantitative drug susceptibility testing of Mycobacterium tuberculosis by use of MGIT 960 and EpiCenter instrumentation. J. Clin. Microbiol, 47: 1773–1780.

Tostmann A, Boeree MJ, Aarnoutse RE, de Lange WC, van der Ven AJ, Dekhuijzen R. (2008). Antituberculosis drug-induced hepatotoxicity: concise up-to-date review. J Gastroenterol Hepatol, 23(2):192-202.

Vázquez-Gallardo R, Anibarro L, Fernández-Villar A, Díaz-Cabanela D, Cruz-Ferrro E, ML Pérez del Molino, Tuñez V, Samper S, Iglesias MJ. (2007). Multidrug-resistant tuberculosis in a low-incidence region shows a high rate of transmission. Int J Tuberc Lung Dis, 11(4): 429–435.

Wandwalo E, Kapalata N, Egwaga S, Morkve O. (2004). Effectiveness of community-based directly observed treatment for tuberculosis in an urban setting in Tanzania: a randomised controlled trial. Int J Tuberc Lung Dis, 8(10): 1248-54.

WHO. Resolution WHA53.1. Stop Tuberculosis Initiative. In: Fifty-third World Health Assembly. Geneva, 15-20 May 2000. Resolutions and decisions. Geneva, 2000. WHA53/2000/REC/1, Annex: 1-2.

WHO. Global tuberculosis report 2012. 1.Tuberculosis – epidemiology. 2.Tuberculosis, Pulmonary – prevention and control. 3.Tuberculosis – economics. 4.Directly observed therapy. 5.Treatment outcome. 6.National health programs – organization and administration. 7.Statistics. I.World Health Organization. ISBN 978 92 4 156450 2.

WHO. Global tuberculosis control: surveillance, planing and financing. WHO Report 2006. World Health Organization Document, 2006. WHO/HTM/TB/2006.362.

WHO. Stop TB Partnership. The Stop TB Strategy. Building on and enhancing DOTS to meet the TB-related Millennium Development Goals. Geneva, 2006. WHO/HTM/TB/2006.368.

WHO. Global tuberculosis control: surveillance, planning, financing: WHO report 2008. WHO/HTM/TB/2008.393".

WHO. Anti-tuberculosis drug resistance in the world : fourth global report. The WHO/IUATLD Global proyect on Antituberculosis drug resistance surveillance 2002-2007. WHO/HTM/TB/2008.394.

WHO. The Global Plan To Stop TB 2011-2015. World Health Organization Document, 2010. Availabe in: http://www.stoptb.org/global/plan/

Wright J, Walley J, Phillip A, Pushpananthan S, Dlamini E, Newell J, et al. (2004). Direct observation of treatment for tuberculosis: a randomized controlled trial of community health workers versus family members. Tropical Medicine and International Health, 9(5):559-65.

Ziganshina LE, Squire SB. (2008). Fluoroquinolones for treating tuberculosis. Cochrane Database Syst Rev.Jan 23;(1):CD004795.

Directly Observed Treatment in Santiago de Compostela (Galicia): Cost Analysis

Beatriz Mejuto
Pharmacy Department
Hospital da Costa, Burela, Spain

Victoria Tuñez
Tuberculosis Unit , Preventive Medicine Department
Complexo Hospitalario Universitario de Santiago, Santiago de Compostela, Spain

Pilar Gayoso
Clinical Epidemiology Department
Complexo Hospitalario Universitario de Santiago, Santiago de Compostela, Spain

María Luisa Pérez del Molino
Microbiology Department
Complexo Hospitalario Universitario de Santiago, Santiago de Compostela, Spain

Rosario García-Ramos
Pharmacy Department
Complexo Hospitalario Universitario de Santiago, Santiago de Compostela, Spain

1   Introduction

Healthcare is a fundamental human right and, therefore, one of the priority commitments that governments must approach in political actions. Pharmacological therapies are an essential element of healthcare programs because of their impact on the prognosis of many diseases. Diseases have effects on health and resource use, either in health care or social services. Therefore, in addition to the health relevancy, diseases have a significant economic impact.

Cost of illness studies together with epidemiological studies of morbidity and mortality allow to know the magnitude of the problem. Globally, infectious diseases are considered to be of moderate costs, although there are exceptions, such as AIDS or hepatitis C which are considered more expensive by the high consumption of costly therapies and the indirect costs involved (Domínguez-Gil, 2009).

The aim of economic assessments of health care technologies and interventions is to promote more rational choices and to select the options with health benefits at lower costs. The real costs of a disease are not always easy to quantify. Direct costs (diagnostic tests, staff wages, costs of stay, etc.) are easier to measure than indirect costs and other consequences, such as pain or disability. For tuberculosis (TB), significant indirect costs are generated for society due to loss of productivity by morbidity and premature death, especially in developing countries (WHO Stop sign TB iniciative, 2000; WHO Stop sign TB Partnership, 2013).

The essential factor for controlling TB consists of ensuring sufficient adherence to antituberculous chemotherapy. A high percentage of patients discontinue treatment prematurely. The Stop TB Strategy, launched by WHO in 2006, builds on and enhances directly observed treatments (DOT) to address new challenges and to expand access to the most vulnerable populations. It also requires addressing TB/HIV, MDR-TB and the needs of the poor and vulnerable; contributing to strengthening health systems; engaging all health- care providers; empowering people with TB and their communities and promoting research. In addition to its positive impact on the health status of patients with TB, DOT provide economic benefits, direct savings generated by lower use of complex and expensive health services, and indirect savings by increasing productivity through patients quality of life improvements.

Economic assessments offer a way to compare different options of treatment regarding their costs and health outcomes. There are diverse strategies of assessment and practice measures to value the costs of DOT programs. Retrospective studies, case-control, prediction-forecast and cost-effectiveness analyses are the most widely used. Cost effectiveness studies can be used to compare the cost impact of different therapeutic strategies in a specific disease. For TB, DOT has been shown to be more cost-effective than self-administered therapy (SAT) (Chaulk *et al.*, 2000). In addition to the quality of the DOT programs, two key factors associated with the cost-effectiveness of DOT are the low treatment dropout rate and relapse rate (Snyder & Chin, 1999; Sanz, 2001).

Most of the economic studies related to DOT have been performed in low income countries or middle income countries, where TB is a major problem and WHO has targeted their efforts more intensely (Jacquet *et al.*, 2006, Vassall *et al.*, 2009; Cerda *et al.*, 2011). The present study was conducted in Santiago de Compostela, where healthcare is public and the management of TB, including DOT, is performed by the unit of tuberculosis (UTB) (Mejuto B *et al, 2010*; Garcia Ramos R *et al.*, 2001). After each DOT prescription the supply of TB drugs is performed individually per patient at the hospital pharmacy service. The DOT program model in this area is described by Mejuto (Mejuto *et al.*, 2014).

This study aims, firstly, to assess the costs of the DOT program considering its various components and to assess its results; and secondly, to determine where the same patients would be compared to a theoretical model of self-administered treatments (SAT) with the assumption of the same treatment outcomes.

2   Economic Assessment Study

We studied the costs of DOT introduced by the UTB in Santiago de Compostela (453.068 population) between 1996 and 2006. There were 2455 cases of TB diagnosed in this area between 1996 and 2006, among these, 255 DOT were applied. Following the guidelines of the Galician Program for Prevention and Control of Tuberculosis (PGPCTB) (PGPCTB, 1995), those patients constituted the study population. The study was approved by the Clinical Research Ethics Committee of Galicia. Definitions by type of TB are defined by WHO (Global Tuberculosis Report, 2012).

2.1   Estimated Costs

The perspective used was that of the Spanish Health Care System. It included direct healthcare costs per patient. The costs of diagnostic tests, consultations and hospital stays related to TB was estimated based on costs of health services provided by the health administration for 2006 (DOGA, num. 141, do 21 xullo 2006[1]). Microbiological determinations costs (smear, culture and antibiogram) are represented by the real costs spent by the Microbiology Department.

	Unitary cost (Euros)	Nº	Cost (Euros)
Mantoux	3.6	1	3.6
Smear	1.8	3	5.4
Culture (with identification)	31.2	3	93.6
Antibiogram	61.6	1	61.6
Radiography	29.0	1	29.0
CBC	2.2	1	2.2
Biochemistry	4.1	1	4.1
Medical consultation	141.1	1	141.1
Nurse consultation	11.7	2	23.4
First total			364.1

Monthly cost	Unitary cost (Euros)	Nº/Month	Cost (Euros)
Smear	1.8	3	5.4
Culture (without identification)	14.4	3	43.1
Radiography	29.0	0.5	14.5
CBC	2.2	1	2.2
Biochemistry	4.1	1	4.1
Medical consultation	47.0	1	47.0
Nurse consultation	11.7	1	11.7
Monthly cost			128.1

Table 1: Costs of first consultation and follow-up for an initial TB case.

---

[1] http://www.xunta.es/dog/Publicados/2006/20060721/Anuncio14BAA_gl.pdf

1) First consultation diagnosis cost of an initial case and follow-up

The costs of diagnosis at the first visit after the initiation are identical for standard cases, chronic or relapsing cases, but are higher in MDR-TB.

2) Drug therapy costs

We used the actual purchase prices for the hospital in 2006 based on official manufacture sale price (OMSP) minus trade discounts applied to each drug by provider plus value added tax (VAT).

3) Costs for drug dispensation from the hospital pharmacy (HPh)

Unit dose system of medication distribution and pharmaceutical care were used to prepare TB drugs for patients. To calculate dispensation costs relative value units (RVU), listed in Table 2, were applied. (TECNO Group, 2009, JR Glass & Anderson KP., 2002).

RVU	Value
Unit dose system dispensing line	1
1st Pharmaceutical care consultation	39.58
Pharmacist dispensing time per line	0.4180
Technician dispensing time per line	0.6000
Orderly dispensing time per line	0.0680

Table 2: Values of Relative Value Units (RVU) to calculate dispesing cost.

The personnel costs were calculated considering average salary for each staff member involved (pharmacist, technician, administrative and orderly) and minutes worked per year, to get the cost per minute. Multiplying these costs by the RVU corresponding to the time unit dose dispensing (in minutes) we obtained the cost per line dispensed for each category of staff. The total dispensing line cost was obtained by summing all the previously estimated costs.

Depending on the duration of the treatment and the particular subsequent treatment line, specific costs were obtained. To calculate the total costs, the costs of pharmaceuticals at the first consultation (AF) were added for the whole study and patient treatment planning.

4) Supervision cost

Costs per month and total treatment were calculated for the professional (physician, nurse or social worker) assuring drug intake, according to the time involved and the professional wage. We calculated this activity as a lump-sum of a three minutes commitment (preparation, observation and recording of drug administration) and the costs per minute were calculated for each supervisor category.

5) Costs of hospital stays

The days of hospital stays were collected based on the hospital health information system-history-(HIS). The costs of hospital stays were calculated by multiplying the days of hospitalization by the cost of one day stay.

2.2   Cost Analysis of Directly Observed Treatment (DOT) in Comparison to Self-administered Treatment (SAT)

For each case of DOT evaluated applying the above criteria we calculated the cost of a SAT based on a theoretical model. Thus, for each case, we assumed that monitoring cost (the number of consultations and diagnostic tests) would be the same as for the equivalent SAT. Drug therapy costs in case of SAT corresponded to the official fixed price sale to the public (PSP) without pharmacy discount because, in this case, the medication would be administered at the community pharmacy. Since they are drugs prescribed on official recipe and the Spanish health care system assumes the whole cost, we considered the whole rate. The cost of dispensing to be hold at the community pharmacy is included in the final price of the drug. The prices applied were those at the Catálogo Oficial de Medicamento del Consejo Oficial de Farmacéuticos del 2006. Therefore it is assumed that the cost differences are related to the costs of dispensing, acquisition and supervision, and that health outcomes would be the same for DOT and SAT, why it is considered a cost-minimization study.

2.3   Statistical Analyses

The Statistical Package for Social Sciences (SPSS) for the Windows version 15.0 (SPSS, Chicago, IL, USA) and Microsoft Excel were used for data analysis. Quantitative variables were characterised by mean and standard deviation (SD). Quantitative variables were compared using Student's t-test or its non-parametric equivalent, the Mann Whitney U-test and bivariate analysis (ANOVA and chi-square) to compare quantitative variables of more than two groups and qualitative variables. Categorical variables expressed as absolute frequency and percentage and were compared using the χ^2 or Fisher's exact test, and the Mann Whitney U test for non-normally distributed continuous variables. Differences with a p value < 0.05 were considered statistically significant.

3   Economic evaluation

3.1   Disease Costs

The total costs of the program were € 2,412,172: 19.8% clinical follow-up, 2.5% drugs, 0.3% dispensing and pharmaceutical care, 1.6% supervision/ observation, and 75.8% hospitalization (Table 3). The average cost per case is € 16,326 (SD 20,509). The average total cost of treatment was € 9,455 DOT (SD 16,102).

Whereas 112 cases (43.9%) were hospitalized, we examined the average cost of DOT treatment. Excluding, hospitalization, the average cost was € 2,280.0 (SD: 1,406.8). Hospitalization costs were higher in the first study period (1996 – 2000) than in the second (2001 – 2006); these differences were statistically significant (p < 0.05).

3.2   Cost analysis of DOT compared to self-administered treatment (SAT)

The results of the costs for the theoretical SAT cohort and the cost difference with the corresponding DOT are shown in Table 4 according to the type of TB.

Cases with relapse are supposed to cause the highest difference in average between DOT and a theoretical SAT, in favour of the first one. This difference is lower in the case of the new TB cases, however also in favour of the DOT.

According to type of TB, treatments of initial TB cases were the least expensive and chronic ones the most costly	New TB cases	Treatment after default	Relapsed	Chronic	Entire cohort	%
Nº Cases	176	30	45	4	255	
Clinical follow-up cost (Euros)	312,000.7	53,600.8	91,506.4	19,982.3	477,090.2	19.8
Mean (SD)	1,772.7 (766.7)	1,786.7 (669.6)	2,033.5 (1,112.1)	4,995.8 (1,423.9)	1,870.9 (927.6)	
Acquisition medication cost (Euros)	33,678.0	3,081.4	17,131.5	7,411.2	61,302.2	2.5
Mean (SD)	191.4 (554.5)	102.7 (74.3)	380.7 (895.1)	1,851.8 (1,452.9)	231.8 (616.7)	
Dispensing cost (Euros)	4,555.6	754.4	1,299.0	233.1	6,842.1	0.3
Mean (SD)	25.9 (6.4)	25.1 (2.9)	28.9 (9.4)	58.2 (13.4)	26.8 (8.0)	
Supervision cost (Euros)	24,046.4	3,921.9	8,327.9	2,076.0	38,372.2	1.6
Mean (SD)	136.6 (106.2)	130.7 (81.7)	185.1 (120.4)	519.0 (270.1)	150.5 (117.8)	
Hospitalization cost (Euros)	926,219.5	239,546.9	525,127.7	137,675.5	1,828,569.6	75.8
Mean (SD)	12,864.2 (10.930.5)	15,969.8 (18.705.3)	23,869.5 (34.914.3)	45,891.8 (38.532.5)	16,326.5 (20.509.0)	
Total cost (Euros)	1,300,500.2	300,905.4	643,392.4	167,374.1	2,412,172.2	100
Mean (SD)	7,389.2 (9,549.7)	10,030.2 (15,307.8)	14,297.0 (27,147.3)	41,843.5 (38,936.3)	9,455.0 (16,102.0)	

Mean: mean cost per case; SD: standard deviation

Table 3: Cost of TB treatment in the DOT cohort.

4   Discussion

The rational behind economic analysis is the notion of scarcity, as inevitability the growing needs of society outweigh the resources, which are limited. Due to the significant growth of need economic assessments are important when deciding what resources to use in the field of health. The purpose is also an important decision when representing an opportunity cost, which is not being able to devote those resources to other activities with potential health benefit. The economic concept of cost and benefit is derived from this principle. It is not to spend as little as possible but to make the best use of available resources. In short, health economic analyses are about choices, and their consequences (Marco, 2006). The purpose of DOTS strategy is to improve cure rates in TB patients, to eliminate sources of infection, to avoid resistance development and to interrupt the chain of transmission (Altet & Alcaide, 2006).

The costs analysis was based on the assessment of the direct costs of health care resources used for DOT programs. This analysis was based on the diagnosis and monitoring protocol in the UTB where dispensing is at the hospital pharmacy service and management oversight is different depending on the origin and status of the patient.

	N	DOT	SAT	DOT with respect to SAT
				Type of TB
New TB cases	176	7,389.2 (9,549.7)	7,451.2 (9,698.9)	- 62.0 (477.0)
Treatment after default	30	10,030.2 (15,307.8)	10,138.6 (15,393.0)	- 108.4 (761.5)
Relapse	45	14,297.6 (27,147.3)	14,553.1 (27,255.3)	- 255.4 (779.8)
Chronic	4	41,843.5 (39,426.9)	42,016.2 (40,316.3)	- 172.7 (1.684.8)
Entire cohort	255	9,455.0 (16,102.0)	9,562.8 (16,244.1)	- 111.9 (587.4)
p value		0.072	0.067	0.214
				Monitoring criteria
Retreatment	81	13,776.2 (24,429.3)	13,966.9 (24,575.7)	- 190.6 (810.5)
Risk of abandonment	151	7,642.5 (9,610.2)	7,643.4 (9,671.6)	- 0.9 (231.1)
Resistance H and/or R	10	9,260.9 (13,935.3)	10,409.6 (14,945.8)	- 1.148.7 (1.459.3)
Previous Therapeutic failure	6	3,978.6 (3,225.6)	3,920.9 (3,225.0)	57.7 (5.6)
Medical reasons	7	3,686.1 (2,563.2)	3632.9 (2,610.9)	53.3 (116.3)
Entire cohort	255	9,455.0 (16,102.0)	9,562.8 (16,244.1)	- 111.9 (587.4)
p value		0.458	0.307	0.002
				Final status of the treatment
Complete	134	7,913.3 (12,621.6)	7,951.9 (12,698.2)	- 38.6 (374.0)
Modification of the treatment	92	9,121.7 (12,950.3)	9.273.8 (13.181.9)	- 152.1 (780.3)
Interruption of the treatment	29	17,676.0 (31,121.8)	17,923.2 (31,272.5)	- 247.3 (799.0)
Entire cohort	255	9,455.0 (16,102.0)	9,562.8 (16,244.1)	- 111.9 (587.4)
p value		0.820	0.884	0.051
				Final status of the case
Satisfactory	222	8,428.4 (12,842.8)	8,513.6 (12,986.6)	- 85.2 (581.4)
Death	15	29,615.6 (39,868.7)	29,831.2 (40,028.9)	- 215.6 (377.5)
Potentially unsatisfactory	18	5,379.9 (5,550.5)	5,612.4 (6,094.8)	- 232.5 (970.3)
Entire cohort	255	9,455.0 (16,102.0)	9,562.8 (16,244.1)	- 111.9 (587.4)
p value		0.016	0.014	0.005

(H=Isoniazide, R=Rifampicine) Data: mean cost per case in Euros; standard deviation in brackets

Table 4: Cost-minimization study (n=255).

The average cost per case was € 9,455. The composition of the overall cost is dominated by hospital costs (75.8%) although less than half of patients have hospital admissions. It is followed by the costs of clinical follow-up (19.8%), then the acquisition of drugs (2.5%), the monitoring (1.6%) and finally the dispensing and pharmaceutical care (0.3%). These data are slightly higher than those published by other authors (Iseman *et al.*, 1993; Porco *et al.*, 2006, Menzies *et al.*, 2008).

Although it is desirable to keep the tuberculosis patient in the community to avoid the dreaded nosocomial transmission and costs rise, in our series we found that the hospital costs involve more than 75% of the costs. We attribute this to the different drug prices and the lower health care costs, while there is a good agreement in the cost of laboratory and radiological tests (Iseman *et al.*, 1993, Rubio-Terres & Dominguez-Gil, 2005). We investigated different variables to deepen the factors associated with costs. Depending on the type of tuberculosis different average costs were obtained, including costs of hospital admissions, ranging from almost € 7,000 for the initial cases to more than € 40,000 for chronic patients. The deviation in the initial cases from theory, for six months of standard therapy, is mainly due to the extension of some treatments, mainly with immunosuppression regimes and the establishment of nine months therapies. We only had eleven cases with intermittent treatments; if it had been extended to more patient that would have lowered the average of the initial costs.

This proportion is similar to other published estimates (Sanz Granda, 2001) and greater than 50% based on American studies (Menzies *et al.*, 2008). These costs are directly proportional to the duration stays generated and the average income has dropped over the recent years when compared with 1994 data available in our area, staying in about a month (García Ramos *et al.*, 1995 Montes-Santiago *et al.*, 2009). In terms of magnitude, it is similar to that in Canada (Menzies *et al.*, 2008) and well below the estimated U.S. data (Porco *et al.*, 2006). Hospital costs of initial cases lead to a 71.2% expenditure which would probably not be necessary and could be avoided for most of the patients, because the TB alone is not a criteria for hospitalization, except for complications. Conclusion obtained by American authors also point out that a partnership with the local health jurisdiction would be required to control patients in outpatient treatment and emphasize that health professionals should make efforts to treat TB patients as outpatients, including those who are infectious, because it may represent savings for the society and patients (Thomas *et al.*, 2010). The Implementation of the Galician Program for Prevention and Control of Tuberculosis (PGPCTB) in Galicia (Spain) has made a clear effort in this regard (PGPCTB, 2012). A study conducted in Baltimore (Chaulk *et al.*, 2000) using the forecasting technique to estimate the number of TB cases prevented by DOT estimated that if the trend of Baltimore between 1978 and 1992 would have been similar to the United States during this period, there would have been 1,577 cases of TB, with an additional cost of $ 18.8 million. If the trend of TB in that city had been similar to that of the other major American cities in this period, there would have been 2,233 cases, with an additional cost of $ 27.1 million. It should be noted that the DOT was the only significant change in Baltimore during this period (Chaulk *et al.*, 2000, 2008).

The average cost of medication of a chronic patient was almost ten times higher than that of an initial case and the overall average cost was five times higher, due to the prolongations of the treatment.

The use of second-line drugs, such as fluoroquinolones, increases the average cost of medication. It could be established almost fifty DOT in intermittent treatment regimen twice a week in the theoretical supervisory conditions (no income) for each chronic patient treated. A Canadian study on the costs of care in TB concluded that the costs associated with this disease were significant, accounting for 60% curative services and the remaining 40% to the prevention and control activities. As mentioned above, a large part of the cost of the disease corresponds to the hospital, which can be increased in low incidence countries due to a delay in diagnosis. (Menzies *et al.*, 2008).

Interestingly, the results obtained in relation to the costs of dispensing and monitoring among cases with hospitalization and receiving all the treatment on an outpatient basis, since no statistically significant differences were found, enhance the smooth operation of the DOT system, as the cost differences between these patients are only due to hospitalizations.

The current structure of the UTB allows to establish domiciliary DOT and intermittent regime, not being necessary in all the cases that the treatment is administered by sanitary personnel. Thus we can establish more DOT with lower costs. This conclusion, which is supported by other authors (Aspler *et al.*, 2008; Goodchild *et al.*, 2011), assures the therapeutic compliance. In our study there is a decrease of nursing time in preparing doses to administer as this is done in the hospital service pharmacy, in individual unit doses per patient per day, thus doing more advantageous the supervision system and, consequently making the cost dispensing only 0.3% of the total, which is significantly lower than that estimated in a study that assessed the cost to the nursing staff in an area of the United States (Rubado *et al.*, 2008).

Since we did not include indirect costs in the analyses, our estimates are lower than those of other studies which considered cases of treatment after default, localization patient costs and management to achieve their incorporation into a DOT program, including judicial proceedings for hospitalization (Iseman *et al.*, 1993, Brown *et al.*, 1995; Mangura, 2002; Porco *et al.*, 2006, Menzies *et al.*, 2008).

PGPCTB established that DOT should at least be implemented in patients belonging to previously defined groups (Mejuto *et al.*, 2010; PGPCTB, 2012). For this reason, it has not been possible to conduct a comparative study against a real SAT in our health area.

In recent years other original DOT programs were initiated in Spain. The Valencian Community started a pilot program in which DOT is based on drug taking at the community pharmacy. Early results indicate that it may be a good alternative for the future (Juan *et al.*, 2006). The costs are similar as compared to ours, but the patients in their cohort are less complex and the Valencian study does not analyse the costs of hospitalizations of patients or the logging of diagnostic tests. Moreover, other studies consider the contribution of pharmacists to the control of TB, especially MDR-TB, showing an increase of patient adherence to treatment, with consequent benefits in cure rates (Clark *et al.*, 2007; Manzor, 2008).

In conclusion, the comparative analysis between the average cost of DOT and the theoretical SAT, assuming similar conditions, yields in favour of DOT management system in our health area, as both the final case status as in the monitoring reason are more profitable for the system under this scheme. This indicates that the model influences the management of drug procurement and the cost of health care. In the cost analysis regarding the type of tuberculosis, the highest average of the overall cost was in chronic cases, and the lowest average cost in initial cases, all variables were statistically significant, except the costs of hospital admissions.

Our DOT program optimizes health resources by using hospital pharmaceutical care and dispensing from a public health centre with a distribution system in unit dose. Also improves quality and efficiency of treatment supervision.

References

Altet Gómez MN, Alcaide Megíasa J. *Control y eliminación de la tuberculosis en España: las estrategias para el siglo XXI. An Pediatr (Barc) 2006; 64(1): 66-73.*

Aspler A, Menzies D, Oxlade O, Banda J, Mwenge L, Godfrey-Faussett P, Ayles H. *Cost of tuberculosis diagnosis and treatment from the patient perspective in Lusaka, Zambia. Int J Tuberc Lung Dis. 2008 Aug; 12(8): 928-35.*

Brown RE, Miller B, Taylor WR, Palmer C, Bosco L, Nicola RM, Zelinger J, Simpson K. *Health-care expenditures for tuberculosis in the United States. Arch Intern Med 1995; 155(15):1595-600.*

Cerda R, Muñoz M, Zeladita J, Wong M, Sebastian JL, Bonilla C, Bayona J, Sanchez E, Arevalo J, Caldas A, Shin S. *Health care utilization and costs of a support program for patients living with the human immunodeficiency virus and tuberculosis in Peru. Int J Tuberc Lung Dis 2011; 15(3):363-368.*

Chaulk CP Kazandjian VA, Vallejo P. *Evaluación en salud pública: lecciones aprendidas de la gestión de la tuberculosis pulmonar. Gac Sanit 2008; 22(4): 362-70.*

Chaulk CP, Friedman M, Dunning R. *Modeling the epidemiology and economics of directly observed therapy in Baltimore. Int J Tuberc Lung Dis 2000;4:201-7.*

Clark PM, Karagoz T, Apikoglu-Rabus S, Vehbi Izzettin F.*Effect of pharmacist-led patient education on adherence to tuberculosis treatment. Am J Health Syst Pharm 2007; 64(5):497-505.*

Consejo General de Colegios Oficiales de Farmacéuticos. Catálogo de Especialidades Farmacéuticas. Barcelona; 2006.

Domínguez-Gil Hurlé, A. Impacto económico de la terapéutica. El gasto en medicamentos. Eficacia y efectividad. Calidad y coste de la terapéutica. Monografías de la Real Academia Nacional de Farmacia, 2009.

García Ramos R, Pérez del Molino ML, Túñez V, Martí Mallén M, Guerrero E. Utilización de medicamentos Antituberculosos en un hospital. Aproximación a la morbilidad tuberculosa hospitalaria. Farm Hosp 1995; 19(4): 199-204.

García Ramos R, Túñez Bastida V, Golpe Gómez A, Pérez del Molino ML. Evaluation of 6 years of directly observed treatment of tuberculosis. Int J Tuber Lung Dis 2001; 5 (suppl):S193.

Glass KP, Anderson JR. Relative Value Units: from A to Z (Part I of IV). Journal of Medical Practice Management 2002; 17 (5): 225-8.).

Glass KP, Anderson JR. Relative value Units and productivity: Part 2 of 4. Journal Medical of Practice Management 2002; 17 (6): 285-90.

Goodchild M, Sahu S, Wares F, Dewan P,. Shukla RS, Chauhan LS, Floyd K. A cost-benefit analysis of scaling up tuberculosis control in India. Int J Tuberc Lung Dis 2011 Mar;15(3):358-62.

Grupo TECNO. Sociedad Española de Farmacia Hospitalaria. Base de datos de información para el cálculo automático de URVs y facturación. Ed. SEFH 2009. Disponible en: http://www.sefh.es/sefhgrupotrabajo/grupodetrabajo_descargas.php 14-12-2010.

Iseman MD, Cohn DL, Sbarbaro JA. Directly Observed Treatment of Tuberculosis. New Engl J Med 1993; 328: 576-578.

Jacquet V, Morose W, Schwartzman K, Oxlade O, Barr G, Grimard F, Menzies D. Impact of DOTS expansion on tuberculosis related outcomes and costs in Haiti. BMC Public Health 2006, 6:209.

Juan G, Lloret T, Perez C, Lopez P, Navarro R, Ramón M, Cortijo J, Morcillo EJ. Directly observed treatment for tuberculosis in pharmacies compared with self- administered in Spain. Int J Tuberc Dis   2006; 10: 215–221

Mangura B, Napolitano E, Passannante M, Sarrel M, McDonald R, Galanowsky K, Reichman L. Directly observed therapy (DOT) is not the entire answer: an operational cohort analysis. Int J Tuberc Lung Dis. 2002; 6 (8):654- 661

Manzor B. Treatment of extensively drug-resistant tuberculosis and role of the pharmacist. Pharmacotherapy 2008; 28(10):1243-1254

Marco A. Farmacoeconomía de los tratamientos para la infección por el VIH y para la tuberculosis. Enf Emerg 2006; 8 (4): 154-165.

Mejuto B, Tunez V, Perez del Molino ML, Garcia R: Characterization and evaluation of the directly observed treatment for tuberculosis in Santiago de Compostela (1996–2006). Risk Management and Healthcare Policy 2010:3 21–26, 70.

Mejuto, B., Tuñez, V., Perez del Molino, M.L. & García-Ramos, R. (2014). Directly observed treatment: implementation and validation of an original model. Tuberculosis - A Comprehensive Clinical Reference. ISBN:XXX . iConcept Press. Retrieved from http://www.iconceptpress.com/books/tuberculosis--a-comprehensive-clinical-reference

Menzies D, Lewis M, Oxlade O. Costs for Tuberculosis Care in Canada. Can J Public Health 2008 Sep-Oct; 99(5):391-6.

Montes-Santiago J, Rey-García G, Mediero-Domínguez A, Del Campo V, Felpeto I, Garet E, González- Fernández E. Tendencias seculares en la morbimortalidad y costes de hospitalización por tuberculosis en Galicia. Galicia Clin 2009; 70 (1): 19-24.

Porco TC, Lewis B, Marseille E, Grinsdale J, Flood JM, Royce SE. Cost-effectiveness of tuberculosis evaluation and treatment of newly-arrived immigrants. BMC Public Health 2006; 6 :157.

Programa galego de prevencion e control da tuberculose (PGPCTB). Documentos Tecnicos de Saúde Pública. Xunta de Galicia. Consellería de Sanidade e Servicios Sociais. Direccion Xeral de Saude Pública. Santiago de Compostela, 1995. ISBN: 84-453-1379-7.

Programa galego de prevencion e control da tuberculose (PGPCTB) Documentos Tecnicos de Saúde Pública. Xunta de Galicia. Consellería de Sanidade e Servicios Sociais. Direccion Xeral de Saude Publica. Santiago de Compostela, 2012.

Rubado DJ, Choi D, Becker T, Winthrop K, Schafer S. Determining the cost of tuberculosis case management in a low-incidence state. Int J Tuberc Lung Dis 2008 Mar;12(3):301-7.

Rubio-Terrés C, Domínguez-Gil, A. Análisis farmacoeconómico del tratamiento de pacientes con exacerbación aguda de la bronquitis crónica con cefditoren pivoxilo o cefuroxima axetilo. Pharmacoeconomics-Spanish Research Articles 2005: 2 (2):45-54.

Sanz A. Evaluación farmacoeconómica de la prevención de tuberculosis. Panorama Actual Med 2001; 25 (241): 213-215.

Sanz Granda A. Farmacoeconomía de la tuberculosis pulmonar. Farmacoeconomía 2001:160-162.

Servicio Galego de Saúde. SERGAS. www.sergas.es

Snyder D, Chin D. Cost-effectiveness analysis of Directly Observed Therapy for patients with tuberculosis at low risk for treatment default. Am J Respir Care Med 1999; 160: 582-6.

Thomas JA, Laraque F, Munsiff S, Piatek A, Harris TG. Hospitalizations for tuberculosis in New York City: how many could be avoided? Int J Tuberc Lung Dis 2010 Dec; 14(12):1603-12.

Vassall A, Chechulin Y, Raykhert I, Osalenko N, Svetlichnaya S, Kovalyova A, van der Werf MJ, Turchenko LV, Hasker E, Miskinis K, Veen J, Zaleskis R. Reforming tuberculosis control in Ukraine: results of pilot projects and implications for the national scale-up of DOTS. Health Policy and Planning 2009; 24:55-62.

WHO. Resolution WHA53.1. Stop Tuberculosis Initiative. In: Fifty-third World Health Assembly. Geneva, 15-20 May 2000. Resolutions and decisions. Geneva, 2000. WHA53/2000/REC/1, Annex: 1-2.

WHO. Global tuberculosis control: surveillance, planning and financing. Who Report 2006. World Health Organization Document, 2006. WHO/HTM/TB/2006.362.

WHO. Global tuberculosis report 2012. 1. Tuberculosis – epidemiology. 2. Tuberculosis, Pulmonary – prevention and control. 3. Tuberculosis – economics. 4. Directly observed therapy. 5. Treatment outcome. 6. National health programs – organization and administration. 7. Statistics. I.World Health Organization. ISBN 978 92 4 156450 2.

WHO Stop TB Partnership, 2013 GLOBAL PLAN TO STOP TB 2011-2015. Transforming the Fight towards elimination of Tuberculosis.

Multidrug-Resistant Tuberculosis – An Emerging Challenge: Timely Diagnosis the Key to Prevention

Amita Raoot
Directorate of Family Welfare
Government of National Capital Territory of Delhi, India

Geeta Dev
Department of Pathology
University College of Medical Sciences, Delhi, India

1   Introduction

Tuberculosis (TB) is a disease of great antiquity. The oldest evidence of TB infection in humans was discovered in human remains from the Neolithic era dating from 9,000 years ago, in a settlement in the eastern Mediterranean (Hershkovitz *et al.*, 2008). Hippocrates (460-370 BC) described this disease as 'pthisis sylivas' meaning "wasting away" (Appling & Miller., 1981). Lucas Schoenlein first coined the term "tuberculosis" in 1832. The causative agent of tuberculosis was discovered by Robert Kochs on 24th March 1882. Tuberculosis continues to be a global health problem and having serious repercussions on the health and economic infrastructure of any country. Tuberculosis displays all the characteristics of a global epidemic. It is believed that every second someone, somewhere in the world is infected with TB (WHO, 2003). TB was declared a "global emergency" by WHO in 1993 because of its toll on the health of individuals and wider social and economic impact on the overall progress of a country (*WHO/* IUATLD Report 3, 2004). Despite availability of highly effective drugs and potent vaccine, TB continues to be a major cause of morbidity and mortality in the world. In 2011, an estimated 8.7 million new cases of TB were reported and about 1.4 million people died from TB. TB was also one of the top killers of women in 2011, with 300,000 deaths among HIV-negative women and 200,000 deaths among HIV-positive women. Geographically, the burden of TB is highest in Asia and Africa. India and China together account for almost 40% of the world's TB cases (WHO, 2012).India alone accounts for one-fifth of the global TB incidence and ranks highest in the world (GOI, RNTPC Annual Status Report 2012).

2   Drug Resistance in Tuberculosis

A major setback in the treatment and cure of TB has been the emergence of mutated strains of *Mycobacterium tuberculosis (MTB)* that are resistant to the major anti-tuberculosis drugs, posing new challenges for both clinical management and control programmes. The story of anti-tuberculosis chemotherapy is a miniature of the history of anti-infective chemotherapy as MTB is an ancient human pathogen with mechanisms for survival. After Robert Koch's discovery of the Tubercle bacilli in 1882, there was no breakthrough in the treatment of TB for a long time until Streptomycin and Para-aminosalicylic acid (PAS) were first introduced in the 1940s.As said by Paul Ehrlich 'Drug resistance follows the drug like a faithful shadow", the phenomenon of Drug resistance to Streptomycin was soon observed in the 1950s (Sharma & Mohan, October 2004). Isoniazid (INH) and Thiacetazone were the next anti-TB drugs introduced in 1950s. INH became the most effective drug at killing the actively dividing bacilli. This gave global impetus for treatment and control of TB. In the 60s, new and perhaps the most important drug in the treatment of TB was identified i.e. Rifampicin (Rfm) which could kill even the very slowly dividing bacilli. Its introduction ushered the era of short course–chemotherapy (Prahlad, 2005). Directly Observed Treatment Short Course (DOTS) became an internationally recommended strategy for TB control. It is based on a 6-month treatment regimen with first-line drugs i.e. isoniazid, rifampicin, pyrazinamide, and ethambutol for new patients and an 8-month treatment regimen with isoniazid, rifampicin, pyrazinamide, ethambutol, and streptomycin for re-treatment patients. But with the emergence of strains that are resistant to the two most important drugs for any anti-TB regimen, INH & Rfm the treatment of TB has suffered a major setback.

Drug Resistance in MTB occurs by random, single step spontaneous mutation at a low but predictable frequency, in large bacterial population. The probability of incidence of drug resistant mutants is 10^{-8}

for rifampicin, while for isoniazid and some of the other commonly used drugs it is 10^{-6} (Paramasivan & Venkataraman, 2004). Recent studies have demonstrated that the drug resistant mutants are equally infectious and can cause severe disease in an individual exposed to the same (Telenti *et al.*, 1993).

2.1   Definition of Drug Resistance (DR)

Drug Resistance can be innate or acquired. In the innate drug resistance, a bacterial species may be naturally resistant to a drug before its introduction. More serious is acquired resistance where bacteria that were initially sensitive to a drug become resistant (Ebrahim, 2010). The capacity of disease-causing microorganisms to withstand exposure to drugs previously toxic to them; acquired either through spontaneous mutation or by gradual selection of relatively resistant strains after drug exposure is defined as drug resistance. As per the WHO classification (2013) MTB DR is classified in categories based on drug susceptibility testing (DST) of clinical isolates confirmed to be M. tuberculosis as given below:

  i.   Monoresistance: resistance to one first-line anti-TB drug only.
  ii. Polydrug resistance: resistance to more than one first-line anti-TB drug (other than both isoniazid and rifampicin).
  iii. Multidrug resistance: resistance to at least both isoniazid and rifampicin.
  iv. Extensive drug resistance: Resistance to any fluoroquinolone and to at least one of three second-line injectable drugs (capreomycin, kanamycin and amikacin), in addition to multidrug resistance.
  v.   Rifampicin resistance: Resistance to rifampicin detected using phenotypic or genotypic methods, with or without resistance to other anti-TB drugs. It includes any resistance to rifampicin, whether monoresistance, multidrug resistance, polydrug resistance or extensive drug resistance.

These categories are not all mutually exclusive.

2.2   Causes of Drug Resistance

Drug resistant tuberculosis including multi-drug resistance is predominantly a man-made problem. (WHO, 2008) The sources and causes are multi-factorial that may be related to health provider, patient and programmatic errors (World Health Organization, 2003 TB Fact Sheet). In addition the inherent property of MTB to undergo spontaneous mutations naturally which are transmitted vertically also contribute to DR. Factors like poor case detection, inadequate/irregular treatment, use of anti-TB drugs for indications other than TB, laboratory delays in identification and susceptibility testing of MTB, massive bacillary load in patient, non-compliance, illiteracy and low socio-economic status of patient etc. play an important role in emergence of DR.

2.3   Molecular Mechanism of Drug Resistance to Rfm

Rifampicin is a bactericidal agent that was introduced as an anti-tuberculosis drug in 1972, and thereafter it has been a key component of DOTS therapy. Rifampicin is important in killing *mycobacteria* that are metabolizing slowly, killing the persisters and sterilizing the patient's sputum, thereby greatly shortening the duration of chemotherapy. Rifampicin is believed to target the *mycobacterial* RNA polymerase and kills the organism by interfering in the transcription process. *Mycobacterial* RNA polymerase is a complex oligomer composed of 4 different sub units, each coded by 4 different genes (rpoA, rpoB, rpoC, rpoD). However, with respect to acquisition of resistance to Rfm, rpoB coded sub-unit plays the most important role. Mutations in the rpoB locus lead to resistance to Rfm because with structural changes in this unit, Rfm is unable to bind with RNA polymerase and exert its bactericidal effect (Jin & Gross, 1988). Moreover, virtually all mutations that occur in this region result in Rfm resistance. Rifampicin resistance is considered an excellent surrogate marker for MDR-TB, since 90% of Rfm-resistant strains are also resistant to INH and hence, are classified as multidrug resistant (Telent *et al.*, 1993). Rifampicin resistance is also amenable to detection by rapid genotypic assays, because approximately 95% of all Rfm-resistant strains contain mutations localized in an 81-bp "Rifampicin Resistance Determining Region" (RRDR) of the bacterial rpoB gene corresponding to 507-533 codons (Musser, 1995; Riska *et al.*, 2000).

2.4   Molecular Mechanism of Drug Resistance – Resistance to INH

The mechanism of action of INH on MTB is that INH inhibits the biosynthesis of cell wall mycolic acid, thereby making *mycobacteria* susceptible to reactive free oxygen radicals. For exerting its bactericidal effect on MTB, activation of INH to an unstable electro-philic intermediate is necessary. This activation is brought about by the *mycobacterial* enzyme catalase – peroxidase which is coded by the gene called Kat G. Thus any mutation of this gene (partial or total deletions, point mutations, or insertions) leads to the abolition or diminution of catalase activity and activation of INH to an unstable electro-philic intermediate does not take place. A deficiency in the enzyme activity produces high-level resistance and is found in more than 80% of Isoniazid-resistant strains (Ramaswamy & Musser, 1998). There are other proposed mechanisms for INH resistance including point mutations in the regulatory region of inhA operon, point mutations in the regulatory region of ahpC, but they are known to confer low-level resistance (Heym *et al.*, 1999).

3   Multi-Drug Resistance Tuberculosis (MDR-TB)

Emergence of MDR is posing a serious threat to the effectiveness of TB control programme. There were an estimated 0.31million MDR-TB cases among notified pulmonary TB patients in 2011. Almost 60% of these cases were in India, China and the Russian Federation. Globally 3.7% (2.1–5.2%) of new cases and 20% (13–26%) of previously treated cases are estimated to have MDR-TB. Though MDR-TB has been observed in all regions of the world but its prevalence varies considerably throughout the world. Levels of MDR-TB have been found to be worryingly high in some parts of the world, notably countries in Eastern Europe and Central Asia. In several of these countries, 9–32% of new cases and more than 50% of previously treated cases were diagnosed to have MDR-TB. Though the number of MDR-TB cases notified in the 27 high MDR-TB burden countries has doubled between 2009 and 2011, however it represents only one in five (19%) of the MDR-TB cases estimated to exist among notified TB patients. In the two countries (India & China) with the largest number of MDR-TB cases, the notification of these cases is less than one in ten (WHO, 2012). The estimated proportion of MDR-TB in India is 2.1% (1.5% – 2.7%) in new TB cases and 15% (13% – 7%) in previously treated cases. In India, the estimated number of MDR-TB patients out of notified Pulmonary TB cases is 21,000 (range 15,000 to 27,000) among new cases and 45,000 (range 40,000 to 50,000) in pre-treated cases as per the WHO Global TB Report 2012.

3.1   Consequences of MDR-TB

Presence of MDR gene in the non-responders is a serious challenge not only from the public health point of view but also in context of its economic burden, especially in the absence of diagnostic and treatment facilities for MDR-TB at national level programmes in most of the countries. From the patient's point of view, presence of MDR prolongs the treatment duration from the standard six months to 18-24 months. The second line drugs used in the treatment of MDR cases have serious side effects that may need hospitalization. These drugs are 50-200 times more expensive than the first line ATT drugs (WHO, 2010). Furthermore, patients with MDR-TB have lower cure rates and higher mortality than do patients with drug-susceptible TB (Shin *et al.*, 2006). It is also known that some strains of MDR-TB e.g. Beijing Strain are more infectious and is likely to cause large outbreaks of TB (Munsiff *et al.*, 2003; Ignatova, 2006) Patients infected with MDR-TB continue to have active TB despite optimal treatment and may even die of it.

3.2   MDR-TB and HIV

The accelerating and amplifying influence of HIV on TB is well established. Clinically it has been seen that HIV infection alters the immunity and increases susceptibility to TB infection and MDR-TB. Institutional outbreaks of MDR-TB were reported among HIV-infected patients in USA, Argentina and some European countries (WHO/ IUATLD Report 3, 2004). These outbreaks resulted in high mortality, generally more than 70% among those with HIV infection within a very short time of 4-8 weeks (Well *et al.*, 2007). In controlled clinical trials, acquired mono-resistance to Rfm has been reported to be associated with HIV infection. (Jenny, 2002) Although the catastrophic association of HIV-associated MDR-TB is not clearly understood, there are likely explanations for this association. In patients suffering from AIDS MTB replicates in the continuous phase, which results in exposure of bacilli to Rfm alone because INH has a shorter half-life and there are no other supporting drugs. In addition, acquisition of Rfm resistance in patients of HIV undergoing treatment for TB may also result from the malabsorption of anti-TB drug, which has been documented in patient cohorts in settings of high HIV prevalence (Nelson *et al.*, 2002).

India is estimated to have the third highest number of people living with HIV/AIDS, after South Africa and Nigeria (UNAIDS, 2010). Though only 5% of TB patients are HIV infected, in absolute terms it ranks 2nd in the world and accounts for about 10% of the global burden of HIV associated TB (TB India, Annual report, 2012) There has been quadrupling of TB cases in several Asian countries over past the ten years as a direct result of HIV (WHO/IUATLD Report 3, 2004). Clearly, to block further convergence of the HIV infection and MDR-TB epidemics the need of rapid diagnostic test(s) for detection of drug resistance in the clinical samples cannot be overstressed.

3.3   DOTS-Plus

The revised treatment regimen for MDR-TB which has been endorsed by WHO in 2000 is known as DOTS-Plus. The DOTS-Plus strategy includes additional measures like continuous drug resistance surveillance, culture, drug susceptibility testing for TB patients, and individualization of drug regimen through the use of first and second-line drugs. The regimen uses 5 to 6 drugs (kanamycin, ofloxacin, ethionamide, pyrazinamide, ethambutol, and cycloserine) to which the MTB is likely to be susceptible for the initial 6 months, and then 3 to 4 drugs (ofloxacin, ethionamide, ethambutol, and cycloserine) subsequently (Grover & Takkar, 2008).

3.4   Extensively Drug-resistant Tuberculosis (XDR TB)

The term "Extensively drug-resistant tuberculosis" (XDR TB) was first introduced in March 2006 by the US CDC and the World Health Organization. The WHO XDR TB Task Force in October 2006 defined XDR TB as those strains of TB that are resistant to at least rifampicin and isoniazid (which means that it is MDR -TB), and also resistant to a fluoroquinolone and to at least one of the three injectable TB drugs, capreomycin, kanamycin and amikacin (WHO, Geneva, 2006) By 2012 at least one case of XDR TB has been reported from 84 countries, however it is believed that in absence of effective XDR TB surveillance and lack of laboratory capacity for testing of resistance to second line drugs many XDR TB cases remain undiagnosed. (WHO, Global Tuberculosis Report 2012). As per WHO estimate 5% of people with MDR TB may actually have XDR TB. Hence XDR TB cases can be presumed to be quite high. (WHO, Global Report WHO 2010) Owing to insufficient laboratory capacity and inadequate policies to detect drug-resistant TB patients accurately and in a timely manner, the actual incidence and prevalence rate of XDR-TB in India is not available, except for a few scattered reports (Mondal & Jain, 2007; Paramasivan *et al.*, 2012).

4   Diagnosis of Tuberculosis

There are many traditional methods of laboratory diagnosis of TB including smear microscopy, culture, tuberculin test, and characteristic histopathology of tissue samples, radiological examination and other imaging methods. Smear microscopy with Ziehl-Neelsen (ZN) staining for Acid Fast Bacilli (AFB) of clinical material is the most frequently used cost effective preliminary detection test for TB. However, smear microscopy which requires 10,000 to 100,000 organisms/ ml, exhibits low sensitivity (10% – 20%) and cannot determine drug-susceptibility or viability status of bacilli. Conventional fluorescence micros-copy uses quartz-halogen or high-pressure mercury vapour lamps and allows scanning of larger smear area at a lower magnification objective and therefore taking less time than ZN microscopy. The smears are stained with fluorescent stains like auramine instead of ZN stain. The salient features of WHO rec-ommended techniques for microscopic diagnosis of tuberculosis are listed in Table 1.

Culture still remains the yardstick for diagnosis of TB. Though culture of this fastidious organism is specific but is time consuming with results available only after 4-8 weeks and is not very sensitive (<50%) (Thwaites *et al.*, 2002). Culture techniques also require viable organisms (10 to 100 viable organ-isms per sample), and this is often a problem in partially treated patients and pauci-bacillary cases (Hob-by *et al.*, 1973).

The diagnosis of extra-pulmonary TB is more difficult as it frequently requires invasive or semi-invasive methods for sample procurement (Thwaites *et al.*, 2002). Samples may not have adequate num-ber of bacilli. Characteristic histopathology may be difficult to obtain due to lack of representative speci-men, and non-specific histologic features. Insufficient sample amounts or volume leading to non uniform distribution of bacilli while allocating the small amount of samples for various diagnostic tests (histo-cytology, biochemical tests, culture based tests, and molecular assays etc.), non availability of uniform sample processing technique and poor performance of conventional microbiological techniques in extra-pulmonary specimens make diagnosis of extra-pulmonary TB all the more challenging (Soumitesh Chakravorty *et al.*, 2005). Immunoassay based approaches are often non-conclusive as antibodies and delayed type hypersensitivity response persists long after the subsidence of sub-clinical or clinical disease (Katoch, 2004).

S.No	Technique	Principle	Advantage	Disadvantage
1	Conventional Light Microscopy	Examination of ZN-stained direct smears prepared directly from sputum / clinical samples The thick lipid-containing cell-walls of MTB retain stains despite de-colourisation by acid-containing reagents (so-called 'acid fastness').	1. Most widely available test 2. Cost effective 3. Simple 4. Useful in resource-limited settings. 5. 5. Highly specific	1. Variable sensitivity (20–80%). 2. Not sensitive for extra-pulmonary TB 3. Cannot distinguish be-tween: MTB from non-tuberculous mycobacte-ria (NTM)s, viable from non-viable organisms, drugs susceptible from drug-resistant strains.
2	Conventional Fluorescence Microscopy	Examination of fluoro-chrome-stained smears using quartz-halogen or high-pressure mercury vapour lamps as light sources. The fluorescent commonly used are au-ramine-O and rhodamine	1. 10% more sensitive than ZN 2. Takes less time	1. High cost of mercury vapour light sources 2. Regular maintenance 3. Needs dark room 4. Considerable technical expertise
3	LED Microscopy	Examination of fluoro-chrome-stained smears with help of LED	1. Less expensive 2. Requires less power 3. Can run on batteries 4. Bulbs have long half-life 5. Can be used in resource-limited settings 6. Overall sensitivity was 93% (95% CI, 85–97%), & the overall specificity was 99% (95% CI, 98–99%).	Relatively expensive

Table 1: WHO recommended techniques of Microscopic diagnosis of Tuberculosis. (Source: Fluorescent light-emitting diode (LED) microscopy for diagnosis of Tuberculosis: Policy statement, WHO 2011 WHO/HTM/TB/2011.8 http://whqlibdoc.who.int/publications/2011/9789241501613_eng.pdf)

4.1   Laboratory Methods for Drug Susceptibility Testing (DST)

Drug Susceptibility Testing is a crucial step in initiating the right anti-infective chemotherapy. DST provides a definitive diagnosis of drug-resistant TB. Determination of Drug susceptibility of MTB is carried out by either examination of growth or inhibition of a defined metabolic activity in a medium containing anti tuberculosis drug or detection of genetic mutations conferring drug resistance, at the molecular level. The following two broad categories of DST techniques are available:

i. Phenotypic methods involve culturing of MTB to detect the growth of the bacilli in drug containing media.

ii. Genotypic methods target specific molecular mutations associated with resistance against individual drugs.

4.2   Phenotypic Methods

Phenotypic DST (Culture-based method): Culture of MTB remains the gold standard for both diagnosis and drug sensitivity testing. Technically, phenotypic methods for DST are based on growth (or metabolic activity) inhibition due the presence anti-TB drugs which is interpreted by macroscopic observation of growth in drug-free and drug-containing media, detection/ measurement of the metabolic activity or products and use of mycobacteriophage. Conventional DST involves culturing of MTB in the presence of anti-TB drugs to detect growth (indicating drug resistance) or inhibition of growth (indicating drug susceptibility). Phenotypic DST methods are performed as direct or indirect tests on solid or liquid media. In direct testing, a set of drug-containing and drug-free media is inoculated directly with a concentrated patient's specimen. Indirect testing involves inoculation of drug-containing media with a pure culture growth from the original specimen. Initially DST is carried out with a primary set of drugs, consisting of the front-line drugs isoniazid, rifampicin, ethambutol and, optionally, streptomycin. It is a common practice to test an extended spectrum of antimicrobial compounds, if resistance to one or several of these drugs is detected. Three different growth-based laboratory methods have been accepted for determining antimicrobial susceptibility of *MTB* (1) the resistance ratio method, (2) the absolute concentration method, and (3) the proportion method (C.B. & Nash, 1996). The proportion method of detecting DR in MTB is based on calculating the "proportion of resistant bacilli" presents in a strain. The strain is assumed to be resistant when the growth detected on culture media containing a defined concentration of drug is more than the "critical proportion" of the inoculums. The *"critical proportion" is defined as* the percentage of tubercle bacilli in the inoculums whose growth on culture media containing the critical concentration of an anti-TB drug signifies the clinical ineffectiveness of that drug. (Elvira *et al.*, 2009)

Most laboratories in the Western hemisphere utilize a modified proportion method on solid medium, according to the proposed standard of the National Committee for Clinical and Laboratory Standards. Conventional culture methods using solid media [Lowenstein-Jensen (LJ) or 7H11 medium] are cheap and simple but have the major disadvantage of being very slow. LJ cultures take 20 – 56 days for diagnosis and four to six weeks after initial culture for DST. Since DST on solid media requires three weeks of incubation; hence testing is preferentially done in liquid media now days. To overcome the long turnaround time, one of the major disadvantages of conventional DST, various new tests have been developed for rapid detection of resistance. A number of commercial systems are available for culture and DST, some of which may have slight advantages in certain settings.

In addition to primarily culture-based approaches, assessment of drug susceptibility can now also be achieved by identifying alternative markers of drug-resistant metabolic activities. Some of these alternative methods also require culture as preliminary step. Among these are colorimetry (Yajko *et al.*, 1995), flow cytometry (Norden *et al.*, 1995) bioluminescence assay of *mycobacterial* adenosine triphosphate (Nelson *et al.*, 1998), quantitation of *mycobacterial* antigens (Drowart *et al.*, 1997), and mycobacteriophage-based methods like luciferase reporter phages which appear to have potential for future use. However, the complexities of these technologies and high cost have largely hampered their wider application in the clinical mycobacteriology laboratory. The table below summarizes a few new rapid systems available for culture and DST.

S. No	Technique & Company	Principle	Advantage	Disadvantage
	New rapid commercial methods for diagnosis and DST			
1	BACTEC 460-TB® Becton Dickinson (US)	The MTB presence is detected based on its metabolism by detecting radiolabelled ^{14}C production in the tube when growth occurs in the tube.	Faster than solid media	1. Expensive Technology 2. Requires appropriate laboratory infrastructure 3. Proper nuclear waste Disposal. *The use of radioisotopes & cost of equipment precludes use.
2	BACTEC MGIT 960® (Fully Automated) Becton Dickinson (US)	Consumption of O_2 by MTB produces fluorescence in a glass tube containing modified Middlebrook 7H9 which has fluorescence quenching-based oxygen sensor that is detected by a UV lamp. It is a non-radiometric, noninvasive system	1. High throughput capacity 2. Standardized automated sample reading. 3. MTB detection in 7 days for sputum positive, up to 42days for Sputum negative & DST in 8 to 12 days of culture	1. Technology more expensive. 2. Specific training of technical personnel. 3. Liquid media are technically limited.
3	MGIT (manual) Becton Dickinson (US)	Same as Above	1. MGIT machine not required. 2. More samples can be processed than conventional culture 3. Diagnosis in 7 to 42days. DST in 8 to 12 days of culture.	1. Tubes are expensive. 2. Manual MGIT requires reagents, manipulations & use of handheld UV lamp. 3. Liquid media are known to have a high %of contaminations leading to unreliable results
4	MB/Bact T®system Organon Teknika (Netherlands)	Based on detection of CO2 as an indicator of bacterial growth in cultures in a closed and a fully automated system	Increased flexibility of use	1. Relatively slow: diagnosis 17 days, DST 8 to 12 days. 2. Needs expensive and non-robust machine. 3. Complicated and cumbersome
5	E Test AB Biodisk (Sweden)	Based on determination of DST using strips (E Test strip) containing gradients of impregnated antibiotics. These are placed on the surface of the solid culture medium and MICs are determined by interpreting the point at which the ellipse of inhibition crosses the strip	1. Simple 2. Minimal training required. 3. Accurate & reproducible. 4. Relatively fast (5-10 days after primary culture. 5. Allows the reading of MIC directly on agar plates	Requires high bacterial concentration for inoculums i.e. needs to start from a culture.

6	MB redox® Biotest (Germany)	Based on the reduction of a tetrazolium salt indicator in liquid Medium (red to violet) MB Redox® allowing macroscopic visualization of the bacterial growth.	1. Simple 2. Can be read by eye or simple spectrophotometer	1. Cannot be used to measure DST on initially positive samples as dye is toxic; 2. Visualization is not easy; very few reports available 3. Relatively slow
	**New rapid noncommercial methods for diagnosis and DST** These tests have shown initial promise as being rapid & inexpensive. Their performance found to be acceptable under stringent laboratory protocols, as assessed by WHO recently. The salient features are summarized below:			
1	Microscopically observed drug susceptibility (MODS)	Performed in liquid medium (7H9) with or without drug incorporation, followed by observing microcolony growth & typical cord formation of MTB in sealed microtitre plates, using an inverted microscope	1. Quicker than solid culture, & MGIT as volumes are smaller. 2. Cheaper, non-commercial, adaptable method. 3. Highly sensitive (Pooled estimate, 98%; 95% CI, 95–99%) & pooled specificity estimate, 99%; 95% CI , 96–100%) for the detection of Rfm resistance &for INH (pooled sensitivity, 91%; 95% CI, 87–95%).	1. MODS is a delicate method that requires experienced personnel 2. Bio-safety risk for laboratory staff 3. Laborious & time-consuming
2	Nitrate reductase Assay	Direct or indirect method based on the ability of MTB to reduce nitrate, which is detected by a colour reaction. Performed on solid media. Microplate nitrate reductase assay (MNRA): Can also be performed in well plates using liquid Middlebrook 7H9 culture broth.	1. Minimal training & no special equipment required. 2. Relatively rapid results (10 days). 3. Results read out visually, without opening the tubes therefore safer 4. Highly sensitive (pooled estimate, 97%; 95% CI, 95–98%) & pooled specificity estimate, 100%; 95% CI, 99–100%) for Rfm resistance detection & pooled sensitivity for INH resistance, 97%; 95% CI, 95–98%; pooled specificity, 99%; 95% CI, 99–100%).	1. Only for DST for first-line drugs. 2. Low throughput
3	Thin Layer Agar (microcolony detection)	For diagnosis of MTB, plates with thin layer of 7H11 agar medium are incubated & examined microscopically. Micro colonies of MTB can be detected in < 7 days	1. Test can be done with a standard light microscope. 2. Uses solid media which is safer than liquid media. 3. Faster conventional culture. Diagnosis 5-10 days; DST 10-15 days.	1. Requires a CO_2 incubator 2. Not as fast as liquid culture

4	Colorimetric redox indicator metods(CRI)	Indirect methods based on the reduction of a colored indicator (reazurin RE-MA) added to liquid culture medium on a microtitre plate after exposure of *M. tb* strains to anti-TB drugs in vitro. Resistance is detected by a change in colour (blue to pink means a growth of the isolate) of the oxidation-reduction indicator, which is directly proportional to the number of viable mycobacteria in the medium.	1. Test requires small volume of liquid . 2. Easy to implement in resource-limited & field settings . 3. No special equipment and training required. 4. Rapid results in 8-10 days (especially for DST). 5. Results determined visually by a colour change. 6. Highly sensitive (pooled estimate, 98%; 95% [CI], 96–99%) and specific (pooled estimate. 99%; 95% CI, 99–100%) for the detection of Rfm resistance & also INH resistance (pooled sensitivity, 97%; 95% CI, 96–98%; pooled specificity, 98%;95% CI, 97–99%).	1. Only for DST (requires prior identification of MTB from culture) 2. Risk to the laboratory personnel 3. More standardization needed.
Phage-based tests				
Phage tests are based on the ability of viable MTB to support the replication of an infecting mycobacteriophage.				
1	FASTPlaque TB test and Fast laqueTB-RI Biotec	Replication of MTB-specific phage D29 can be determined by counting the viral particles	1. Speed (2-3 days). 2. For in-house systems: relatively cheap 3. Sensitivity & specificity of 70.5% & 86.2%, respectively	1. Technically complex 2. Require well functioning. Bacteriology laboratory, a strict incubation protocol & well-trained technicians. 3. Labor intensive 4. High contamination rate
2	Luciferase reporter phages	Recombinant phage (phage incorporated with gene luciferase gene) In the presence of luciferin substrate, infected bacteria emit light that can be detected with luminometer	Rapid result (2 days post culture).	1. Under development; only limited reports of clinical application are available. 2. High contamination rate.

Table 2: New rapid commercial and non-commercial methods for diagnosis and DST. Source: 1) Guillerm M, Usdin M, Arkinstall J.October 2006 Tuberculosis diagnosis and drug sensitivity An overview of the current diagnostic pipeline. 6-16 (www.accessmed-msf.org) 2) World Health Organization. The World health report 2003: changing history. Geneva,Switzerland: 200. http://www.who.int/tb/laboratory/policy_statements/en/index.html.

4.3   DST for Second-Line Anti-Tubercular Drugs

Second-line DST is complex, expensive and remains a global challenge due to lack of reliability and re-producibility of these tests The absolute concentration/resistance ratio DST on solid medium have not been validated , however commercial liquid methods and the proportion method on solid medium have shown promising results.DST results for Aminoglycosides, polypeptides, and fluoroquinolones have shown to relatively good reliability and reproducibility, allowing a quality-assured diagnosis of XDR-TB. With only few laboratories worldwide having the required capacity and expertise to reliably test for all classes of available anti-TB drugs, routine DST for second-line drugs (ethionamide, prothionamide, cy-closerine, terizidone, *P*-aminosalicylic acid, clofazimine,amoxicillin-clavulanate, clarithromycin, linezol-id) is not recommended Currently automated liquid culture systems have been recommended by the WHO as the "Gold Standard" for second-line DST (WHO, 2008).

4.4   Genotypic Methods (Molecular Methods)

In the past few years, genetic and molecular insights have unraveled the mechanisms involved in the de-velopment of drug resistance by MTB. Further characteristically drug resistance in MTB always results from genetic mutations. And unlike other bacteria these mutations appear to be confined to chromosomal DNA and do not involve mobile genetic elements (such as plasmids). These characteristics features and the knowledge about specific gene sequences of MTB have led to focus on development of large array gene probes/gene amplification systems. Molecular methods are genetic procedures that make use of ge-netic materials (DNA or RNA) to detect specific proteins or genes of the test organism using specific probes or short stranded oligonucleotides (primers) complementary to the test DNA strand. These molec-ular methods are not only useful in confirmation of identity of the isolates, direct detection of gene se-quences from the clinical specimens but also for molecular detection of drug resistance (Katoch, 2003). The methods include; conventional Polymerase Chain Reaction (PCR), single-stranded conformation polymorphism (SSCP)-PCR, nested PCR, reverse PCR, Real-Time PCR, DNA Microarrays, sequencing and Restricted Fragment Length Polymorphism (RFLP) analysis. The sequencing and hybridization-based assays directly detect mutations and can define the precise mutations involved, whereas electropho-retic assays provide an indirect method of detecting the existence of mutations without having the ability to define the exact nucleotidic substitution involved.

4.5   Nucleic Acid Sequence-based Amplification (NASBA)

Nucleic acid hybridization probes are single-stranded or double-stranded DNA/RNA fragments comple-mentary to a target DNA or RNA sequence which are labeled with a radioactive, chemi-luminescent or a fluorescent marker. (Wetmur, 1991) In clinical microbiology, nucleic acid hybridization probes often tar-get ribosomal RNA (rRNA) as it is available in larger number in organisms growing in culture. Of the many nucleic acid based amplification tests only a few have been evaluated by clinical laboratory. Those evaluated are Transcription Mediated Amplification (TMA) and NASBA. Using the enzyme RNA poly-merase, rRNA is transcribed by the process of reverse transcription. The advantages of this technique include isothermal amplification, greater sensitivity (rRNA is more abundant than DNA) and gives addi-tional information regarding viability of organism as compared to DNA based amplification methods that may pick up non-vaible organisms.

4.6   PCR Methods for Detection of Mycobacterium Tuberculosis

The technique of PCR is a rapid, inexpensive and simple way of making virtually unlimited copies of specific DNA fragments from minute quantities of the source DNA. During the last decade, primer sequences of specific regions in the MTB genome have been designed for detection, identification and typing of the bacteria from clinical samples and cultures using PCR technique. The usefulness of PCR for detection of tubercle bacilli in clinical specimens has been confirmed in several recent studies, with sensitivities and specificities ranging from 60% to 100% (Jain, 1997) In conventional PCR which is the most basic and simple PCR technique, the reaction products are separated by gel electrophoresis. Depending on the quantity produced and the size of the amplified fragment, the reaction products are visualized directly by staining with ethidium bromide or a silver-staining protocol, or by means of radioisotopes and autoradiography at the end of the PCR (end point PCR). Low sensitivity, short dynamic range < 2 logs, low resolution (about 10 fold difference), Non – Automated, size-based discrimination only, results are not expressed as numbers, Ethidium bromide for staining is not very quantitative and post PCR processing leading to risks of carry over and cross contamination have been cited as disadvantages of conventional agarose gel PCR by Parashar *et al.* (October2006).

PCR Sequencing: Sequencing is considered the "gold standard" for detecting mutations as it is accurate and reliable. It has been widely used for characterizing mutations in the rpoB gene in Rfm resistant strains and to detect mutations responsible for resistance to other anti-tuberculosis drugs. Hybridization based assays: Hybridization can be carried on solid phase (Line Probe Assay, DNA chip technology) or on liquid phase (hetero-duplex analysis, mismatch cleaving assay, molecular beacon). The two popular Solid-phase Hybridization Techniques include the Line Probe Assay ((INNO-LiPA) that detects Rfm resistance and the GenoType MTBDR assay (Hain's test) that simultaneously detects INH and Rfm resistance (based on the detection of the most common mutations in the katG and rpoB genes respectively). WHO in 2008 has endorsed Line Probe Assays (LPA) for molecular detection of drug resistance from smear-positive patients who are at the risk of developing MDR-TB. LPAs use PCR/hybridization technique to indentify members of MTB while simultaneously identifying drug-resistant strains by detecting the most common single nucleotide polymorphisms (SNPs) associated with resistance. The major advantage of LPAs is that the drug susceptibility results are available within approximately 5 hours as this technique can be performed directly on smear-positive sputum samples without the need for culture. Many laboratories have now replaced phenotypic DST with the LPAs as the primary method for DST (Pai *et al.*, 2009). The disadvantages of LPAs are that they are labor intensive and require highly trained personnel and dedicated laboratory space and equipments (Nicol, 2010). Phenotypic DST methods for MTB are inexpensive and accurate but time consuming. Genotypic DST methods for MTB are rapid and accurate but expensive. Thus molecular methods have certain benefits as in they can play an important role in scaling-up programmatic management of drug-resistant TB, in particular with regard to speed, standardization of tests, reduction in turnaround time, potential for high throughput, and reduced biosafety needs.

4.7   Real-time PCR

PCR technology has advanced from detection at the end point of reaction in conventional PCR to Real-time PCR where the detection is done while the reaction is taking place. Real-time PCR methods are based on hybridization of amplified nucleic acids with fluorescent-labeled probes spanning DNA regions of interest and monitored inside thermal cyclers (Ruiz *et al.*, 2004). The fluorescent signal increases in direct proportion to the amount of amplified product inside the reaction tube. Real-time PCR detects the PCR amplification during the early phases of the reaction, and measures the kinetics of the reaction, omitting the post PCR detection by electrophoresis or hybridization giving rapid results. This ability to generate results in very short time gives Real-time PCR an added edge over conventional agarose gel PCR (Parashar *et al.*, October2006). Monitoring the fluorescence intensities during the PCR run (i.e. in real time) allows detection and quantitation of the accumulating product without having to re-open reaction tubes after the PCR run. The simultaneous monitoring of the amplification of PCR product also lowers the risks of carry over and cross contamination since both reaction and detection occurs in a single tube giving more precise results (Parashar *et al.*, October2006). Real time PCR has better resolution than conventional PCR with the ability to detect even two fold changes. Real-time PCR is a quantitative method unlike conventional PCR. Real-time PCR can quantify *mycobacterial* load by template quantification in the clinical samples. [7] The reported sensitivity of Real-time PCR in clinical specimens has ranged from 71.6 to 98.1 per cent (Van, Coppenraet *et al.*, 2004) and specificity close to 100% (Broccolo *et al.*, 2003). Being highly sensitive, these assays can play a very useful role in early confirmation of diagnosis in paucibacillary and very early stages of *mycobacterial* diseases (WHO, 2008). Also viable bacteria are not a prerequisite for this technique. This feature can be helpful in detection of MTB in partially treated patients. Real-time PCR has been applied successfully in clinical samples directly (Mateu *et al.*, 2005; Ruiz *et al.*, 2004) for the detection of various micro-organisms including MTB (Lemaitre *et al.*, 2004). Several Real-time PCR based detection chemistries are available like FRET (fluorescent DNA dye–binding technique; SYBR Green1), hydrolysis probe (taqman probes), dual hybridization probes, molecular beacons and scorpion probes (Arya *et al.*, 2005).

Real-time PCR compares favorably with culture with respect to direct detection of MTB. There is a need to adequately validate the protocols for Real-time PCR on MTB containing specimens. It has also been shown by several studies that the identification of MTB and differentiation between MTB and Non Tubercular Mycobacterium (NTM) can be obtained faster than with any other Nucleic Acid Assays based technique (Arya *et al.*, 2005).

4.8   Role of Rifampicin Resistance in Timely Detection of MDR-TB

The fundamental role of Rfm in the treatment of patients with active TB cannot be overemphasized. Rfm is the most effective bactericidal drug that has not only helped in shortening the duration of Anti-TB treatment but also reduces its recurrence (Prahlad, 2005). The following points highlight the importance of Rfm resistance in MDR-TB:

1. WHO recommends Rfm resistance as a "surrogate marker" for detecting MDR-TB. Whereas mono-resistance to INH is quite common, mono-resistance to Rfm is rare. At least 90% of all Rfm-resistant clinical isolates are also resistant to INH (WHO/ IUATLD Report 3, 2004).
2. Although detection of MDR-TB is of utmost importance, Rfm mono-resistance has also been linked with treatment failure and thus is of clinical and public health relevance (WHO/ IUATLD Report 3, 2004). Rfm resistance is particularly suitable for genotypic DST because of two important reasons, firstly resistance to Rfm in MTB mostly occurs via genetic mechanism (Siddiqi *et al.*, 2002) and secondly 95% of Rfm resistance associated mutations are localized in an 81 bp region of the rpoB gene known as the Rifampicin Resistance Determining Region (RRDR).
3. Further molecular resistance to other anti-TB drugs like INH is more complicated and demands assessment of mutations in multiple genes for good correlation with phenotypic DST results. Ac-

curate genotypic DST for first-line and second-line anti-TB drugs is technically more challenging.

4. Molecular DR tests for Rfm resistance are much more developed than the tests for other anti-TB drugs. For example Xpert/MTB RIF (Cepheid, Sunnyvale, California, USA) is one of the most upcoming point-of-care (POC) diagnostic tests to be developed in recent years. This fully automated test is based on simultaneous detection of MTB and Rfm resistance using Real-time PCR. Results are available in less than 2 hours with a very high specificity and sensitivity (Grady *et al.*, 2011). This rapid, sensitive and simple test which has been endorsed by WHO (World Health Organization, 2012) is robust enough to be introduced outside conventional laboratory settings.

Thus Rfm resistance can be used as a proxy for MDR TB, saving the cost of analyzing the status of INH resistance in suspected cases. In a study by Payanandan *et al* the incidence of MDR-TB in Thailand was found to be same as incidence of Rfm resistance, further proving that Rfm resistance can be effectively used as surrogate marker for MDR-TB. Missense mutations at codons 526 to 531 (RRDR) have been reported to be crucial in conferring a high degree of resistance to Rfm (Mateu *et al.*, 2005). The reported frequencies of mutations in rpoB are 41% in codon 531, 32-36% in codon 526, and 7-9% in codon 516 (Ramaswamy & Musser, 1998; Williams et al.. 1994) By using Real-time PCR directly on FNA samples of patients with tubercular lymphadenitis we were also able to detect 17 of 30 (56.7%) Rfm resistant isolates with a probe that covered codons 526 and 531, the most frequent site for mutations (RRDR) of rpoB (Raoot & Dev, 2012).Earlier studies from South India have also shown that codon 531 and codon 526 are most frequently involved in mutations (Mani *et al.*,2001; Mercy *et al.*, 2009).

Real-time PCR, being very rapid, powerful, accurate and sensitive method, holds immense potential for detection of MTB, identification of *mycobacterial* species, quantitation of MTB load in patient, monitoring the efficacy of drug therapy and detection and genotyping of drug resistance .T h e use of PCR based genotypic DST methods, like Real-time PCR for the assessment of status of rpoB gene in MDR-TB patients is a very logical, economical and time saving approach over the traditional nonmolecular culture based methods. WHO endorsed Xpert MTB/RIF test which detects both MTB and rifampicin resistance in a single test is an appropriate example of the above fact. This test can be used as a stand-alone diagnostic test in individuals at risk of MDR-TB (WHO 2013). Based on heminested PCR technology the new Xpert MTB/RIF (Cepheid AB, Bromma, Sweden) test uses 5 molecular probes to confirm MTB detection and targets the *rpoB* gene of wild-type MTB strains. This real-time PCR test consists of a single-use multi chambered cartridge preloaded with the buffers and reagents required for sample processing, amplification, and detection. A barcode on each cartridge enables test details to be completed automatically by the software. Xpert MTB/RIF assay is currently the only established technology representing a new generation of automated molecular diagnostic platforms that satisfies all the demands of being 'quick', 'cheap' 'easy' and high specific. (Manuel Causse *et al.*, 2011) In August 2012, a publicprivate partnership announced between the United States President's Emergency Plan for AIDS Relief (PEPFAR), the United States Agency for International Development USAID), UNITAID, and the Bill & Melinda Gates Foundation allowed for a drop in price of the Xpert MTB/RIF test cartridge from 16.86 USD to 9.98 USD for the public sector of 145 high-burden and developing countries plus NGOs and other non-profit agencies in these countries. (USAID PRESS Release 6th August 2012)

4.9   Timely Diagnosis-the Key to Prevention of MDR TB

As discussed above, the diagnosis of MDR-TB by traditional methods can take up to 3 months considering the maximum incubation period of cultures and DST. In view of the grave consequences of MDR-TB, timely diagnosis of resistance is the most critical step in prevention and reduction of further transmission of the resistant strains. Timely identification of drug resistance is especially important to avoid exposing patients to standard first-line treatment for months till the DST results become available. Such exposure to inadequate therapy would result in amplified drug resistance and ongoing transmission, adding to the ever growing pool of drug resistant strains. In addition, the longer the resistant clones are allowed to evolve within infected individual the more they become difficult to treat and are associated with higher mortality. Prompt diagnosis and timely initiation of appropriate therapy in MDR-TB patient's leads to sputum culture conversion to negative in half of patients within 3 months and improves the overall outcome (Yagui *et al.*, 2006).The availability of DOTS Plus further necessitates timely detection of DR however detection of drug resistance still remains a major challenge. In 2011, only 12% of the estimated MDR-TB cases were reported to the WHO. (*WHO Global Report 2012*) indicating that the vast majority of patients went undiagnosed and could not be treated according to internationally recognized standards. Capacity building of laboratories to ensure high-quality performance standards and high bio-safety levels is one of the most needed measures of scaling up of MDR-TB control strategy for better case detection.

In the absence of an "ideal TB diagnostic test" which would be point–of–care (POC) test, simple, rapid, sensitive, accurate, based on easy technology, and would simultaneously identify drug resistance, the currently available DST methods cannot effectively meet the urgent need of providing timely and accurate diagnosis to HIV associated and MDR-TB patients. The knowledge gained from advancement in mycobacterial genomics, deciphering of molecular mechanisms of drug resistance and development of newer DST techniques will give the required momentum to the TB control programmes across the globe and help meet the challenge of timely diagnosis and decrease the catastrophic effect of MDR-TB and XDR-TB on universal TB control programmes.

Reference

Appling, D., Miller, R.,H.(1981). MTB Cervical Lymphadenopathy.1981 update Laryngoscope, 91:1259-1266.

Arya, M., Shergill, S.,I., Willamson, M. et al.(2005). Basic Principles of real-time quantitative PCR . Expert rev. Mol. Diagn. 5(2):209-219.

Broccolo, F.,F., Scarpellini, P., Locatelli, G.(2003). Rapid diagnosis of mycobacterial infections and quantitation of Mycobacterium tuberculosis load by two real-time calibrated PCR assays. J Clin Microbiol 41: 4565-4572.

C.,B., Nash, K.,A.(1996). Antimicrobial agents: In vitro susceptibility testing, spectra of activity, mechanisms of action and resistance, and assays for activity in biologic fluids. Antibiotics in Laboratory Medicine. Baltimore, Md: Williams & Wilkins; 127-175.

Drowart, A., Cambiaso, C.,L., Huygen, K. et al(1997). Detection of rifampicin and isoniazid resistance of M. tuberculosis by particle counting immunoassay (PACIA). Int J Tuberc Lung Dis 1:284-288.

Ebrahim (2010). Bacterial resistance to antimicrobials. J Trop Pediatr, 56 (3): 141-143.

Elvira, Richter., Sabine, Rüsch-Gerdes.,& Doris, Hillemann.(2009) Drug-susceptibility Testing in TB: Current Status and Future Prospects Elvira Richter, Sabine Rüsch-Gerdes, Doris Hillemann Expert Rev Resp Med. 3(5):497-510.

Espasa, M., Salvadó, M., Vicente, E. et al., (February 2012). Evaluation of the VersaTREK System Compared to the Bactec MGIT 960 System for First-Line Drug Susceptibility Testing of Mycobacterium tuberculosis. J. Clin. Microbiol; vol. 50 no. 2 488-491.

Government of India (2012). TB INDIA , Revised National TB Control Programme: Annual Status Report: 8 (http://www.tbcindia.nic.in).

Grady, O.,J., Maeurer,M., Mwaba, P. et al.(2011). New and Improved diagnostics for detection of drug resistant pulmonary tuberculosis. Clinical Opinion in Pulmonary Medicine. 17:134-141.

Hershkovitz, I., H. D. Donoghue, et al. (2008). "Detection and molecular characterization of 9,000-year-old Mycobacterium tuberculosis from a Neolithic settlement in the Eastern Mediterranean." PLoS One 3(10): e3426.

Heym, B., Saint-Joanis B., Cole, S., T. (1999). The molecular basis of isoniazid resistance in Mycobacterium tuberculosis. Tuber. Lung Dis. 79:267–271.

Hobby, G.,L., Holman, A.,P., Iseman, M., D. et al.(1973). Enumeration of tubercle bacilli in sputum of patients with pulmonary tuberculosis. Antimicrob Agents Chemother 4:94-104.

Ignatova, A,. Dubiley, S., Stepanshina, V., Shemyakin, I. (2006). Predominance of multi-drug-resistant LAM and Beijing family strains among Mycobacterium tuberculosis isolates recovered from prison inmates in Tula Region, Russia. J Med Microbiol. 55(Pt10):1413-1418.

Jain, N., K.(1996). Laboratory Diagnosis of Pulmonary Tuberculosis: Conventional and Newer Approaches. Ind. J. Tub 43:107.

Jenny-Avital, E.R.(2002) Acquired rifampin resistance in AIDS-related TB. AIDS Clin Care 14:72-3.

Jin, D., & Gross, C. (1988).Mapping and Sequencing of Mutation in E coli Rpo -B gene that leads to Rfm resistance. J.Mol Biol 202:45-58.

Katoch, V.,M., Guest Column: Advances in Molecular Diagnosis of Tuberculosis. (2003).MJAFI 59 : 182-186.

Katoch, V.,M.(October 2004) .Review Article: Newer diagnostic techniques for tuberculosis. Indian J Med Res 120: 418-428.

Lemaitre, N., Armand, S., Vachee, A.(2004). Comparison of the real-time PCR method and the Gen-Probe amplified Mycobacterium tuberculosis direct test for detection of Mycobacterium tuberculosis in pulmonary and nonpulmonary specimens. J Clin Microbiol 42: 4307-4309.* Comparative study of real-time PCR with the amplified MTD method in clinical samples.

Mani, C., Selvakumar, N., Sujatha, N., Narayanan, P., R.(2001). Mutations in the rpoB Gene of multidrug-resistant Mycobacterium tuberculosis Clinical Isolates from India. J. Clin. Microbiol 39: 2987-2990.

Manuel, Causse., Pilar, Ruiz., Juan, Bautista., et al., (2011). Comparison of Two Molecular Methods for Rapid Diagnosis of Extrapulmonary Tuberculosis. Clin. Microbiol. vol. 49 no. 8;3065-3067.

Mateu, Espasa¹,. Julián, González-Martín¹,. Fernando, Alcaide. et al .(2005). Direct detection in cliniical samples of multiple gene mutations causing resistance of Mycobacterium tuberculosis to isoniazid and rifampicin using fluorogenic probes .Journal of Antimicrobial Chemotherapy. 55(6) :860-865.

Mercy, A., Lingala, L., Srikantam, A., Jain, S., Rao, KVSM, Rao, PVR. (2010).Clinical and geographical profiles of rpoB gene mutations in Mycobacterium tuberculosis isolates from Hyderabad and Koraput in India. Journal of Microbiology and Antimicrobials; 2(2):13-18.

Mondal R. & Jain A, (2007). Extensively Drug-Resistant Mycobacterium tuberculosis, India. Emer Infectious Dis, 13: 1429–31.

Munsiff, S.,S., Nivin, B., Sacajiu, G., Mathema, B., Bifani, P., Kreiswirth, B.,N. (2003). Persistence of a highly resistant strain of tuberculosis in New York City during 1990-1999. J Infect Dis. 188(3):356-363.

Musser, J. M. (1995 Oct). Antimicrobial Agent Resistance in Mycobacteria: molecular Genetic Insights. Clin Microbiol Rev 8(4):496–514.

National Committee of Clinical and Laboratory Standards (NCCLS).(1995). Antimycobacterial susceptibility testing for Mycobacterium tuberculosis; Tentative Standard M24-T. Villanova, Pa: NCCLS.

Nelson, L. J., Talbot, E.A., Mwasekaga, M.J., et al. (2002). Antituberculosis drug resistance and anonymous HIV surveillance in tuberculosis patients in Botswana. Lancet 366:488-490.

Nicol, M., P. New developments in the laboratory diagnosis of tuberculosis. (2010). Continu Med Educ 2010; 28: 246–250.

Nilsson, L.,E., Hoffner, S.,E., Ansehn, S. (1998). Rapid susceptibility testing of M. tuberculosis by bioluminescence assay of mycobacterial ATP. Antimicrob Agents Chemother 32:1208-1212.

Norden,M.,A., Kurzynski,T.,A., Bownds,S.,E. et al(1995). Rapid susceptibility testing of Mycobacterium tuberculosis (H37Ra) by flow cytometry. J Clin Microbiol 33:1231-1237.

Pai, M., Minion, J., Sohn, H. et al. (2009). Novel and improved technologies for tuberculosis diagnosis: progress and challenges. A critical review of new TB diagnostic. Clin Chest Med 30:701–716.

Paramsivan, C. N. &Venkataraman, P.(2004) .Drug Resistance in Tuberculosis in India. Indian J Med. Res,120, 377-386.

Parashar, D., Chauhan, D.,S., Sharma, V., D., Katoch, V.(October2006). Review article Applications of real-time PCR technology to mycobacterial research. Indian J Med Res 124: 385-398.

Payananda, V., Kladphuang, B., Somsong, W., Jittimanee, S.(1999). Thailand tuberculosis programme report, (Battle against TB). Bangkok: Thai Agricultural Cooperative Press.

Prahlad, Kumar,.(April 2005) Guest Lecture, Journey of TB Control Movement in India: NTP to RNTCP. Ind J Tuberc, 52:68-71.

Ramaswamy, S., & Musser, J., M.(1998). Molecular genetic basis of antimicrobial agent resistance in Mycobacterium tuberculosis. Tuber. Lung Dis; 79:3–29.

Raoot,A., Dev. G. (2012). Assessment of Status of rpoB Gene in FNAC Samples of Tuberculous Lymphadenitis by Real-Time PCR. Tuberculosis Research and Treatment :Article ID 834836, 5.

Riska, P.,F., Jacobs, W.,R., Alland, D., Jr.(Feb 2000). Molecular determinants of drug resistance in tuberculosis. Int J Tuberc Lung Dis. 4(2 Suppl 1):S4-10.

Ruiz, M., Torres, M.J., Llanos, A.,C. et al.(2004). Direct detection of rifampin- and isoniazid-resistant Mycobacterium tuberculosis in auramine-rhodamine-positive sputum specimens by real-time PCR. J Clin Microbiol 42:1585-1589.

Sharma ,S.K. & Mohan, A. (October 2004).Review Article-Multi Drug Resistant Tuberculosis. Indian J Med Re, 120,354-376.

Shin, S.S., Pasechnikov, A.D., Gelmanova, I.Y., et al.(2006) Treatment outcomes in an integrated civilian and prison MDR-TB treatment program in Russia. Int J Tuberc Lun Dis 10:402-408.

Siddiqi, N., Shamim, M., Hussain, S. et al. (February 2002). Molecular Characterization of Multidrug-Resistant Isolates of Mycobacterium tuberculosis from Patients in North India. Antimicrob Agents Chemother. 46(2): 443–450.

Singh, Gagandeep. Grover. & Takkar. Jaspreet (2008). Recent Advances in Multi-Drug-Resistant Tuberculosis and RNTCP Indian J Community Med, 33(4): 219–223.

Soumitesh, Chakravorty., Manas, Kamal., Sen., & Jaya, Sivaswami., Tyagi.(2005.) Diagnosis of Extrapulmonary Tuberculosis by Smear, Culture, and PCR Using Universal Sample Processing Technology J Clin Microbiol;43(9) 4357-4362.

TB India (2012).Revised National Tuberculosis Control Program Annual report 2012 (http://www.tbcindia.nic.in).

Telenti, A., P. Imboden, F. Marchesi, D. Lowrie, S. Cole, M. J. Colston, L .Matter, K. Schopfer, and T. Bodmer. (1993). Detection of Rifampicin Resistance Mutations in Mycobacterium tuberculosis. Lancet 341: 647–50.

Thwaites, G.,.E., Chau, T.,T., Stepniewka, K. et al.(2002). Diagnosis of adult tuberculous meningitis by use of clinical and laboratory features. Lancet 360: 1287-1292.

UNAIDS (2010). Report on the Global AIDS epidemic.

USAID (2012). Public-Private partnership announces immediate 40 percent cost reduction for rapid TB test; USAID PRESS Release 6 [th] August 2012.

Van, Coppenraet., E.,S.,B., Lindeboom, J.,A., Kuijper, J. et al.(2004). Real-time PCR assay using fine needle aspirates and tissue biopsy specimens for rapid diagnosis of mycobacterial lymphadenitis in children. J Clin Microbiol 42: 2644-50.

Wells, C.D., Cegielsk,I P., Nelson, L.J., et al. (2007) HIV Infection and Multidrug-Resistant Tuberculosis—The Perfect Storm. J Infect Dis. 196(Supplement 1): S86-S107.doi: 10.1086/518665.

World Health Organization (2003). Tuberculosis fact sheet. (url:http://www.who.int/gtb/publications/fact sheet/index.htm.2003).

World Health Organization (2003). Treatment of tuberculosis: guidelines for national programmes. 3rd ed.Geneva: The Organization; (WHO/CDS/2003.313). http://www.who.int/tb/publications/cds_tb_2003_313/en/index.html).

World Health Organization/International Union Against Tuberculosis and Lung Disease (IUATLD) (2004) Anti-tuberculosis drug resistance in the world: Report 3. WHO Geneva: WHO/HTM/TB/2004: 343.

WHO, Geneva, (2006).Extensively drug-resistant tuberculosis (XDR-TB): recommendations for prevention and control", Weekly epidemiological record, 81 www.who.int.

World Health Organization. (2008).Molecular line probe assays for rapid screening of patients at risk of multidrug-resistant tuberculosis (MDR-TB). Geneva: World Health Organization.

WHO (2010.)Multidrug and extensively drug-resistant TB (M/XDR-TB) 2010 Global Report on Surveillance and Response", WHO, Geneva, 15 www.who.int/tb/publications.

WHO (2012). Global Tuberculosis Report, WHO Geneva, 201 www.who.int/tb/publications/global_report.

World Health Organization (2013).Definitions and reporting -framework for tuberculosis (1-40) WHO/HTM/TB/2013.2: www.who.int/tb.

World Health Organization/International Union Against Tuberculosis and Lung Disease (IUATLD) (2004) Anti-tuberculosis drug resistance in the world: Report 3. WHO Geneva: WHO/HTM/TB/2004: 343.

Williams, D.,L., Waguespack, C.,Eisenach, K. et al.(1994). Characterization of rifampin resistance in pathogenic mycobacteria. Antimicrob Agent Chemother 38 : 2380-2386.

Yagui, M., Perales, T.,M., Asencios, L. et al. (2006). Timely diagnosis of MDR-TB under program conditions: is rapid drug susceptibility testing sufficient. Int J Tuberc Lung Dis 10(8):838–843.

Yajko, D., M., Madej, J.,J., Lancaster, M.,V. et al. (1995). Colorimetric method for determining MICs of antimicrobial agents for Mycobacterium tuberculosis. J Clin Microbiol 33: 2324-2327.

Tuberculosis-related Uveitis

Ozlem Sahin
Department of Ophthalmology/Uveitis
DunyaGoz Hospital Ltd., Ankara, Turkey

Alireza Ziaei
Ophthalmology Department
Boston University, USA

1 Review of Tuberculosis Related Uveitis

Tuberculosis (TB) infection is considered common worldwide affecting one-third of the world's population especially in developing economies, immigrant populations, and immunocompromised patients in developed nations (Bloom & Murray, 1992). According to the World Health Organization, the highest prevalence has been reported in Southeast Asia (Department of Health of the Philippines, National Tuberculosis Control Programme). The incidence of tuberculosis has reported to increase with the increase in the HIV infected population (Tollefson *et al.*, 2013). TB is a chronic infection caused by Mycobacterium tuberculosis (M. Tuberculosis) which is a particularly aggressive microorganism. The host's defense is based on the induction of cellular immunity, in which the creation of a granulomatous structure is considered to have an important role (Bloom & Murray, 1992). M. tuberculosis is regarded the most insidious microbial human pathogen known. This bacillus is able to induce an infection in the human body, the so-called latent tuberculosis infection (LTBI), which is considered persist for a long period of time, even, for the whole life (Bloom & Murray, 1992). It is currently reported that around a third of the world's population (2.5 billion people) has an LTBI (Guimaraes *et al.*, 2012). 10% of people with LTBI are disclosed to develop active TB, contributing to 9 million new cases and 2 million deaths every year (Guimaraes *et al.*, 2012). This is considered as a catastrophic process with no apparent end in sight as all these TB infections constantly generate new LTBI cases (approximately 100 million a year) (Rivest *et al.*, 2013). The incidence of tuberculosis-related uveitis (TRU) is also shown to have a rising trend (Campos *et al.*, 2008; Mathur & Biswas, 2012). In a Western urban multi-ethnic population, patients from Asia, TB history or contact in the past are considered at higher risk of TRU (Rodriquez *et al.*, 1996). The purpose of this chapter is to review the pathogenesis of tuberculosis, ocular manifestations, diagnosis and differential diagnosis of TRU. Furthermore, this chapter addresses the new diagnostic criteria for intraocular tuberculosis specifically, IFN-gamma Release Assays (IGRAs) and polymerase chain reactions.

2 Pathogenesis of Tuberculosis-related Uveitis

The natural history of LTBI is considered to start with inhalation of an infected aerosol, which allows the bacilli to reach the alveolar spaces and subsequently to be phagocytosed by the alveolar macrophages (Cordero-Coma *et al.*, 2010). The bacilli avoid the phagolysosome union, and reported to grow until they destroy the macrophage, which in most cases results in necrosis if the macrophage has not previously induced its own apoptosis (Cordero-Coma *et al.*, 2010). This rupture of the infected macrophage temporarily stops bacillary growth by releasing them into the stressful extracellular milieu, where it is thought that cannot grow (Cordero-Coma *et al.*, 2010). These bacilli can potentially remain embedded in the necrotized environment for a long period of time until they are phagocytosed by another macrophage (Cordero-Coma *et al.*, 2010). The presence of natural killers (NK) plays a relevant role at this stage as they can activate macrophages and cause a small amount of bacillary destruction (Abebe, 2012). Neutrophils, which were previously thought to have a bactericidal effect when apoptotic also contribute this process by inducing necrosis in the extracellular matrix, and curtailing bacterial dissemination, contributing to the formation of a granulomatous structure that is regarded to support sudden cellular entrance (Abebe, 2012). In this granulomatous structure, approximately 10% of monocytes are disclosed to become dendritic cells (DCs), which, once infected, migrate towards the regional lymph nodes where they present M. tuberculosis antigens and induce the proliferation of specific T lymphocytes (Chen & Kolls, 2013). These lymphocytes, mainly type 1 CD4 with some type 1 CD8, then migrate towards the infection site, where they are considered to recognize the infected macrophages and activate them by IFN γ or cause their death by necrosis or apoptosis, thus controlling the bacillary load. This process is regarded to be faster for immune hosts as they already have memory T lymphocytes, thus allowing a faster generation of effector T cells (Chen & Kolls, 2013). Another process, which is considered the removal of cellular debris by macrophages, which progressively become filled with lipid bodies to become foamy macrophages (FMs), takes place simultaneously (Silva Miranda et al., 2012). The slow pace of bacillary growth is disclosed in a discrete pathological process at the beginning of the infection (Silva Miranda et al., 2012). In the experimental murine model, where infection is induced with a low-dose aerosol, infected lungs are shown to have a very limited and transient localized increase in the cellularity between the epithelia and the lamina propria rather than granulomatous lesions in the first three weeks post-infection despite the fact that the bacillary load increases up to 105 CFU (Calderon et al., 2013). Granuloma formation is considered to depend entirely on TNF production by the infected macrophages and T cells, as well as the integrity of all ligands and receptors of the TNF family (Heuts et al., 2013). Sustained TNF signaling is disclosed to maintain the necessary local chemokine gradients to hold the cells in close apposition, thus favoring the activation of infected macrophages (Allie et al., 2013). Aqueous cytokine and chemokine analyses have shown that subjects with TRU who respond to anti-TB therapy do not have an active ocular tuberculosis infection, but rather an autoimmune-related ocular inflammation that may be triggered by TB (Ang et al., 2012a). Higher levels of interleukin-6, interleukin-8, interferon-gamma, and interferon-gamma-induced protein 10 have been disclosed in the aqueous analysis of the patients with TRU (Ang et al., 2012a).

3 Clinical Manifestations of Tuberculosis Related Uveitis

TB in the eye is considered to associate with a wide spectrum of clinical manifestations (Bouza et al., 1997; Rodriquez et al., 1996). Definitive diagnosis of confirmed ocular tuberculosis is reported to be daunting due to the difficulty of getting ocular samples for microbiologic or histologic evaluation. High awareness of ocular manifestations is considered as important for the diagnosis of ocular tuberculosis (Vyas, 2009). The diagnosis of presumed ocular tuberculosis (POTB) is based on the clinical signs of tuberculosis uveitis associated with a history or signs and symptoms of pulmonary or extra pulmonary tuberculosis (Lara & Ocampo, 2013). The common clinical presentations are reported as anterior granulomatous uveitis, vitritis, choroiditis, choroidal tubercles, multifocal choroiditis, occlusive vasculitis, rarely serpiginous-like choroiditis, subretinal abscesses or suspected ocular tumors (Manousaridis et al., 2013). Anterior uveitis associated with tuberculosis has also been reported as non-granulomatous with broad-based posterior synechia formation (Lara & Ocampo, 2013). Anterior granulomatous uveitis might be associated with bilateral central interstitial keratitis (Kamal et al., 2013). POTB might also present only with low grade anterior chamber activity (Manousaridis et al., 2013). Rarely hypopyon associated anterior uveitis might occur (Chatziralli et al., 2012). Focal, nodular, diffuse or necrotizing scleritis with or without keratitis have also been disclosed in patients with POTB (Manousaridis et al., 2013). Although scleritis is considered as a rare condition associated with POTB, anterior nodular non-necrotizing scleritis is revealed as the most common scleral involvement. Anterior scleritis has also been reported as associated with extensive posterior synechia (Ang et al., 2012b).

Nodular episcleritis with pain, redness and blurred vision has been disclosed in POTB (Bathula *et al.*, 2012). Necrotizing scleritis associated with recurrent erythema nodosum related to an immune reaction of delayed hypersensitivity type IV to various antigenic components of mycobacteria has been reported in patients with no history of pulmonary or systemic disease, and 50% of no evidence of pathology on chest X-ray (Pedroza *et al.*, 2010). Necrotizing scleritis might also be associated with peripheral ulcerative keratitis in POTB (Gupta *et al.*, 2008). Isolated posterior scleritis is reported as a rare condition associated with POTB (Gupta *et al.*, 2003; Sharma *et al.*, 2010). Very rarely, posterior scleral granuloma mimicking choroidal melanoma has been reported in POTB (Velasco e Cruz *et al.*, 2011). Posterior segment inflammation associated with POTB is reported to include intermediate, posterior, or panuveitis (Chu & Hui, 2010). Multifocal chorioretinitis presented with transient visual disturbances is another manifestation of posterior segment inflammation due to tuberculosis (Baha *et al.*, 2009; Anna *et al.*, 2013). Multifocal serpiginoid choroiditis is described in patients particularly from TB-endemic regions presenting fundus changes similar to serpiginous choroiditis but also showing evidence of active TB and/or the presence of mycobacterial DNA in the aqueous humor (Nazari Khanamiri & Rao, 2013). Multifocal outer retinal and inner choroidal inflammation is considered as a marker of intraocular TB even in a non-endemic area. The lesions are described as multifocal, irregular in shape, very numerous, widespread, noncontiguous to the optic disc, often asymmetrical and often demonstrating both active and resolved areas simeltenously (Gan & Jones. 2013). Tubercular serpiginous-like choroiditis is reported predominantly affecting the young to middle-aged man, and it is associated with moderate to severe vitreous inflammation unlike serpiginous choroiditis (Bansal *et al.*, 2012). Retinal periphlebitis in multiple quadrants of the retina and choroiditis lesions might occur simultenously (Nayak *et al.*, 2011). Choriocapillaritis is regarded as another posterior segment manifestation of POTB. It has similar features of acute multifocal posterior placoid pigment epitheliopathy (APMPPE), but it shows smoldering relentless evolution monitored by indocyanine green angiography (De Luigi *et al.*, 2012). Isolated retinal vasculitis with pulmonary tuberculosis characterized by multiple retinal hemorrhages, vascular sheathing, and a yellowish retina associated with the sign of xanthopsia has also been described (Roh *et al.*, 2011). Macular edema in patients with POTB is reported to cause significant visual impairment (Al-Mezaine *et al.*, 2008). Three patterns of macular edema: diffuse, cystoid and serous retinal detachment which is the most common type were described. Optical coherence tomography is considered useful in monitoring the efficacy of treatment in patients with macular edema (Al-Mezaine *et al.*, 2008). Patients who are immunosuppressed or HIV infected are reported to develop active mycobacterial disease in the eye leading to rapid destruction of the ocular structures (Babu *et al.*, 2006; Nwosu, 2008). Ocular TB in AIDS is considered to occur even at CD4+ cell counts greater than 200 cells/microl (Babu *et al.*, 2006). Choroidal tuberculosis characterized by choroidal granuloma has been reported in patients with HIV and miliary tuberculosis.

4   Diagnosis and Differential Diagnosis of Tuberculosis Related Uveitis

With absence of proper diagnostic standard, it usually leads to missed diagnosis, misdiagnosis, and delayed diagnosis of POTB which is considered to result in severe consequences such as vision loss, blind, and even eye enucleation (Tabbara, 2013). However, POTB is considered a diagnostic challenge (Vos *et al.*, 2013). A history of TB contact, abnormalities on chest X-ray, extraocular manifestations of TB associated with good response to anti-tuberculosis therapy (ATT) are marked as helpful parameters for the diagnosis of POTB (Vos *et al.*, 2013). Tuberculosis skin test (TST) is considered to determine the immune response to the Bacille Calmette Guerin (BCG) substrain of Mycobacterium (American Thoracic Society, 2000). This immune response is reported to develop if the individual has active TB or had exposure to TB in the past or received the BCG vaccine against TB. The immune response is considered a delayed type sensitivity reaction of memory T-cells sensitized prior to the purified protein derivatives of the bacterium (American Thoracic Society, 2000). The TST test is reported to be in clinical use primarily to identify latent TB infection in persons at risk of progression to active disease, and to support the diagnosis of active TB disease (Huebner *et al.*, 1993). However, the TST might be an imperfect marker of TB infection since it has been reported that 10-25 % of persons with active TB have a negative TST result (Holden *et al.*, 1971; Nash & Douglass, 1980). On the other hand, persons with a positive TST are considered less likely to have a disseminated disease (Colditz *et al.*, 1994). In general, it has been found that persons with TST $\geq$ 15 mm were less likely to have military or combined pulmonary and extrapulmonary disease, and more likely to have cavitary pulmonary disease relative to the non-cavitary pulmonary disease (Auld *et al.*, 2013). TST is also reported to be influenced by the HIV status and birth place of the person. Persons with HIV, and US-born persons without HIV who have a TST $\geq$ 15 mm are considered to have more likely cavitary pulmonary disease while foreign-born persons without HIV who have a TST $\geq$ 15 mm are significantly less likely to have cavitary pulmonary disease (Auld *et al.*, 2013). The TST is reported to be insensitive in immunocompromised persons because of the high rates of anergy, and false-positive results in persons who have BCG vaccination (Ahmed & Karter, 2004). *In vitro* assays that measure effector T cell response to stimulation of early secretory antigen target-6 (ESAT-6) and culture filtrate protein-10 (CFP-10) antigens from Mycobacterium tuberculosis, called interferon gamma release assays (IGRAs) are reported to be more effective in immunosuppressed population, and also reported that they are not affected by previous vaccination with BCG (Mori, 2009). There are three commercially available IGRAs including T-SPOT.TB (Oxford Immunotec United Kingdom), Quantiferon Gold (Celletis USA) and Quantiferon In-tube (Celletis USA) (Winthrop *et al.*, 2008). T-SPOT.TB is considered a type of ELISPOT assay which counts the number of anti-mycobacterial effector T-cells that produce interferon (IFN) gamma in a sample of blood (Meier *et al.*, 2005). T-SPOT.TB assay is regarded to give an overall measurement of the host immune response against mycobacteria which might reveal the presence of either active or latent infection with Mycobacterium tuberculosis (Huebner *et al.*, 1993). This test is reported to be not effected by the previous BCG vaccine and previous infections with non-tuberculous mycobacterium (Ang *et al.*, 2013). Based on these facts, T-SPOT.TB test is considered more specific but less sensitive than TST that is recommended to use in preference to the TST in low-TB prevalence populations (Holden *et al.*, 1971). It has been also recommended to use both T-SPOT.TB and TST in conjunction to increase the likelihood diagnosis of POTB (Lalvani & Pareek, 2010). T-SPOT.TB is considered helpful either to rule-in or to rule-out active TB in immunocompromised patients from intermediate TB burden regions (Jung *et al.*, 2012). The Quantiferon-TB Gold test is considered as an enzyme linked immunosorbent assay (ELISA) which measures the amount of IFN gamma in the sample of blood after the effector T- cells are stimulated with ESAT-6 and CFU-10 antigens (Bellete *et al.*, 2002). A combination of the Quantiferon-TB Gold and TST tests rather than solo test are recommended in endemic areas for TB, such as India, Asia, and Western urban multi-ethnic population (Babu *et al.*, 2013). The sensitivity (S) and specificity (Sp) of the TST and Quantiferon–TB Gold are disclosed not differentiating significantly as S 87% vs. 90% and Sp 85% vs. 82% (Liorenç *et al.*, 2013). The limiting factors for the combining the tests in these areas are reported the higher cost, technical issues, and inability to distinguish active and latent TB (Babu *et al.*, 2013). The use of 18(F) fluorodeoxyglucose positron emission tomography/CT in quantiferon-TB Gold positive patients with POTB is recommended to identify the size and metabolic activity of the hilar and mediastinal lymph nodes and pulmonary lesions and to find out whether these lesions are appropriate for biopsy (Doycheva et al., 2011). The Quantiferon-TB Gold In-tube (QFT-G-IT) test is considered as a third generation of IGRAs which measures the IFN gamma concentration of blood in tube after stimulating the effector T-cells by ESAT-6, CFP-10 and Tb7.7 (p49) peptide antigens (Streeton et al., 1998). It has been reported that QFT-G-IT has a consistent specificity of > 99% in low risk individuals and a sensitivity as high as 92% in individuals with active disease, depending on setting and extend of disease (Moon & Hur, 2013). QFT-G-IT is considered to have advantages when combined with TST in immunosuppressed patients especially in older patients with a negative TST and in BCG vaccinated patients with a positive TST (Garcia-Gasalla et al., 2013). It is reported to prevent unnecessary treatments and toxicities related to a false-positive TST result (Garcia-Gasalla et al., 2013). The sensitivities of QFT-G-IT, T-SPOT-TB and TST to rule out active TB in immunosuppressed patients are revealed as 11.1%, 40% and 25% respectively (Jung et al., 2012). Since the IGRAs have limitations to differentiate latent TB from active infection nucleic acid amplification techniques (NAAT) have emerged as an important tool for rapid and accurate diagnosis of TB (Boehme et al., 2007). NAAT-based diagnostic methods mostly use a single target Mycobacterium genome (IS6110) for the amplification and detection of tuberculosis (Sarmiento et al., 2003). It has been reported that IS6110 is absent in 10-40% Mycobacterium tuberculosis isolates in endemic areas like India that likelihood increases the false-negative tests (Das et al., 1995; Sarmiento et al., 2003).

A low sensitivity (37.7) has been reported with NAAT (IS6110) in ocular samples from POTB patients (Arora et al., 1999). An alternative approach is considered to use multi-targeted PCR using three targeted genes specific including IS6110, MPB64 and Pab which are specific for Mycobacterium tuberculosis (Sharma et al., 2013). Presence of TB DNA in the ocular fluid is considered suggesting presence of Mycobacterium infection within the eye, but does not differentiate the clinical picture from an immune response to mycobacterial antigens being loaded from the retina pigment epithelial (RPE) cells or somewhere else from the body. Thus, multi-targeted PCR cannot differentiate between active and latent TB infection. Besides, multi-targeted PCR positivity has been reported in POTB patients groups with both active and latent TB infections (Sharma et al., 2013). Several acid-fast bacteria localized within the necrotic RPE cells has been demonstrated (Rao et al., 2006). This finding is considered to support the possibility of tubercular uveitis as an immune response to these sequestered bacteria within the RPE cells (Rao et al., 2006). Several studies revealed the presence of Mycobacterium tuberculosis genome in the vitreous samples of patients with retinal vasculitis so-called Eales' disease and chronic or recurrent choroiditis (Bhuibhar et al., 2012, Singh et al., 2012). Multifocal serpiginoid choroiditis characterized by multifocal lesions that are noncontagious to the optic disc and showing serpiginoid spread associated with vitreous inflammation has been described (Bansal et al., 2012; Nazari Khanamiri & Rao, 2013; Vasconcelos-Santos et al., 2010). The distinction between serpiginous choroiditis and multifocal serpiginoid choroiditis is considered crucial to avoid unnecessary ATT for serpiginous choroiditis (Bansal et al., 2012; Nazari Khanamiri & Rao, 2013).

5   Therapeutic Approach of Presumed Ocular Tuberculosis

ATT is considered highly effective and for both confirming the diagnosis and resolving the inflammatory process, and it is recommended to be initiated for cases with a clinical suspicion of POTB. It is also reported that ATT has additional advantages, such as preventing latent-tuberculosis reactivations due to immunosuppressive therapy, and decreasing the number and /or severity of uveitis relapses (Cordero-Coma *et al.*, 2013). Early referral is recommended for patients who are not responding appropriately to anti-inflammatory therapy (Patel *et al.*, 2013). Patients diagnosed after 500 days after initial ocular symptoms are reported to be more likely losing their vision (Patel *et al.*, 2013). The initial prescribed ATT is reported to include 4 drugs: isoniazid, rifampicin, pyrazinamide and ethambutol (Blumberg *et al.*, 2005). The minimum length for the treatment of drug-susceptible TB with a rifampin-based regimen is revealed 6-9 months (Blumberg *et al.*, 2005). The recommendations for treatment of LTBI in both HIV-infected and HIV-uninfected patients are reported to include isoniazid for 9 months as the preferred regimen, or isoniazid for 6 months based on the local program condition, rifampin and pyrazinamide for 2 months or rifampin for 4 months (Cohn, 2000). In patients with either proven or POTB in the absence of constitutional or respiratory symptoms, elevated inflammatory markers, or an abnormal chest X-ray, a minimum of 6 month of ATT is suggested (Manousaridis *et al.*, 2011; Sanqhvi *et al.*, 2011). However, it is reported that it may not be effective in patients having complications such as, retinal vasculitis with vitreous hemorrhage, branch retinal vein occlusion, persistent macular edema, choroidal scar and optic atrophy (Yasaratne *et al.*, 2010). Topical or systemic anti-inflammatory therapy in conjunction with ATT is indicated for patients with hypopyon uveitis, interstitial keratitis, phylectenular keratitis, tubercular serpiginous-like choroiditis, tuberculosis-related choriocapillaritis, focal choroiditis and choroidal and brain tuberculoma associated with miliary tuberculosis (Bansal *et al.*, 2012; Bogadhi & Le Hoanq, 2000; Chatziralli *et al.*, 2012; De Luigi *et al.*, 2012; Kamal *et al.*, 2013; Manousaridis *et al.*, 2013; Takakura *et al.*, 1998). Paradoxical worsening of patients condition after initiating ATT are described as Jarisch-Herxheimer reaction to the therapy (Bogadhi & Le Hoanq, 2000; Takakura *et al.*, 1998). The prompt resolution of this allergic reaction with systemic steroid treatment has been reported in these patients (Cheung & Chee, 2009; Neunhöffer *et al.*, 2013). Anti-inflammatory therapy in conjunction with ATT is considered to prevent worsening of the existing lesion in the eye, recurrence of the disease, and paradoxical reactions (Basu & Das, 2010).

References

Abebe F. (2012). Is Interferon –gamma the right marker for bacille calmette-Guerin-induced immune presentation? The missing link in our understanding of tuberculosis immunology. Clin Exp Immunol 2012;169:213-9.

Ahmed AT, Karter AJ. Tuberculosis in California dialysis patients. (2004). Int J Tuberc Lung Dis 2004;8:341-5.

Al-Mezaine HS, Al-Muammar A, Kanqave D, et al. (2008). Clinical and optical coherence tomographic findings and outcome of treatment in patients with presumed tuberculous uveitis. Int ophtahlmol 2008;28:413-23.

Allie N, Grivennikov SI, Keeton R, et al. (2013). Prominent role for T-cell derived tumor necrosis factor for sustained control of Mycobacterium tuberculosis infection. Sci Rep 2013;3:1809.

American Thoracic Society. (2000). Diagnostic standards and classification of tuberculosis in adults and children. Am J Respir Crit Care Med 2000;161:1376-95.

Ang M, Cheung G, Vania M, et al. (2012a). Aqueous cytokine and chemokine analysis in uveitis associated with tuberculosis. Mol Vis 2012;18:567-73.

Ang M, Hedayaftar A, Zhang R, et al. (2012b). Clinical signs of uveitis associated with latent tuberculosis. Clin Experiment Ophtalmol 2012;40:689-96.

Ang M, Wong WL, Li X, et al. (2013). Interferon gamma release assay for the diagnosis of uveitis associated with tuberculosis: a Bayesian evaluation in the absence of gold standard. Br J Ophthalmol 2013;97:1062-7.

Anna TK, Tomasz Z, Aqnieszka JS, et al. (2013). Clinical picture of multifocal chorioretinitis caused by mycobacterium tuberculosis: case report. Klin Oczna 2013;115:51-2.

Arora SK, Gupta V, Gupta A, et al. (1999). Diagnostic efficancy of polymerase chain reaction in granulomatous uveitis. Tuberc Lung Dis 1999;79:229-33.

Auld SC, Click ES, Heilig CM, et al. (2013). BMC Infectious Diseases 2013;13.460.

Babu K, Philips M, Subbakrishna DK. (2013). Perspectives of Quantiferon TB Gold test among Indian practitioners: a survey. J Ophthalmic Inflamm Infect 2013;11:9.

Babu RB, Sudharshan S, Kumarasamy N, et al. (2006). Ocular tuberculosis in acquired immunodeficiency syndrome. Am J Ophthalmol 2006;142:413.

Baha A, Benhaddur R, Hajj I et la. (2009). Choroidal tuberculosis: Reports of 3 cases. Bull Soc Belge Ophthalmol 2009;313:31-7.

Baha Ali T, Benhaddou R, Haji I, et al. (2009). Choroidal tuberculosis: report of 3 cases. Bull Soc Belge Ophthalmol 2009;313:31-7.

Bansal R, Gupta A, Gupta V, et al. (2012). Tubercular serpiginous-like choroiditis presenting as multifocal serpiginoid choroiditis. Ophtahlmology 2012;119:2334-42.

Basu S, Das T. (2010). Pitfalls in the management of TB-associated uveitis. Eye 2010;24:1681-4.

Bathula BP, Pappu S, Epari SE, et al. (2012). Tubercular nodular episcleritis. Indian J Chest Dis Allied Sci 2012;54:135-6.

Bellete B, Coberly J, Barnes GL, et al. (2002). Evaluation of a whole blood interferon gamma release assay for the detection of Mycobacterium tuberculosis infection in two study populations. Clin Infect Dis 2002;34:1449-56.

Bhuibhar SS, Biswas J. (2012). Nested PCR- positive tubercular ampiginous choroiditis: a case report. Ocul Immunol Inflamm 2012;20:303-5.

Bloom BR, Murray JL. (1992). Tuberculosis: commentary on a re-emergent killer. Science 1992; 257: 1055-64.

Blumberg HM, Leonard MK Jr, Jasmer RM. (2005). Update on the treatment of tuberculosis and latent tuberculosis infection. JAMA 2005;8:2776-84.

Boehme CC, Nabeta P, Henostroza G, et al. (2007). Operational feasibility of using loop-mediated isothermal amplification for diagnosis of pulmonary tuberculosis in microscopy centers of developing countries. J Clin Microbiol 2007;45:1936.

Bogadhi B, Le Hoanq P. (2000). Ocular tuberculosis. Curr Opin Ophthalmol 2000;11:443-8.

Bouza E, Merino P, Munoz P, et al. (1997). Ocular tuberculosis: A prospective study in a general hospital. Medicine (Baltimore) 1997;76:53-62.

Calderon VF, Valbuena G, Goez Y, et al. (2013). A humanized Mouse model of tuberculosis. PLos One 2013;8:e63331.

Campos WR, Henriques JF, KritskiAL, et al. (2008). Tuberculosis uveitis at a referral center in southeastern Brasil. J Bras Pneumol 2008;34:98-102.

Chatziralli IP, Keryttopoulos P, Papazisis L, et al. (2012). Hypopyon in the context of tuberculous uveitis. Clin Exp Optom 2012;95:241-3.

Chen K, Kolls JK. (2013). T-cell mediated host immune defenses in the lung. Annu Rev Immunol 2013;31:605-33.

Cheung CM, Chee SP. (2009). Jarisch-Herxheimer reaction: paradoxical worsening of tuberculosis chorioretinitis following initiation of antituberculous therapy. Eye 2009;23:1472-3.

Chu ZJ, Hui YN. (2010). Recent advances in tuberculosis uveitis. Zhonqhua Yan Ke Za Zhi 2010;46:861-4.

Cohn DL. (2000). Treatment of latent tuberculosis infection: renewed opportunity for tuberculosis control. Clin infect Dis 2000;31:120-4.

Colditz GA, Brewer TF, Berkey CS, et al. (1994). Efficacy of BCG vaccine in the prevention of tuberculosis- meta analysis of the published literature. JAMA 1994;271:698-702.

Cordero-Coma M, CallejaS, Torrey HE, et al. (2010). The value of immune response to M.tuberculosis in patients with chronic posterior uveitis revisited: utility of the new IGRAs. Eye 2010;24:36-43.

Cordero-Coma M, Garzo I, Salazar R, et al. (2013). Treatment of presumed tuberculosis uveitis affecting the posterior segment: diagnostic confirmation and long term outcomes. Arc Soc Esp Ofthalmol 2013;88:339-44.

Das S, Paramasivan CN, Lowrie DB, et al. (1995). IS6110 restriction fragment length polymorphism typing of clinical isolates of Mycobacterium tuberculosis from patients with pulmonary TB in Madras, South India. Tuberc Lung Dis 1995;76:550-4.

De Luigi G, Mantovani A, Papadia M, et al. (2012). Tuberculosis-related choriocapillaritis (multifocal serpiginous choroiditis): follow-up and precise monitoring of therapy by indocyanine green angiography. Int Ophthalmol 2012;32:55-60.

Department of Health of the Philippines. National Tuberculosis Control Programme.

Doycheva D, Deuter C, Hetzel J, et al. (2011). The use of positron emission tomography/CT in the diagnosis of tuberculosis-associated uveitis. Br J Ophthalmol 2011;95:1290-4.

Gan WL, Jones NP. (2013). Serpiginous-like choroiditis as a marker for tuberculosis in a non-endemic area. Br J Ophthalmol 2013;97:644-7.

Garcia-Gasalla M, Fernandez-Baca M, Juan-Mass A, et al. (2013). Use of Quantiferon-TB Gold In Tube test for detecting latent tuberculosis in patients considered a s candidates for anti-TNF therapy in routine clinical practice. Enferm Infecc Microbiol Clin 2013;31:76-81.

Guimaraes RM, Lobo Ade P, Siqueira EA, et al. (2012). Tuberculosis, HIV, and poverty: temporal trends in Brazil, the Americas and worldwide. J Bras Pneumol 2012;38:511-7.

Gupta A, Gupta V, Pandav SS, et al. (2003). Posterior scleritis associated with systemic tuberculosis. Indian J Ophthalmol 2003;51:347-9.

Gupta N, Chawla B, Venkatesh P, et al. (2008). Necrotizing scleritis and peripheral ulcerative keratitis in a case of Sweet's syndrome found culture-positive for Mycobacterium tuberculosis. Ann Trop Med Parasitol 2008;102:557-60.

Heuts F, Gavier-Widen D, Carow B, et al. (2013). CD4+ cell-dependent granuloma formation in humanized mice infected with mycobacterium. Proc Natl Acad Sci USA 2013;110:6482-7.

Holden M, Dubin MR, Diamond PH. (1971). Frequency of negative intermediate-strenght tuberculin sensitivity in patients with active tuberculosis. N Eng J Med 1971;285:1506-9.

Huebner RE, Schein MF, Bass JB. (1993). The tuberculin skin test. Clin Infect Dis 1993;17:968-75.

Jung JY, Lim JE, Lee HJ, et al. (2012). Questionable role of interferon gamma release assays for smear-negative pulmonary TB in immunocompromised patients. J Infect 2012;64:188-96.

Kamal S, Kumar R, Kumar S, et al. (2013). Bilateral Interstitial keratitis and granulomatous uveitis of tubercular origin. Eye Contact Lens 2013; March 27.

Lalvani A, Pareek M. (2010). Interferon gamma release assays: principles and practice. Enferm Infecc Microbiol Clin 2010;28:245-52.

Lara LP, Ocampo V Jr. (2013). Prevalence of presumed ocular tuberculosis among pulmonary tuberculosis patients in a tertiary hospital in the Philippines. J Ophthalmic Inflamm Infect 2013;3:1

Liorenç V, Gonzalez-Martin J, Keller J, et al. (2013). Indirect supportive evidence for diagnosis of tuberculosis-related uveitis: form the tuberculin skin test to the new interferon gamma release assays. Arch Ophthalmol 2013;91:99-107.

Manousaridis K, Onq A, Stenton C, et al. (2013). Clinical presentation, treatment, and outcomes in presumed intraocular tuberculosis: experience from Newcastle, Tyne, UK. Eye 2013;27:480-6.

Mathur G, Biswas J. (2012). Ssytemic ssociations of anterior uveitis in a tertiary care center in South India. Int Oph 2012;32:417-21.

Meier T, Eulenbruch H, Wrighton-Smith P, et al. (2005). Sensitivity of a new commercial enzyme linked immunospot assay (T-SPOT.TB) for diagnosis of tuberculosis in clinical practice. European Journal of Clinical Microbiology and Infectious Diseases 2005;24:529-36.

Moon HW, Hur M. (2013). Interferon-gamma release assays for the diagnosis of latent tuberculosis infection: un updated review. Ann Clin Lab Sci 2013;43:221-9.

Mori T. (2009). Usefulness of interferon-gamma release assays for diagnosis TB infection and problems with these assays. J Infect Chemotr 2009;15:143-55.

Nash D, Douglass J. (1980). Anergy in active pulmonary tuberculosis. A comparison between positive and negative reactors and an evaluation of 5 TU and 250 TU skin test doses. Chest 1980;77:32-7.

Nayak S, Basu S, Singh MK. (2011). Presumed tubercular retinal vasculitis with serpiginous-like choroiditis in the other eye. Ocul Immunol Inflamm 2011;19:361-2.

Nazari Khanamiri H, Rao N. (2013). Serpiginous choroiditis and infectious multifocal serpiginoid choroiditis. Surv Ophtahlmol 2013;58:203-32.

Neunhöffer H, Gold A, Hoerauf H, et al. (2013). Isolated ocular Jarisch-Herxheimer reaction after initiating tuberculostatic therapy in a child. Int Ophthalmol 2013;11 (e-pub ahead of print)

Nwosu NN. (2008). HIV/AIDS in ophthalmic patients: the Guinness Eye center Onitsha experience. Niger Postgrad Med J 2008;15:24-7.

Patel SS, Saraiya NV, Tessler HH, et al. (2013). Mycobacterial ocular inflammation: delay in diagnosis and other factore impact morbidity. JAMA Ophthalmol 2013;131:752-8.

Pedroza Garcia EM, Reynoso-von Dratein C, Marquez-Perez P, et al. (2010). Necrotizing scleritis and recurrent erythema nodosum: a diagnostic challenge. Rev Med Inst Mex Sequro Soc 2010; 48:331-5.

Rao NA, Saraswathy S, Smith RE. (2006). Tuberculous uveitis: distribution of mycobacterium tuberculosis in the retina pigment epithelium. 2006;124:1776-9.

Rivest P, Street MC, Allard R. Completion rates of treatment for latent tuberculosis infection in Quebec, Canada from 2006 to 2010. Can J Public Health 2013;104:e235-9.

Rodriquez A, calogne M, Pedroza-Seres M, et al. (1996). Referral patterns of uveitis in a tertiary eye care center. Arch Ophtahlmol 1996;114:593-9.

Roh YR, Woo SJ, Ahn J, et al. (2011). Pulmonary tuberculosis associated retinal vasculitis presenting as xanthopsia. Ocul Immunol Inflamm 2011;19:121-3.

Sanqhvi J, Bell C, Woodhead M, et al. (2011). Presumed tuberculous uveitis: diagnosis, management and outcome. Eye 2011;25:475-80.

Sarmiento OL, Weigle KA, Alexander J, et al. (2003). *Assessment of meta-analysis of PCR for diagnosis of smear-negative pulmonary tuberculosis. J Clin Microbiol 2003;41:3233-40.*

Sharma K, Gupta V, Bansal R, et al. (2013). *Novel multi-targeted polymerase chain reaction for diagnosis of presumed tubercular uveitis. J Ophthalmic Inflamm Infect 2013;3:25.*

Sharma R, Marasini S, Nepal BP. (2010). *Tubercular scleritis. Khatmandu Univ Med J 2010;8:352-6.*

Silva Miranda M, Breiman A, Allain S, et al. (2012). *The tuberculosis granuloma: an unsuccessful host defense mechanism providing a safety shelter for the bacteria? Clin Dev Immunol Epub 2012 Jul 3.*

Singh R, Toor P, Parchand S, et al. (2012). *Quantitative polymerase chain reaction for mycobacterium tuberculosis in so-called Eales disease. Ocul Immunol Inflamm 2012;20:153-7.*

Streeton JA, Desem N, Jones SL. (1998). *Sensitivity and specificity of a gamma interferon blood test for tuberculosis infection. Int J Tuberc Lung Dis 1998;2:443-50.*

Tabbara KF. (2007). *Tuberculosis. Curr Opin Ophthalmol 2007;18:493-501.*

Takakura S, Tanaka E, Kimoto T, et al. (1998). *A case of miliary tuberculosis with brain tuberculoma following intraocular tuberculosis. Kekaku 1998,73:591-7.*

Tollefson D, Bloss E, Fanning A, et al. (2013). *Burden of tuberculosis in indigenous people gllobaly: a sytemic review. Int J Tuberc Lung Dis 2013; Jul 12.*

Vasconcelos-Santos DV, Rao PK, Davies JB, et al. (2010). *Clinical picture of tuberculous serpiginouslike choroiditis in contrast to classic serpiginous choroiditis. Arch Ophthalmol 2010;128:853-8.*

Velasco e Cruz AA, Chahud F, Feldman R, et al. (2011). *Posterior scleral tuberculoma: case report. Arq Bras Oftalmol 2011;74:53-4.*

Vos AG, Wassenberg MW, deHong J, et al. (2013). *Diagnosis and treatment of tuberculosis uveitis in a low endemic seting. Int J Infect Dis 2013 May 22.*

Vyas S. (2009). *Role of an ophthalmologist in early diagnosis and management of ocular tuberculosis. AIOC Proceedings 2009;370-2.*

Winthrop KL, Nyendak M, Calvet H, et al. (2008). *Interferon gamma release assays for diagnosing Mycobacterium tuberculosis infection in renal dialysis patients. Clin J Am Soc nephrol 2008;3:1357-63.*

Yasaratne BM, Madeqedara D, Senanayake NS, et al. (2010). *A case series of symptomatic ocular tuberculosis and the response to anti-tubercular therapy. Ceylon Med J 2010;55:16-9.*

Complications of Pulmonary Tuberculosis

H. J. Gayathri Devi

Department of Respiratory Medicine
M.S. Ramaiah Medical College, Bangalore, India

1   Introduction

Tuberculosis is an ancient disease which continues to be a major health problem in most developing countries. In developed countries, it is gaining importance with the emergence of HIV pandemic. Pulmonary tuberculosis (TB) is caused by the bacteria *Mycobacterium tuberculosis*. According to the defenses of the host and virulence of the organism tuberculosis can occur in the lungs or extrapulmonary organs. Various forms of sequelae and complications may result from primary and post-primary pulmonary tuberculosis in both treated and untreated patients (Kim *et al.*, 2001). *Mycobacterium tuberculosis* can affect almost every organ in the body. Major manifestations of the disease usually occur in the lung. Pulmonary tuberculosis can manifest for the first time as a complication (SatyaSri, 2009). A variety of complications can occur in pulmonary tuberculosis. They can be categorized as follows: (*a*) Parenchymal lesions which include thin walled cavity (open negative syndrome), aspergilloma, end stage lung destruction and scar carcinoma. (*b*) Airway lesions which include tuberculous laryngitis, bronchiectasis, tracheobronchial stenosis, anthracofibrosis and broncholithiasis. (*c*) Vascular lesions such as Rasmussen aneurysm. (*d*) Pleural lesions which include dry pleurisy, pleural effusion, empyema, bronchopleural fistula and pneumothorax (Kim *et al.*, 2001). (*e*) General complications include cor pulmonale, secondary amyloidosis and chronic respiratory failure (see Table 1). This chapter describes the pathogenesis, clinical manifestations, diagnostic criteria and management of complications of pulmonary tuberculosis.

Parenchymal lesions
Thin walled cavity (Open negative syndrome)
Aspergilloma
End stage lung destruction
Scar carcinoma
Airway Lesions
Tuberculous Laryngitis
Bronchiectasis
Tracheobronchial stenosis
Anthracofibrosis
Broncholithiasis
Vascular Lesions
Rasmussen aneurysm
Pleural Lesions
Dry pleurisy
Pleural effusion
Empyema & Bronchopleural fistula
Pneumothorax
General Complications
Cor-pulmonale
Secondary amyloidosis
Chronic respiratory failure

Table 1: Complications of Pulmonary Tuberculosis

2   Parenchymal lesions

2.1   Open Negative Syndrome

Cavitation is a hallmark of pulmonary tuberculosis. Residual thin walled cavities may be seen in both active and inactive disease. The cavity may disappear after antituberculous chemotherapy. Occasionally the wall becomes thin and remains as an air filled cystic space even after a bacteriological cure, when it is called as open negative syndrome. Tuberculous cavities heal by two processes, open and closed depending on the status of the draining bronchus. In the open form, the wall of the cavity becomes free of tubercle bacilli with chemotherapy and wall undergoes fibrosis with subsequent epithelialization. The lumen of the draining bronchus usually remains patent (Hermel & Gershon-Cohen, 1954).

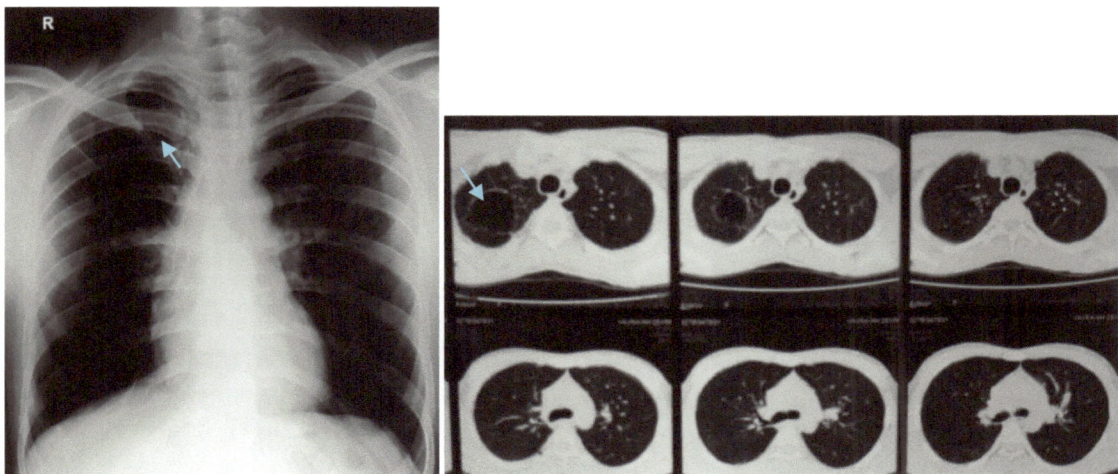

Figure 1: Chest X-ray PA and HRCT Thorax showing right upper lobe thin walled cavity (see arrow marks)

These are thin walled cavities with epithelialization extending from bronchioles. The wall may be smooth and the thickness varies from 1 cm to less than 1mm. These cavities may be associated with complications such as haemoptysis, secondary infection with pyogenic organisms resulting in a lung abscess. Aspergilloma can form in a cavity. Rupture of the cavity can give rise to a spontaneous pneumothorax. Rarely relapse of tuberculosis can occur. In the closed type, the draining bronchus gets occluded and the cavity undergoes atelectasis and scar formation (Hermel & Gershon-Cohen, 1954).

2.2   Aspergilloma

The most common cause of human aspergillosis and pulmonary aspergilloma is Aspergillus fumigatus. Published data indicate that saprophytic colonization of the lung that has been destroyed by tuberculosis, sarcoidosis, bronchiectasis, lung abscess & neoplasms lead to intracavitary aspergilloma. Of these tuberculosis is the most common. Most patients are asymptomatic. Symptomatic patients present with fever, cough and haemoptysis. Haemoptysis could be life threatening. The source of bleeding is usually the bronchial blood vessels. Dyspnea, malaise and weight loss may be there due to the underlying pulmonary disease. Physical examination may be normal or signs of the underlying lung disease may be present. The diagnosis is based on the characteristic radiological finding. Chest radiography reveals a mass in a pre-existing cavity with a crescent of air outlining the mass called as 'air crescent sign' (Felson, 1988), seen usually in the upper lobe as shown in the image. CT scan images provide better definition of the mass within a cavity.

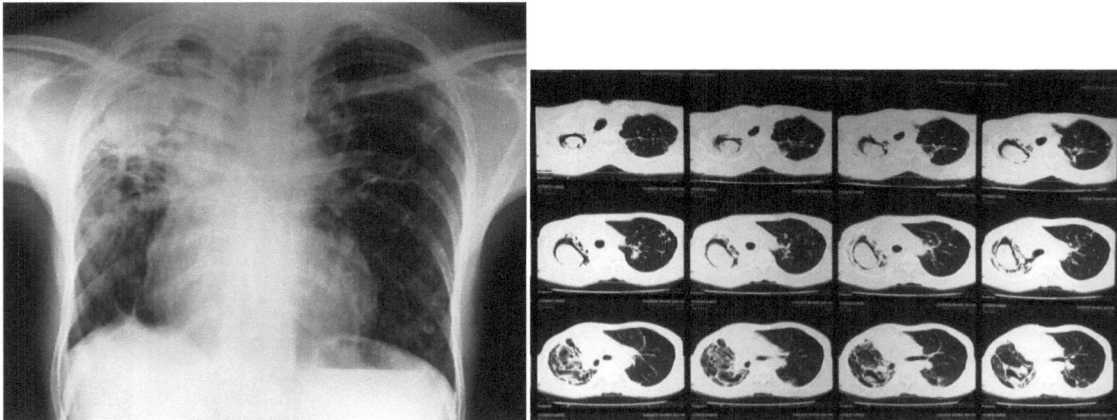

Figure 2: Chest X-ray PA and CECT Thorax showing right upper lobe aspergilloma.

Laboratory abnormalities are uncommon. Aspergillus precipitin antibody test for IgG are usually positive in Aspergilloma (Harman, 2012). Treatment is considered when patients develop symptoms, usually presenting as haemoptysis. Bronchial artery embolization may be used for patients with massive haemoptysis. Prolonged oral itraconazole may provide partial or complete resolution of aspergillomas in 60% of patients. Itraconazole has a high tissue penetration (Kousha *et al.*, 2011). In a small number of patients intracavitary therapy with Amphotericin B has also been used with some success (Klein *et al.*, 1993). Surgical resection is curative and may be considered for patients with recurrent haemoptysis if the patient has adequate pulmonary reserve.

2.3 Destroyed Lung

Unilateral destruction of the lung due to tuberculosis has been a recognized entity. Rajasekaran *et al.* analyzed patients with unilateral lung destruction and found pulmonary tuberculosis as the cause in 83.3% of patients (Rajasekaran *et al.*, 1999). It may occur after primary disease or reinfection. Cicatrization atelectasis is a common finding after postprimary tuberculosis. Marked fibrotic response is seen in up to 40% of patients with post primary tuberculosis (Kim *et al.*, 2001). Reduced lung volume, cavities, bronchiectasis and fibrosis are the predominant findings in destroyed lungs. Fibrotic response manifests as retraction of the hilum and mediastinal shift towards the fibrotic lung. Opposite lung will show compensatory hyperinflation. These patients might seek medical help for the first time for diagnosis or after completion of treatment or referred as non-responders due to treatment failure.

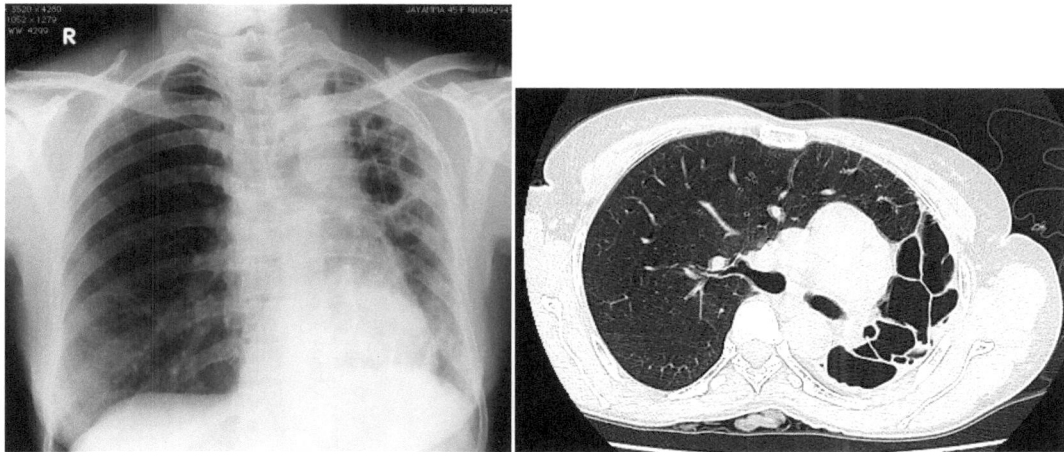

Figure 3: Chest X-ray PA and HRCT Thorax showing destroyed lung on left side with compensatory hyperinflation on the right side.

2.4   Scar Carcinoma

The development of lung cancer in a pulmonary scar was first described by Friedrich as scar or cicatricial cancer of the lung. Scar cancers are associated with high incidence of adenocarcinoma (Ashizawa *et al.*, 2004). Ying U et al studied the relationship between lung cancer risks following detection of pulmonary scarring and found that baseline diagnosis of pulmonary scarring was associated during subsequent follow up with an increased risk of lung cancer (Yu *et al.*, 2008). Lung cancer occurring in pulmonary tuberculosis patients after completing treatment are mistaken for relapse. Although the pathogenesis is unclear uncontrolled epithelial hyperplasia in relation to fibrosis is considered as a possible mechanism. Other possibility is the concentration of carcinogens by scars (McDonnell & Long, 1981). Cigarette smoking contributes to the lung cancer risk associated with scarring.

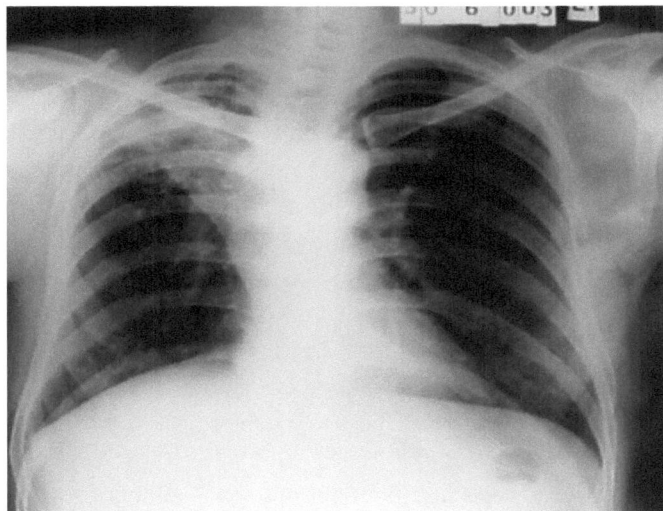

Figure 4: Chest X-ray PA view showing the post tubercular scarring in the (R) upper zone.

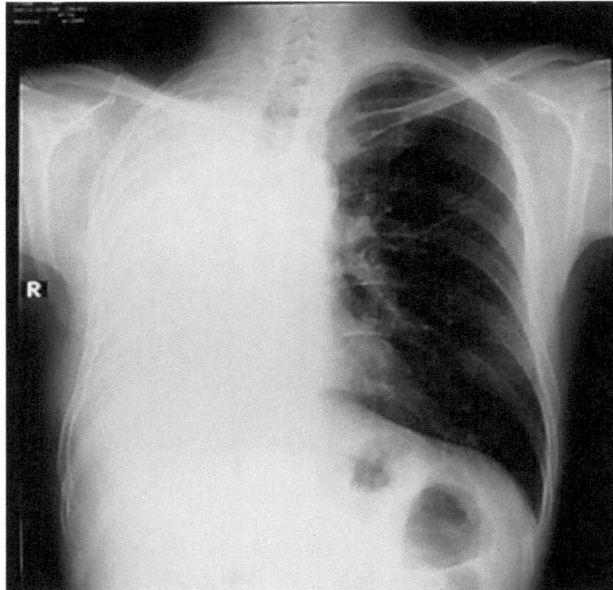

Figure 5: Chest X-ray showing the development of complete collapse of (R) lung due to bronchogenic carcinoma in the same patient.

3 Vascular Lesions

3.1 Haemoptysis

Haemoptysis is defined as expectoration of blood originating from the lungs or tracheo-bronchial tree (Jean-Baptiste, 2005). Haemoptysis is a common symptom of pulmonary tuberculosis (Sharma, 2009). Haemoptysis is most commonly associated with cavitary lesions. Changes in the vasculature of tuberculous lungs are implicated in haemoptysis. Fritz Valdemar Rasmussen, a Danish physician described the aneurysmal dilatation of pulmonary vessels in the wall of tuberculous cavity as the cause for haemoptysis (Rassmussen, 1868). Calmette in 1923 mentioned that branches of pulmonary artery which traverse the wall of tuberculous cavities contain small pedunculated "aneurysms of Rasmussen". Wood & Miller showed that the wall of tuberculous cavities have dilated bronchial arteries (Wood & Miller, 1938).

Haemoptysis may occur in the active stage of tuberculosis or as late sequelae, due to aneurysmal rupture or secondary to bronchiectasis. Aspergillomas can form in pre-existing cavitary lesions and lead to haemoptysis. Erosion of a blood vessel by a calcified lesion can also lead to haemoptysis. Definition of massive Haemoptysis is not clear. It can range from 100 milliliters per day to 1000 milliliters over a few days (Lordan, 2003). Massive haemoptysis can be fatal and lead to asphyxiation. Majority of patients with massive haemoptysis have a poor pulmonary reserve and are not fit for any surgical procedures. The lungs have a dual blood supply. The pulmonary arterial circulation is a low pressure system and bronchial arteries, a high pressure system. The source of massive haemoptysis is most commonly the bronchial circulation (90%) and pulmonary circulation constitutes only 5% (Remy *et al.*, 1992). Patients with mild haemoptysis need a conservative approach. Treatment options available for patients with massive haemoptysis are endobronchial tamponade, single or double lumen intubation, bronchial artery embolization, or surgery (Lordan, 2003). Presently, the main life-saving modality used to control bleeding in massive haemoptysis is angiography and bronchial artery embolization (Sopko *et al.*, 2011). Shin et.al, have retro-spectively analyzed the outcomes of bronchial artery embolization for the treatment of haemoptysis in patients with pulmonary tuberculosis and reported 163 patients out of 169 (96.4%) had significant clinical improvement after the procedure (Shin *et al.*, 2011).

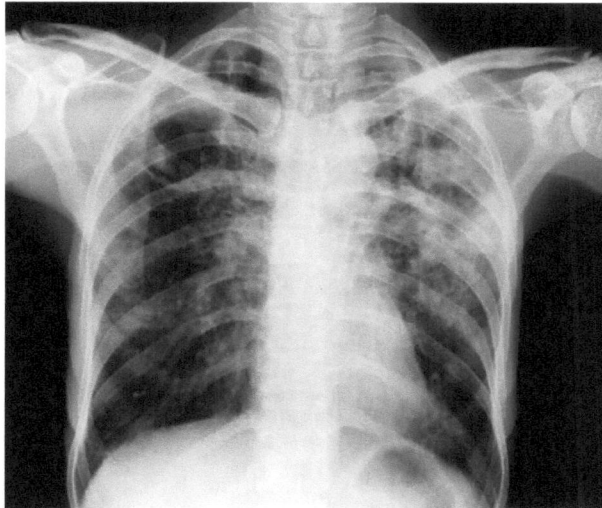

Figure 6: Chest X-ray PA view showing bilateral cavitary lesions.

4 Airway Lesions

4.1 Tuberculous Laryngitis

Laryngeal tuberculosis is usually a complication of pulmonary tuberculosis. The sputum positive rate is 90-95% in patients with active pulmonary tuberculosis with tuberculous laryngitis. Clinical features in-clude hoarseness of voice, odynophagia, cough and dysphagia. The larynx becomes infected either by a direct contact from pulmonary tuberculosis or by a lymphatic/ hematogenous spread from sites other than lungs. It can manifest as edema, hyperemia, ulcerative lesion, nodule or an exophytic mass. Most com-mon site is posterior part of larynx. Laryngeal TB is uncommon in developed countries and authors from developed countries feel that it should be considered as a differential diagnosis in any laryngeal disease in particular laryngeal carcinoma. (Smulders *et al.*, 2009). Antituberculous drugs are the primary treatment for laryngeal tuberculosis. Complications of laryngeal tuberculosis if not treated early can result in sub-glottic stenosis and vocal cord paralysis.

4.2 Bronchiectasis

Bronchiectasis is an abnormal and permanent dilatation of bronchi. Tuberculosis is a major cause of bronchiectasis worldwide. Bronchiectasis may be present in various stages of pulmonary tuberculosis. Bronchiectasis is seen in 30% -60% of patients suffering from active post primary tuberculosis. Various factors may cause bronchiectasis in pulmonary tuberculosis, mainly atelectasis and pulmonary fibrosis. Bronchial stenosis as a consequence of tuberculous inflammation and scarring of the bronchi can lead to retention of secretions. When this is followed by bacterial infection it can lead to destruction and dilatation of the airways.

Compression of the bronchi by enlarged lymph nodes produces consequences similar to intraluminal obstruction. Bronchiectasis may follow as sequelae of healing of pulmonary tuberculosis. Fibrosis of lung parenchyma can lead to bronchial dilatation. Parenchymal retraction due to fibrosis can also cause bronchial dilatation and bronchiectasis. Three types of bronchiectasis have been described, cylindrical bronchiectasis wherein the involved bronchi appear uniformly dilated, varicose bronchiectasis, where the affected bronchi have a beaded pattern of dilatation resembling varicose veins, saccular (cystic) bronchiectasis which shows ballooned appearance of the bronchi ending in blind sacs.

In adults tuberculosis usually occurs in the upper lobes (Crofton, 2000). Other infections often involve dependent parts of the lungs. When upper lobes are involved secretions are drained and superinfection with pyogenic organisms does not usually occur. This is known as dry bronchiectasis or bronchiectasis sicca. Bronchiectasis in the apical and posterior segments of the upper lobe is highly suggestive of tuberculous etiology (Kim *et al.*, 2001).The main complaints are persistent or recurrent cough, purulent sputum, haemoptysis, dyspnea, wheezing, fatigue, fever and failure to thrive. Haemoptysis is a common symptom in 50 – 70% of cases of bronchiectasis and is more common in dry bronchiectasis. On physical examination, clubbing may be present. Coarse crepitation and rhonchi may be heard over the area of bronchiectasis.

Chest radiograph may show nonspecific findings. The definitive diagnosis is made by thoracic CT. HRCT has replaced lipiodol bronchography to establish the presence, severity and distribution of bronchiectasis. HRCT has only 2% false negative and a 1% false positive rate (Young *et al.*, 1991). It is a noninvasive investigation.

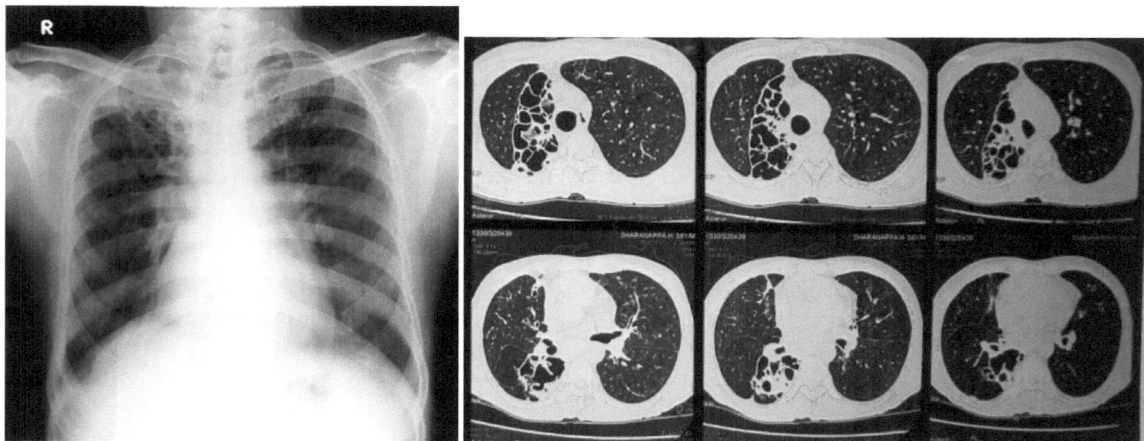

Figure 7: Chest X-ray PA and HRCT Thorax showing right upper lobe bronchiectasis.

Management may be medical or surgical. Medical management is with antibiotics and chest physiotherapy. If the lesion is localized to a resectable area and the medical management fails, elective surgery is indicated.

4.3   Broncholithiasis

The presence of calcified lymph node masses within the bronchi is referred as broncholithiasis (Fishman *et al.*, 2008). This is an uncommon complication of pulmonary tuberculosis (Ann Leung, 1999). Broncholithiasis is caused commonly by erosion and extrusion of a calcified adjacent lymph node into the bronchial lumen. Symptoms may include cough, haemoptysis, lithoptysis or symptoms related to bronchial obstruction (Seo *et al.*, 2002). Chest radiography often does not show the calcification within the bronchus. CT usually provides useful information (Seo *et al.*, 2002). Radiologic findings include calcified peribronchial nodes. In addition to this there may be segmental or lobar atelectasis, obstructive pneumonitis and rarely focal hyperinflation (Seo *et al.*, 2002). If a broncholith is free completely within the bronchus, it can be removed bronchoscopically. Most of the symptomatic broncholiths should be removed at thoracotomy by lobectomy or segmentectomy (Fishman *et al.*, 2008).

4.4   Tracheobronchial stenosis

The most common cause of benign tracheobronchial stenosis is endobronchial tuberculosis in Asian countries (Ryu *et al.*, 2006). Endobronchial tuberculosis is caused either by direct inoculation of the bacilli from the lung parenchymal lesions or by infiltration of the airway by bacilli from adjacent mediastinal lymph nodes (Wan *et al.*, 2002). Despite adequate anti-tuberculosis treatment endobronchial tuberculosis can result in major airway obstruction from stenosis. Studies have found predominance in the female sex (Low *et al.*, 2004). Significant bronchial stenosis of major bronchi is rare (Fishman *et al.*, 2008). Left main bronchus is the common site of stenosis. This could be because the left main stem bronchus is easily compressed by the arch of the aorta and lymph node TB is also more often noted on the left side (Low *et al.*, 2004). CT scans show concentric narrowing of the lumen, uniform thickening of the wall and long bronchial segment involvement (Kim *et al.*, 2001). Flexible bronchoscopy is the most useful modality for diagnosis and assessment of tracheobronchial stenosis (Hoheisel *et al.*, 1994). Minimally invasive endoscopic techniques such as balloon dilation, Nd YAG laser therapy and tracheo-bronchial stent placement are used to establish patency (Verma, 2006). The use of silicone stents could provide an effective means of managing PTTS patients (Ryu *et al.*, 2006). In subjects not responding to interventional bronchoscopic treatment surgical resection may be indicated (Tetikkurt, 2008).

4.5   Anthracofibrosis

Anthracofibrosis is bronchial stenosis due to local mucosal fibrosis that also presents anthracotic pigment in the mucosa. The exact cause has not been well defined. There is a frequent association with tuberculosis and exposure to smoke from biofuel or biomass combustion (Julio *et al.*, 2012). It is a bronchoscopic finding. Hwang J. et al have studied the frequency of anthracofibrosis in foreign born Pulmonary TB patients in Canada. According to them patients from the Indian subcontinent were more likely to have anthracofibrosis compared to patients from other Asian countries. Most of the patients present with cough, sputum and dyspnea. CT and bronchoscopy has to be done to exclude bronchogenic carcinoma if chest radiographs show segmental or lobar atelectasis (Kim *et al.*, 2000).

5   Pleural Lesions

5.1   Pleural Effusion

Inflammation of the pleura is called as pleurisy and when fluid accumulates in the pleural cavity, it is called as pleural effusion. Tuberculous pleural effusion remains as the leading inflammatory pleural disease in countries where tuberculosis is more common. Although tuberculosis is considered as a chronic illness, tuberculous pleuritis can present as an acute illness of less than 1 week duration. In USA, 2% of all effusions are attributed to tuberculosis (Fishman, 2008). In children, effusion may occur as part of primary tuberculosis. It also occurs with increased frequency in middle-aged and elderly people. Pleural effusion usually occurs 3-6 months after the primary infection (Wallgren, 1948). It occurs when the sub-pleural parenchymal focus or a caseating lymph node ruptures into the pleural space. Delayed hypersensitivity plays an important role in tuberculous pleural effusion. Direct contiguous spread to the pleura or haematogenous spread can also lead to pleural effusion (SatyaSri, 2009). The usual presenting symptoms are non-productive cough, fever, pleuritic chest pain and breathlessness in most patients. Patients with chronic infection present frequently with weight loss, malaise and dyspnea. Physical findings reveal dullness on percussion and absence of breath sounds. Tuberculous pleural effusions are usually unilateral and in approximately one-third of patients co-existing parenchymal disease is seen radiologically. Pleural effusions generally appear as dense homogeneous opacities. Chest radiograph will show blunting of the costophrenic angle with small quantities of free pleural fluid. Ultrasonography of the chest detects smaller effusions. Tuberculous pleural effusion is often unilateral and occupies about one-third to half of the hemithorax. Radiologically, it appears as a lateral opacity concave medially extending upwards in the axilla with the base obscuring the hemidiaphragm. It can also present rarely as massive pleural effusion obscuring the whole hemithorax and displacing the mediastinum to the opposite side. Sub-pulmonic effusions may present with fluid collection below the diaphragm in some patients.

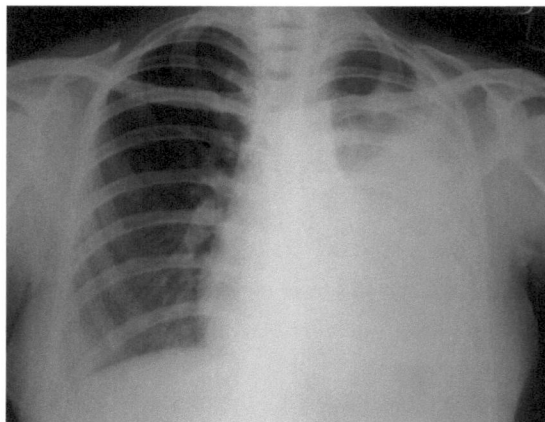

Figure 8: Chest X-ray PA view showing massive left pleural effusion.

A tuberculous pleural effusion is usually a serous exudate with high protein level (>4 gm/ml). The fluid is defined as an exudate if it fulfils one of the Light's criteria such as pleural /serum ratio of total protein >0.5, pleural/serum ratio of LDH >0.6,or LDH greater than 2/3 of the upper limit of serum value. Adenosine deaminase (ADA) level greater than 70 IU/L has been shown to be highly sensitive and specific for the diagnosis of tuberculous pleural effusion. Increased ADA levels have also been found in malignancy or empyema. Low glucose (<60 mg/ml) and low pH (<7.30) are found in approximately 20% of patients (SatyaSri, 2009). Analysis of the pleural fluid for differential cell count shows predominance of lymphocytes in tuberculous pleural effusion. Pleural fluid smear is positive for acid fast bacilli in less than 10% of patients (SatyaSri, 2009). Culture of pleural fluid is often negative for tubercle bacilli. Chances of positive culture increases in proportion to the quantity of fluid sent to the laboratory. Pleural biopsies show granulomas in about two-thirds of patients. Pleural aspiration and pleural biopsy using Abrams punch can be done in one sitting. Treatment involves pleural fluid aspiration and administration of anti-tuberculosis drugs. Therapeutic aspiration of pleural fluid will relieve symptoms of dyspnea. Aspiration should be done relatively slowly. Rapid removal of large quantity of pleural fluid may result in unilateral pulmonary edema due to increased microvascular permeability in the expanded lung.

5.1.1   Empyema

An empyema is pus in the pleural cavity (Light, 2006). In the developing world, tuberculosis remains as the common cause of empyema. Studies done in India have shown tuberculous empyema as the common cause of empyema (Kundu, 2010). Tuberculous empyema occurs usually as a result of the rupture of a subpleural caseous focus into the pleural cavity. Rarely, hematogenous spread from the involved thoracic lymph nodes or from a sub diaphragmatic focus can cause empyema. The presenting clinical symptoms are fever, cough with expectoration, chest pain and breathlessness. On examination, patients might have digital clubbing due to chronic secondary infection by pyogenic organisms. Tenderness of the chest wall is seen in some of the patients. Radiological investigation shows a dense homogeneous opacity of the hemithorax. Broncho-pleural fistula is a common complication in empyemas of tubercular origin, when there is a delay in treatment. Development of bronchopleural fistula is characterized by expectoration of a large quantity of sputum and volume depends on the position of the patient.

If the patient develops bronchopleural fistula, it can present as pyopneumothorax. Pus aspirated from the pleural cavity can be positive for acid fast bacilli. Secondary infection by staph, streptococcus, pseudomonas and K. pneumoniae are common. If tuberculous empyema is not treated properly, it may spontaneously perforate the pleura and extend through fascial planes and collect in the chest wall. This condition is known as 'empyema necessitates'. It is an unusual complication of empyema. Other sites of extension of empyema include the paravertebral soft tissue and retroperitoneum. Rarely, pus can track down posterior to the diaphragm and will accumulate in the groin or lumbar region (Behera, 2010). Chest x-ray shows a soft tissue mass in the chest wall with or without bony destruction in empyema necessitates. Contrast enhanced CT is helpful in identifying the direct communication between the pleural and the chest wall collection. Management consists of appropriate antibiotics and anti-tubercular treatment. Repeated aspirations are attempted in the initial stage, but intercostal tube drainage is required to remove the pus, since the chances of developing pleural thickening are more with empyema. In some patients surgical debridement of the pleura with physical removal of loculation, fibrous septae and thick exudate is required. Minimal access surgery using video-assisted thoracoscopy techniques have succeeded in achieving equivalent results to open thoracotomy in the past few years (Wait *et al.*, 2007). Surgical procedures like thoracoplasty and decortication are required in some cases. Decortication via thoracotomy is the standard treatment method for chronic empyema. Decortication is an elective surgical procedure, in which fibrous wall of the empyema cavity, the cortex or rind is stripped off the visceral and parietal pleura. This procedure allows the expansion of the underlying lung (Katariya *et al,* 1998). Some patients may require thoracoplasty.

5.2   Spontaneous Pneumothorax

Spontaneous pneumothorax is a well known complication in cavitary tuberculosis. Pneumothorax is defined as the presence of gas in the pleural space (Loscalzo, 2010). The term Pneumothorax was first coined by Itard, a student of Laennec in 1803 and Laennec himself described the clinical picture of pneumothorax in 1819 (Kaya *et al.*, 2009). Pneumothorax may be primary or secondary. Secondary pneumothorax occurs in persons with significant underlying pulmonary disease. Pneumothorax complicating pulmonary tuberculosis can occur at any age (Lichter & Gwynne, 1971). In countries where tuberculosis is a common problem, pulmonary tuberculosis remains the commonest cause of secondary spontaneous pneumothorax (SSP). According to Gupta *et al.*, the commonest cause of spontaneous secondary pneumothorax in India is pulmonary tuberculosis (Gupta *et al.*, 2006). In tuberculosis, the rupture of the sub pleural focus and rupture of a cavity are the common causes for pneumothorax. Other causes are rupture of a bleb or bulla which has developed adjacent to fibrosis.

All the patients will have chest pain and dyspnea. The clinical symptoms are dependent on the degree of collapse of the underlying lung. Cough is also a common symptom. Patients with tension pneumothorax will have acute onset of chest pain and dyspnea. On examination diminished movements of chest and reduced vocal fremitus are found on the affected side. Trachea deviates away from the affected side. The affected side may also be hyper resonant on percussion with diminished or absent breath sounds. Hypotension, tachycardia, hypoxia, jugular venous distension may be present. Radiography of the chest shows hyper-translucent area without bronchovascular markings on the affected side with the lung being compressed towards the hilum.

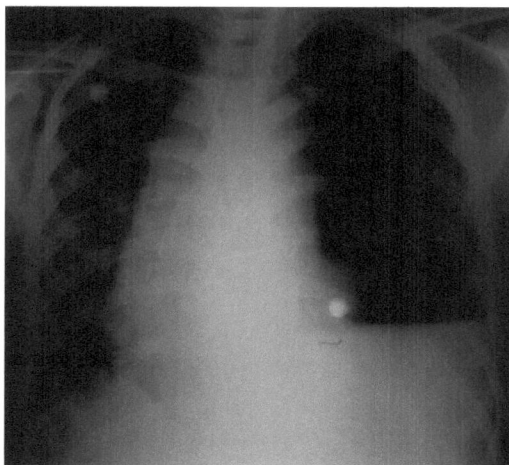

Figure 9: Chest X-ray PA view showing Pyopneumothorax on left side.

In tension pneumothorax the mediastinum will be displaced to the opposite side. Pneumothorax secondary to tuberculosis is frequently associated with untreated empyema, when it is called as pyopneumothorax. Pneumothorax is uncommon in miliary tuberculosis, and thus only few cases have been reported (Khan *et al.*, 2011; Arya *et al.*, 2011).

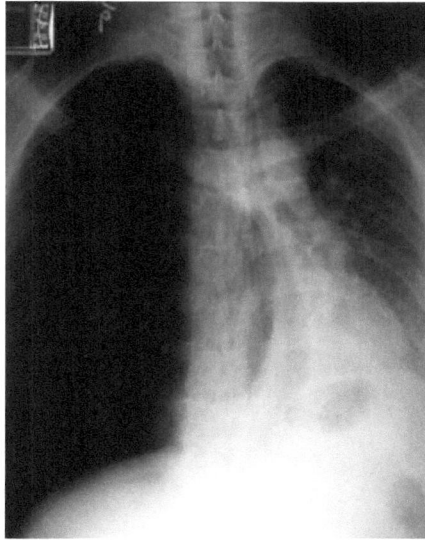

Figure 10: Chest X-ray PA view showing right tension pneumothorax with mediastinal shift to left side.

Management of pneumothorax consists of conservative approach and active management. Both ACCP and BTS guidelines recommend treatment based on the severity of symptoms and the degree of collapse of the underlying lung as determined by chest radiographs (Baumann *et al.*, 2001). Conservative approach is indicated if patient has minimal symptoms and volume of pneumothorax is very small i.e. less than 20% of the hemi thoracic volume. The principle of this approach is based on natural tendency for the gas to get absorbed. The absorption is hastened by giving 100% supplementary oxygen. Patients with pre-existing lung disease are unable to tolerate pneumothorax in which case active management is indicated. Active management consists of simple aspiration or intercostal tube drainage. Aspiration is less likely to be successful in patients with SSP. Blanco et.al studied pneumothorax in active pulmonary tuberculosis. Patients with pulmonary tuberculosis showed a lesser and slower response to catheter aspiration in their study (Blanco-Perez *et al.*, 1998). It can be considered in patients with small pneumothoraces, who are symptomatic in order to avoid chest tube drainage. Otherwise, underwater seal chest tube drainage which allows gradual re-expansion of the lung is recommended. In case of persistent air leak or recurrent pneumothorax surgical intervention is recommended. Surgical intervention consists of limited thoracotomy with pleurectomy or pleural abrasion. Chemical pleurodesis by using sclerosing agents is indicated in patients with recurrent pneumothorax who are unwilling or unable to undergo surgery. Over the past years, widespread use of less invasive video-assisted thoracic surgery (VATS) has been more commonly used in the management of pneumothorax (Ng, 2006).

5.3   Calcification

The term calcification refers to the deposition of the calcium salts in tissues. It may be limited or diffuse. Diffuse can be metastatic calcification where calcium deposits are found in normal tissues. In dystrophic calcification it occurs in injured lung tissues. Dystrophic calcifications are frequently seen in granulomatous infections like tuberculosis, histoplasmosis and coccidiodomycosis. Tuberculous lung lesions heal by calcification. The calcification can either be microscopic or macroscopic (Behra, 2010). In parenchymal disease calcification presents as discrete radio opacities. Sheet like calcification can be seen in pleural disease. Tuberculous pleuritis leaves sequelae ranging from minimal pleural thickening to extensive calcification encompassing and restricting the lung (Choi *et al.*, 2001). Occasionally calcified lymph nodes or concretions can get detached and erode through the bronchial walls or blood vessels causing massive haemoptysis. Extensive calcification can lead to respiratory failure or cor pulmonale.

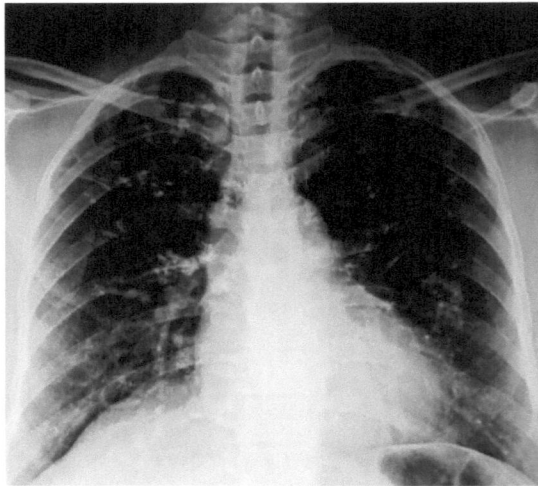

Figure 11: Chest X-ray PA view showing bilateral extensive calcification.

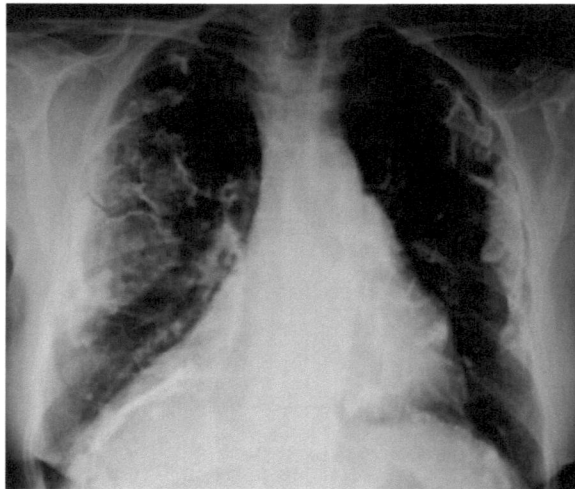

Figure 12: Chest X-ray PA view showing bilateral extensive pleural calcification.

6   General Complications

6.1   Cor Pulmonale

Cor pulmonale is right ventricular dysfunction (enlargement) due to pulmonary hypertension secondary to diseases of the lung, bony thorax, lung ventilation or pulmonary circulation (Rajendran, 2004). Virchow in nineteenth century found changes like right ventricular hypertrophy in autopsies of patients who died of pulmonary tuberculosis (Kapoor, 1994).

Bilateral and extensive tuberculosis can cause pulmonary hypertension due to extensive fibrosis which causes distortion of parenchyma. The basic underlying pathophysiology is increase in the pulmonary vascular resistance and pulmonary hypertension. Clinical diagnosis depends on right ventricular dysfunction, pulmonary hypertension and evidence of primary lung disease. Early treatment prevents this late complication of pulmonary tuberculosis.

6.2   Amyloidosis

Tuberculosis is the commonest underlying cause for renal amyloidosis in developing countries, whereas Rheumatoid arthritis is the most frequent underlying inflammatory disease in developed countries. Amyloidosis is caused by deposition of insoluble fibrillar proteins in various tissues which leads to organ dysfunction or failure. Amyloidosis commonly involves kidneys. Secondary renal amyloidosis is seen in disorders that usually includes chronic inflammatory disease or infectious diseases. Pro-inflammatory mediators /cytokines such as interleukin -1, tumor necrosis factor alpha, and interleukin 6 stimulate the serum amyloid A synthesis in liver and other sites. This accumulates in renal tissue. Proteinuria is the most consistent feature of renal amyloidosis. In patients with tuberculosis, presence of pedal edema, proteinuria and grossly abnormal kidneys on ultrasonography should be evaluated by renal biopsy for amyloidosis. The time interval between the onset of predisposing disease and first evidence of amyloidosis has shown variable results in different studies, varying from one to thirty years (Chug *et al.*, 1981) or two months to seven years (Dixit *et al.*, 2009). Secondary amyloidosis has now become a rarity as a complication of pulmonary tuberculosis due to availability of effective anti-tuberculosis treatment.

6.3   Chronic Respiratory Failure

Chronic respiratory failure may complicate pulmonary tuberculosis (Sharma, 2009). Tuberculosis continues to be a chronic infection with very high rates of morbidity and mortality. Delays in the diagnosis and treatment of tuberculosis can lead to pulmonary sequelae that are characterized by impairments in the bronchial and parenchymal structure. The structural changes include bronchovascular distortions, bronchiectasis, emphysema and fibrosis. This leads to greater ventilation perfusion (V/Q) mismatch (Behra, 2010). Tuberculosis destroyed lung term is used to describe the destructive lung parenchymal changes which occur over many years following pulmonary tuberculosis (WHO Report. 2008) Non- invasive ventilation has greatly improved the outlook for patients with previous tuberculosis who develop chronic respiratory failure (Shneerson, 2004). Acute respiratory failure can occur over a chronic respiratory failure due to respiratory infection with pyogenic organisms (SatyaSri, 2009).

7   Conclusion

Various forms of complications may result from pulmonary tuberculosis. It is important to be aware of the full spectrum of clinical and radiologic features of the sequelae to facilitate diagnosis and management of the complications of pulmonary tuberculosis.

Acknowledgement

Dr. Kiran Joshy, Bangalore, India; for assisting in manuscript preparation.

References

Ann Leung., (1999). Pulmonary Tuberculosis: The Essentials. Radiology, 210: 307-322.

Arya,M., George,J., Dixit, R., Gupta, RC., Gupta, N., (2011). Bilateral spontaneous pneumothorax in miliary tuberculosis. Indian J Tuberc., 58(3):125-8.

Ashizawa, K., Matsuyama, N., Okimoto, T., Hayashi, H., Takahashi, T., Oka, T., et al. (2004). Coexistence of lung cancer and tuberculoma in the same lesion: demonstration by high resolution and contrast-enhanced dynamic CT. British journal of radiology, 77 (923), 959-962.

Baumann, MH., Strange, C., Heffner, JE., et al.,(2001). Management of spontaneous pneumothorax: an American College of Chest Physicians Delphi consensus statement. Chest, 119: 590–602.

Behera, D. (2010). Textbook of Pulmonary Medicine. New Delhi: Jaypee Brothers Medical publications.

Blanco-Perez, J., Bordón, J., Piñeiro-Amigo, L., Roca-Serrano, R., Izquierdo, R., Abal-Arca, J.,(1998). Pneumothorax in active pulmonary tuberculosis: resurgence of an old complication? Respir Med., 92(11):1269-73.

Choi, J., Hong, K.T., Oh, Y., et al., (2001). CT Manifestations of Late Sequelae in Patients with Tuberculous Pleuritis. American Journal of Roentgenology, 176: 441-445.

Chug, K.S., Singhal, P.C., Sakhuja, V., Datta, B.N., Jain, S.K., Dasu, S.C. (1981). Pattern of renal amyloidosis in Indian Patients. Postgrad Med J., 57:31–5.

Crofton and Douglas's Respiratory disease. (2000), 5th ED. Oxford: Blackwell science.

Dixit, R., Gupta, R., Dave, L., Prasad, N., Sharma, S., (2009). Clinical profile of patients having pulmonary tuberculosis and renal amyloidosis. Lung India, 26:41-5.

Felson, B., (1998). Chest Roentgenology, Elsevier Science Health.

Fishman, A. P., et al. (2008). Fishman's Pulmonary Diseases and Disorders. 4th edn. New York: McGraw Hill.

Gupta,D., Mishra,S., Faruqi, S., Aggarwal, AN.,(2006). Aetiology and clinical profile of spontaneous pneumothorax in adults.Indian J Chest Dis Allied Sci., 48(4):261-4.

Harman, M. E., (2012). Aspergillosis.http://emedicine.medscape.com/article/296052-overview.

Hermel, M.B., & Gershon-Cohen, J. (1954). Healing Mechanisms of Tuberculous Cavities. Radiology, 63: 544-549.

Hoheisel, G., Chan, B.K.M., Chan, C.H.S., Chan, K.S., Teschler, H., Costabel, U., (1994) Endobronchial tuberculosis: diagnostic features and therapeutic outcome. Respir Med, 88:593–597.

Jean-Baptiste, E. (2005). Hospital Physician. Review Article: Management of Haemoptysis in the Emergency Department.

Julio, G.S., Irene, P.B., Jordi, G.G., Feliciano, S.N., Iker, F.N., Maria, J.R., (2012). Anthracofibrosis or Anthracostenosis. Arch Bronconeumol, 48: 133-136.

Kapoor, S.C. (1994). Electrocardiology in pulmonary tuberculosis. Ind. J. Tub., 41,129.

Katariya, K.,Thurer, R.J., (1998). Surgical management of empyema. Clin Chest Med., 19(2): 395-406.

Kaya, S.O., Karatepe,M.,Tok, T. Et.al., (2009). Were pneumothorax and its management known in 15th-century anatolia?. Tex Heart Inst J., 36(2): 152–153.

Khan, N.A., Akhtar, J., Baneen, U., Shameem, M., Ahmed, Z., Bhargava, R. (2011). Recurrent pneumothorax: A rare complication of miliary tuberculosis. N Am J Med Sci., 3(9): 428-30.

Kim, H.Y., Im, J.G., Goo, J.M., et al., (2000). Bronchial anthracofibrosis (inflammatory bronchial stenosis with anthracotic pigmentation): CT findings. Am J Roentgenol, 174: 523-527.

Kim, H.Y., Song, K.S., Goo, J.M., & Lee, J.S. (2001). Thoracic sequelae and complications of tuberculosis. Radiographics, 21(4):839-58.

Klein, J.S., Fang, K., Chang, M.C., (1993). Percutaneous transcatheter treatment of an intracavitaryaspergilloma. Cardiovasc Intervent Radiol, 16: 321–324.

Kousha, M., Tadi, R., Soubani, A.O., (2011). Pulmonary aspergillosis: a clinical review. Eur Respir Rev, 121, 156-174.

Kundu, S., Mitra, S., Mukherjee, S., et al.,(2010). Adult thoracic empyema: A comparative analysis of tuberculous and nontuberculous etiology in 75 patients. Lung India, 27: 196-201.

Lichter, I., Gwynne, J.F., (1971). Spontaneous pneumothorax in young subjects: A clinical and pathological study. Thorax, 26(4): 409–417.

Light, R.W. (2006). Parapneumonic effusions and empyema. Proc Am Thorac Soc., 3(1):75-80. Review.

Lordan, J.L., Gascoigne, A., Corris, P.A., (2003). The pulmonary physician in critical care: Assessment and management of massive haemoptysis. Thorax, 58: 814-819.

Loscalzo J. (2010). Harrison's Pulmonary and Critical Care Medicine. New York: The McGraw-Hill Companies, Inc.

Low, S.Y., Hsu, A., Eng, P., (2004). Interventional bronchoscopy for tuberculous tracheobronchial stenosis. Eur Respir J, 24,345-347.

McDonnell, L., Long, J.P. (1981). Lung scar cancer - a reappraisal. J Clin Pathol, 34: 996-999.

Ng, C.S., Lee, T.W., Wan, S., Yim, A.P., (2006). Video assisted thoracic surgery in the management of spontaneous pneumothorax: the current status. Postgrad Med J. 82(965):179-85.

Rajasekaran, S., Vallinayagi,V., Jeyaganesh, D.,(1999).Unilateral Lung Destruction: a computed tomographic evaluation. Ind. J. Tub., 46,183.

Rajendran, S. (2005). Clinical Diagnosis-Cardiovascular System, ISBN: 9788180612541.

Rasmussen, V., (1868). On Haemoptysis, especially when fatal, in its anatomical and clinical aspects. Edinburgh Med J., 14: 385–401.

Remy, J., Remy-Jardin, M., Voisin, C., (1992). Endovascular management of bronchial bleeding. In: Butler, J., eds. The bronchial circulation. New York, NY: Dekker.

Ryu, Y.J., Kim, H., Yu, C.M., Choi, J.C., Kwon, Y.S., Kwon, O.J.,(2006). Use of silicone stents for the management of post-tuberculosis tracheobronchial stenosis. Eur Respir J. 28:1029–1035.

SatyaSri S. & Ashish S. (2009). Text Book of Pulmonary & Extra Pulmonary Tuberculosis, Banginwar: Mehta Pub.

Seo, J. B., Song, K. S., Lee, J. S., Goo, J. M., Kim, H. Y., Song, J. W.,et.al., (2002). Broncholithiasis: Review of the Causes with Radiologic-Pathologic Correlation1. Radiographics, 22(suppl 1), S199-S213.

Sharma, S.K., (2009). Tuberculosis, New Delhi: Jaypee Brothers Medical Publishers (P) Ltd.

Shin, B.S., Jeon, G.S., Lee, S.A., Park, M.H., (2011). Bronchial artery embolisation for the management of haemoptysis in patients with pulmonary tuberculosis. Int J Tuberc Lung Dis., 15(8):1093-8.

Shneerson, J. M.,(2004). Respiratory failure in tuberculosis: a modern perspective. Clin Med., 4(1):72-6.

Smulders, Y.E., De Bondt B.J., Lacko, M. & Hodge J.A. (2009). Laryngeal tuberculosis presenting as a supraglottic carcinoma: a case report and review of the literature. J Med Case Rep, 20; 3:9288.

Sopko, D.R., & Smith, T.P., (2011). Bronchial Artery Embolization for Haemoptysis. Semin Intervent Radiol., 28(1): 48–62.

Tetikkurt, C., (2008). Current perspectives on endobronchial Tuberculosis Pneumon 21(3):239–245.

Verma A, Park HY, Lim SY, Um SW, Koh WJ, Suh GY, et al., (2012) Posttuberculosis tracheobronchial stenosis: Use of CT to optimize the time of silicone stent removal. Radiology, 263:562-8.

Wait, M.A., Becklen D.L., Paul, M., Hotze, M., DiMaio M.J.,(2007). Thoracoscopic management of empyema Thoraces. J Min Access Surg, 4:141-8.

Wallgren, A., (1948). The time table of tuberculosis. Tubercle, 29:245–251.

Wan, I.P., Lee, T., Lam, H.K., Abdullah, V., Yim, A.C., (2002). Tracheobronchial Stenting For Tuberculous Airway Stenosis. Chest, 122(1):370-374.

WHO report 2008: Global tuberculosis control.
http://www.who.int/tb/publications/global_report/2008/annex_3/en/#.UkexkikSLEU.google.

Wood, D. A., & Miller, M. (1938). The role of the dual pulmonary circulation in various pathologic conditions of the lungs, J. thorac. Surg.,7, 649.

Young, K., Aspestrand, F., Kolbenstvedt. (1991). High resolution CT and bronchography in the assessment of bronchiectasis. Acta Radiology, 32:439-441.

Yu, Y.-Y., Pinsky, P. F., Caporaso, N. E., Chatterjee, N., Baumgarten, M., Langenberg, P., et al., (2008). Lung cancer risk following detection of pulmonary scarring by chest radiography in the prostate, lung, colorectal, and ovarian cancer screening trial. Archives of internal medicine, 168 (21), 2326.

Genotypic Diversity among the *Mycobacterium Tuberculosis* Complex

Dorothy Yeboah-Manu
Noguchi Memorial Institute for Medical Research
University of Ghana, Ghana

1   Introduction

Tuberculosis (TB) is an ancient disease and still a worldwide health problem; a third of the world population is infected by the causative agent, and more than eight million get sick of TB and close to two million people die of TB annually (WHO, 2010). The main strategy being used for the control of this disease is by case detection and antimycobacterial treatment which last for at least six months using multiple drugs (WHO, 2008). A threat to this control strategy is the over reliance of an old diagnostic tool that is microscopic detection of acid-fast bacilli using the Ziehl Neelson protocol which lacks sensitivity and specificity, at the same time this diagnostic tool cannot determine drug susceptibility status of the infecting strain (Kent and Kubica, 1985; Daniel, 1990). In addition, there is lack of an effective vaccine for prevention, and more importantly, the major threat to this strategy is the emergence of strains that are resistant to the available drugs for treating TB (Perkins and Cunningham, 2007). Multidrug-resistant tuberculosis (MDR-TB) is defined as resistance to isoniazid and rifampicin, with or without resistance to other first-line drugs (FLD). Extensively drug-resistant tuberculosis (XDR-TB) is defined as resistance to at least isoniazid and rifampicin, and to any fluoroquinolone, and to any of the three second-line injectables (amikacin, capreomycin, and kanamycin) (Gandhi *et al.*, 2006; WHO, 2006 and Velayati *et al.*, 2009). Such cases may either not be cured by the current first-line treatment regimen or have a more expensive and long treatment course (Udwadia, 2009 and WHO, 2012). The tendency to acquire drug resistance may be influenced by the genetic background of the strain (Yeboah-Manu *et al.*, 2011). Potential solutions to this problem include the development of new drugs, simple but sensitive diagnostic tools and an effective TB vaccine.

In this perspective, identification of the mycobacterial components that have important role(s) in the establishment of the infection assumes crucial importance for the development of these needed control tools. The rational design of these control tools requires a better understanding of the pathogen genome, especially the genomic diversity among the various lineages to allow the global applicability of such control tools.

Tuberculosis is caused by a group of closely related gram positive bacteria, together referred to as the *Mycobacterium tuberculosis* complex (MTBC). Even though genetically these species are quite close, they have varying host specificities: *Mycobacterium tuberculosis* sensu sticto (MTB) and *Mycobacterium africanum* (MAF) are the main causative agents of TB in humans (here further referred to as "human MTBC") though *Mycobacterium canettii* (MCT) has occasionally been identified in TB cases from the Horn of Africa, whereas *Mycobacterium bovis* is primarily a pathogen of cattle, (Smith, 1898 and Garnier *et al.*, 2003) *Mycobacterium microti* a pathogen of voles, (Frota *et al.*, 2007;), *Mycobacterium caprae* a pathogen of goats, (Aranaz *et al.*, 2003) and *Mycobacterium pinnipedii* a pathogen of seals and sea lions (Cousins *et al.*, 2003). MAF was first identified in 1968 in Senegal and was described biochemically as having characteristics between MTB and *M. bovis* (Casette *et al*, 1968). Based on biochemical analysis, MAF used to be subdivided into two separate groups, the East-African and West-African sub-species. However, current advancement in molecular biology indicates that the East-African variant is a sub-lineage within MTB, currently known as the "Uganda genotype" (Niemann *et al*, 2002). In this review, MAF is defined as the one originally termed *M. africanum* 1 based on biochemical analysis, which is genetically sub- divided into West-African genotype I and II. In addition to varying host ranges, the members of the MTBC vary in growth requirement and colonial morphology. For example while MTB requires glycerol as a carbon source, *M. bovis* and MAF is reported to grow well using pyruvate as the sole carbon source. In addition, while MTB produces luxuriant growth (eugenic), *M. bovis* produces tiny colonies, termed dysgonic. MCT is the most phenotypically distinct member of the MTBC; together with other members may share a common ancestor, which was likely a human pathogen. MCT is phenotypically characterized by their smooth glossy white colony which is due to the presence of large amounts of lipooligosaccharides in the cell wall. In addition the MTBC seems to vary in virulence, propensity to develop drug resistance and the ability to cause large outbreaks. For example, experimental studies using macrophage and animal models have shown that strains of human MTBC differ in virulence and immunogenicity. Beginning in the first half of the last century, numerous studies carried out in guinea pigs demonstrated that a significant proportion of MTBC strains isolated from TB patients in South India were less virulent compared to strains from the United Kingdom (Mitchison, *et al.*, 1960; Alsaadi and Smith, 1973 and Coscolla and Gagneux, 2010). Similarly, early animal studies comparing MAF from Senegal to *M. tuberculosis* showed that MAF was less virulent (Toure, 1982; de Jong *et al.*, 2010). In another study conducted in Gambia, it was shown that while both MTB and MAF transmit equally, MAF seems to have a longer latency period compared to MTB (de Jong *et al*, 2008). The same group further showed that MAF seems to be less virulent than MTB, as it affects more HIV, and also the affected produces attenuated ESAT6 response (de Jong *et al* , 2005; de Jong *et al*, 2006). In contrast, the MTB strain HN878 caused disease outbreaks in Los Angeles and Houston, has been shown to exhibit a consistent hyper-virulent phenotype in various experimental models, including human monocyte-derived macrophages,(Zang *et al* 1999) mice, (Manca *et al*, 1999, 2001, 2004 & 2005) and rabbits (Tsenova, 2005). It is now known that the HN878 belongs to the MTB Lineage 2, which includes the 'W-Beijing' family of strains. A recent study showed that MTB has a higher propensity to develop drug resistant variants compared to the two lineages of MAF put together (Yeboah-Manu *et al* 2011) (Table 1).

	M tuberculosis (n=92) N (%)	*M africanum(32) N (%)*	*P value**
STR	35 (38%)	4 (12.5.1%)	0.008
INH	14 (15.2%)	2 (6.25%)	0.237
RIF	7 (7.6%)	1 (3.1%)	0.679
EMB	4 (4.3%)	1 (3.1%)	1.000
MDR	4 (4.3%)	0 (0%)	0.572
ANY RESISTANCE	40 (43.5%)	7 (21.9%)	0.030
	Cameroon Sub-lineage (n=47) N (%)	*West-African I (n=26) N (%)*	*P value*
STR	19 (40.4%)	3 (11.5%)	0.015
INH	9 (19.1%)	1 (3.8%)	0.086
RIF	5 (10.6%)	1 (3.8%)	0.412
EMB	4 (8.5%)	1(3.8%)	0.649
MDR	4 (8.5%)	0 (0%)	0.290
ANY RESISTANCE	22 (46.8%)	6(23.1%)	0.046

Table1: The level of resistance obtained from MTBC lineages and sub-lineages from a study conducted in Ghana. The resistance was measured by the proportion method.* Where cells had values 5 or less the P value was computed using the Fisher's exact test. Yeboah-Manu *et al.,* (2011).

Despite their different tropisms, phenotypes and pathogenicities that were revealed very early in TB studies, not much thought has been given to genetic diversity within the human adapted MTBC in terms of development of control tools; most efforts to date have concentrated on finding tools for TB control based on a few laboratory strains of MTB.

The complete genome sequence of the virulent MTB reference strain H37Rv has a size of 4 million base pairs, with 3959 genes (Cole et al). 40% of these genes have had their function characterised, with possible function postulated for another 44%.4,4 Mb GC 65.6% ≈ 4000 genes (http://www.sanger.ac.uk/Projects/M_tuberculosis). The genome contains 250 genes involved in fatty acid metabolism, with 39 of these involved in the polyketide metabolism generating the waxy coat. Such large numbers of lipid-associated genes show the evolutionary importance of the waxy coat to pathogen survival. The genome contains genes for aerobic, micro-aerophilic and anaerobic, abundance of genes involved in lipid metabolism, eukaryotic like Serine/Threonine Protein Kinases and novel gene/protein families e.g. PE/PPE, ESAT-6 (Cole et al, 1998; McEvoy, *et al.*, 2009).

1.1   Genetic Diversity within the MTBC

The species of the MTBC exhibit low DNA sequence diversity. The MTBC share this with other deadly bacterial pathogens, including the causative agents of leprosy, anthrax and plague, are caused by bacterial lineages with extremely low levels of genetic diversity, the so-called 'genetically monomorphic bacteria' (Achtman 2008). These genetically monomorphic bacteria lack genetic events such as horizontal gene transfer (Brosch *et al* 2000, Supply *et al* 2003), which therefore gives them a highly clonal population structure unlike other bacteria like *Helicobacter pylori (Ref)*. Nevertheless, a recent report has provided evidence for lateral gene transfer within the MTB, the PE_PGRS genomic region. On the average these bacteria harbours a single nucleotide difference 2-28kb, when pairs are compared (Table 2). Consequently for a long time, the general dogma was that genetic diversity within the MTBC is negligible and has no phenotypic consequence for host pathogen interaction, propensity to develop drug resistance and antigenic variation which could have implication on the successful global application of control tools including vaccines or diagnostics. This dogma was strengthened by earlier sequencing and other genomic studies that were conducted using limited and often biased strain collections, collected from restricted geographical regions. Despite their remarkable genetic homogeneity, members of the MTBC express very different phenotypes.. Understanding the diversity of bacterial pathogens is important, both for epidemiological and biological reasons. However, because of the low DNA sequence variation in monomorphic bacteria, studying the genetic diversity of these microbes is challenging. Standard sequence-based methods like multilocus sequence typing (MLST) are not applicable because of low phylogenetic resolution. In spite of the conservation of their genomes there are a number of different phenotypic traits, which have been used to distinguish the MTBC (Table 3).

The MTBC nucleotide sequences are 99.9% identical and 16S rRNA sequences do not differ between MTBC members, with the exception of *M. canetti*. DNA-DNA hybridization assay analysis of the members of the MTBC tested were found to share 85 to 100% DNA-DNA relatedness and completely conserved DNA sequences were reported for the 16S rRNA gene (rDNA) and 16S-23S rDNA spacers (Sreevatsan *et al.*, 1997). Furthermore, no significant nucleotide sequence variations either in 26 structural genes or in 24 genes coding for proteins that are targets of the host immune system were found among a diverse group of isolates of MTB (Refs). Hence it has been suggested that the MTBC members have resulted from a recent evolutionary bottleneck with the resulting MTBC being derived from the clonal expansion of a single successful ancestor (Namouchi *et al* 2012).

However, with the advancement in molecular analyses and accessibility to more isolates from diverse geographical regions (especially from Africa and Asia), we now know that genetic diversity

Lineage	SNPs (genomes)	Core genome size (MB)	SNPs per 100kb	Reference
Mycobacterium leprae	222	3.3	7	Monot et al., 2009 Truman et al.,2011
Burkholderia mallei	515	5.7	9	Losada et al. 2010
Bordetella pertussis	471	4.1	12	Bart et al., 2010
Yersinia pestis	1364	4.8	28	Morelli, et al. 2010
Salmonella enterica serovar Typhi	1964	4.4	44	Holt, et al. 2008
Bacillus anthracis	2798	5.5	51	Kuroda,et al., 2010
Mycobacterium tuberculosis	9945	4.4	226	Comas, et al., 2010

Table 2: Single nucleotide polymorphisms (SNPs) in core genomes among genetically monomorphic lineages. Achtmann, 2010.

	M. africanum	*M. tuberculosis* senso scrito	*M. bovis*
Colony Morphology	Dysgonic	Eugonic	Dysgonic
Nitrate reductase	Negative to weakly positive	positive	Negative
Niacin production	Negative to weakly positive	Positive	Negative
Pyrazinamide	Sensitive	sensitive	Resistant

Table 3: Biochemical methods in-use for differentiation of the MTBC. Yeboah-Manu *et al.,* 2011.

within MTBC, especially the human MTBC has been underestimated. Genetic diversity in MTBC is driven mainly by large sequence deletions in the so called region of difference (RD), repetitive elements and insertion sequences, and single nucleotide polymorphisms. Thus allelic variations in bacteria arise from random mutation, which may or may not be subject to selective pressure, horizontal gene transfer or recombination events.

2   Large Sequence Deletions

The availability of the genomes of different members of the MTBC has allowed the comparison of their genomes in the field of comparative genomics. It is recognized that variation in clinical MTBC strains are a result of repeated insertion or deletion events in specific genomic regions known as regions of differences (RDs) (Huard *et al.*, 2006). The deleted regions may be due to transposition and homologous recombination events between adjacent insertion sequence fragments. The work of Behr and colleagues performed comparative hybridization experiments on DNA microarrays containing capture probes for 3902 of the coding sequences present in MTB reference strain H37Rv to assess the relatedness of a set of 13 different BCG substrains. Regions deleted from BCG vaccines relative to the virulent MTB H37Rv reference strain were confirmed by sequencing across the missing segment of the H37Rv genome. Eleven regions (encompassing 91 open reading frames) of H37Rv were found that were absent from one or more virulent strains of *M. bovis*. Five additional regions representing 38 open reading frames were present in *M. bovis* but absent from some or all BCG strain (Behr *et al.*, 1999). Similar studies such as that initially conducted by Mahairas *et al* compared (employing subtractive genomic hybridization) the genomes of virulent MTB and *M. bovis* with avirulent BCG. During this effort three genomic regions of differences (named RD1 to RD3) representing approximately 30 kb of DNA were found to be deleted from the BCG genome (Mahairas et al., 1996; Philipp *et al.*, 1996a). The regions absent from *M. bovis* BCG relative to the MTB H37Rv genome were named RDI to RD16 in the Behr studies. Currently, about seventy RDs have been identified thus far, including those identified from other strains in addition to that from BCG. Some of the deleted segments may containenes that are important for host-pathogen interaction. Example is the RD1 deletion, which was, originally described by Mahairas et al in 1996 (Mahairas *et al.*, 1996), is specific for all BCG substrains (Behr *et aL*, 1999). The deleted region contains eight genes, most of which belong to the ESAT6 gene cluster (Tekaia *et aL*, 1999). ESAT6 has been shown to act as potent stimulator of the immune system and is an extracellular antigen recognised throughout infection (Elhay *et al.*, 1998; Horwitz *et al.*, 1995; Rosenkrands *et al.*, 1998). As this 10-kb region is absent from all BCG strains tested so far, but present in virulent *M. bovis* MTB and MAF, the loss of RD1 could be associated with the attenuation of BCG. Also RD7, which is present in MTB, but also absent from MAF sublineage 2, *M. bovis, M. microti* and *M. bovis* BCG (Gordon *et al.*, 1999; Groenheit R, 2011) contains the *mce3* operon. The *mce* gene was described by Riley and colleagues and codes for a putative invasin-like protein in MTB. In subsequent work, expression of a cloned DNA fragment of this gene from MTB in non-pathogenic *Escherichia coli* strain was shown to confer the ability to invade and survive within macrophages and HeLa cells, and it was named the mammalian cell entry (mce) gene (Arruda *et al.*,1993).

Some of these deletions are not only specific to certain species within the complex but also specific for sub/lineages within the human-specific species of MTB and MAF. Since, deletions tend to be irreversible events in MTBC due to low horizontal gene transfer (Ozcaglar *et al.*, 2011), the pattern of deletions can be used to deduce the phylogeny of MTBC (Figure 1). Thus identification of the presence or absence of these deletions is being used for species, lineage identification and for phylogenetic analysis. Gagneux *et al* used these polymorphic regions to analyse a collection of 875 MTBC isolates from patients originating from 80 countries and divided the global human MTBCs into six main lineages; two from MAF and four from MTB. When the geographic origins of these strains were mapped a strong biogeographical structure became evident (Gagneux *et al.*, 2006, figure 2). One of the major observations was that the two MAF are dominantly found in West-Africa; West-African genotype I (marked by RD711 deletion) and West-African genotype II (RD702 deletion). West-African genotype I is predominantly found around the Gulf of Guinea and West-African genotype II is prevalent in western West-Africa, with countries such as Ghana, Cote d'Ivoire and Benin harbouring both lineages (Gagneux, 2012). These observations were confirmed by a recent RD analysis of 162 MTBC isolates from Ghana (Yeboah-Manu *et al* 2011).

In addition to distinct geographic distributions, these lineages have been tentatively linked to different epidemiologic and clinical profiles. A previous study has suggested that some RD deletions are likely to offer advantages, including escape from the host immune system, antibiotic resistance, curtailing latency and promoting transmission (Malik and Godfrey-Faussett, 2005). A population-based study showed an association between extrapulmonary tuberculosis and infection by strains with deletions of RD105, RD181 and RD142 in Beijing strains (Kong *et al.*, 2005). It has been documented by a number of researchers that the Beijing strain marked by RD207 deletion is associated with high degree of transmission and propensity to develop multiple resistances. In one study it was found that multidrug-resistant (MDR) isolates, rifampicin-resistant isolates (n = and streptomycin (SM) resistant isolates were more common among Beijing genotype strains than among non-Beijing strains. A study by de Jong and colleagues also associated concurrent deletions to RD9 and RD702 to reduced ESAT6 secretion and progression from latency to active disease. Deletion of RD1 from MTB, resulting in attenuation strikingly like that of BCG, suggested the use of RD1 mutant strains for improvement of the tuberculosis (TB) vaccine (Mostowy *et al*, 2002; Lewis *et al.*, 2003). It has been shown that strains with the RD750 deletion are a prominent cause of tuberculosis among Asians in the United Kingdom and in the Indian subcontinent. The RD750 deletion appears to have increased, rather than decreased, the capacity of this lineage of MTB to cause immune deviation and contribute to its persistence and outbreak potential in human populations (Newton *et al.*, 2006).

3   Repetitive Elements

Many repetitive DNA sequences exist in both eukaryotic and prokaryotes genomes, however due to the small size of the bacteria genome and the high pressure of DNA replication and rapid cell division, the size, and number of repeats are limited. Nevertheless, In addition to short sequence repeats (SSR also called microsatellites which are 3-5 bp), few minisatellites like sequences (longer repeats: 50-200 bp) as found in eukaryotes have been described in some bacterial genus. Sharples and Lloyd (1990) reported a repetitive element in enterobacteria; this was named the enterobacterial repetitive intergenic consensus (Eric) sequence. The Eric sequence is a 126bp element that contains highly conserved central inverted repeats located in the extragenic region and appears not to be related to other interspersed elements such as the repetitive extragenic palindromic (Rep) sequence. The Rep sequences, which encompasses repetitive and palindromic sequences with a length between 21 and 65 bases (Gilson *et al.*, 1984 and Gilson *et al.*, 1986) detected in the extragenic space of some bacterial genomes and Box sequences described in *Streptococcus pneumonia*. The functions of these repetitive sequences are not entirely known but it has been considered may be important in the regulation of gene expression, maintenance of chromosomal structure and probably important for evolution. While some of these sequences are direct repeats in a specific region of the genome, others are interspersed throughout the genome.

Sequencing of the MTB reference strain H37Rv genome identified a number of different repeat sequences (Fang *et al*, 1998; Groenen, 1993). Perhaps one of the most intensively investigated repeat is the direct repeat (DR) region which is a member of the Clustered Regulatory Short Palindromic Repeats (CRISPR) sequences family. This region has a unique structure of direct repeat sequences (36 bp): 10 to 50 copies of the repeats, which are separated from one another by spacers that have different sequences (34 to 41 bp). The repeats and the variable spacers together are termed direct variable repeat (DVR) sequences. However, the spacer sequences between any two specific direct repeats are conserved among strains.

While the function of this region of the MTB genome remains to be determined, its preservation throughout the evolutionary history of the MTBC argues for a functionally important domain. In some bacteria, CRISPRs takes about 40% of the genome (http://crispr.u-psud.fr/crispr/CRISPRdatabase.php) and functions as a prokaryotic immune system (Barrangou *et al*, 2007). The CRISPRs have been shown to encode specialized defence mechanisms against extracellular DNA sequences from plasmids and bacteriophages, and changes in the number of spacers have been associated with phage-susceptibility. The spacers are thought to be acquired from external sources, and therefore act as immunological memory for the host bacteria (Cruz and Davies, 2000; Sola *et al.*, 2003; and Barrangou *et al.*, 2007).

The DR shows strain-to-strain polymorphism as the presence or absence of specific spacers is variable between different species and lineages among the MTBC. This polymorphism has been exploited to distinguish the MTBC strains for epidemiological studies and to distinguish the taxons within the group of the MTBC (Kamerbeek *et al.*, 1997). The standard protocol called 'spoligotyping' (spacer oligonucleotide typing), is PCR-based reverse-hybridization blotting technique, uses 43 different spacers. Amplification of the spacers is accomplished by using two primers, DRa and DRb, which enable one to amplify the whole DR region. The obtained PCR product which is labelled as the PCR primers were labelled allows the presence of any of the 43 different spacers be determined by hybridization of the amplified DNA to 43 spacer oligonucleotides, which are covalently linked to a membrane (figure 3). Due to the low discriminatory power of spoligotyping it is used more for phylogenetic analysis, and the congruence between RD and spoligotyping analysis have been reported (Ferdinand *et al.*, 2004 and Brudey *et al.*, 2006). Therefore for epidemiological investigation, it is normally used in conjunction with a second typing method with a higher resolution power. International spoligotype databases that compile the global and local geographical structures of MTBC bacilli populations are available. These include the SpolDB4 (Brudey *et al.*, 2006), which describes 1939 shared-types (STs) representative of a total of 39,295 strains from 122 countries. The most recent database, which was released this year, is named SITVITWEB which include other markers in addition to spoligotypes. The database includes 62,582 clinical isolates corresponding to 153 countries of patient origin (105 countries of isolation). The database report a total of 7104 spoligotype patterns (corresponding to 58,180 clinical isolates)–grouped into 2740 shared-types or spoligotype international types (SIT) containing 53,816 clinical isolates and 4364 orphan patterns (Demay *et al.*, 2012).

Three different studies that analysed clinical MTB isolates, either collected consecutively or as part of outbreak investigation; suggest that the DR region evolves by at least four different mechanisms (Aga *et al*, 2006; van Embden *et al* 2000 and Warren *et al* 2002). These mechanisms include the insertion sequence IS*6110*-mediated mutation, homologous recombination between repeat sequences leading to DVR deletion, strand slippage during replication leading to duplication of DVR sequences, and point mutation. The insertion of IS*6110* into repeat sequences in the DR region resulted in the apparent deletion of DVR sequences according to the spoligotype data. An alternative mechanism was also identified by which the IS*6110* element was inserted into the variable spacer sequence. Homologous recombination between adjacent IS*6110* elements (Warren *et al.*, 2002 and Rodriguez-Campos *et al.*, 2011) could explain the deletion of large portions of the DR region and 5′-flanking region.

Another family of repeats are tandem repeats (TRs). The MTBC's genomes also contain different tandem repeats. These include clusters of short tandem repeats which are 10bp in length, separated by 5bp unique sequences and the 24bp GC rich sequence present in at least 26 loci of the MTB genome. Some TRs are polymorphic in length due to variations in the tandem repeat copy number and therefore these loci are often called variable number tandem repeats (VNTRs) (Nakamura *et al.*, 1987; 1988). Since the numbers of adjacent repeated units varies from strain to strain, VNTRs are therefore thought to be inherently unstable units that undergo frequent variation in the number of copies through slippage strand misalignment during DNA synthesis (Marzars *et al.*,2001; Warren *et al.*, 2002) or double-strand break repair for instance. VNTRs are also invaluable tools for studying various aspects of evolution, ranging from pedigree to evolutionary distant phylogenetic relationships (Richards and Sutherland, 1994; Epplen *et al.*, 1997). The pioneer works done by Supply et al; Magdalena et al identified VNTR elements in the MTBC's, which was also found in *M. leprae* genome and they named the VNTRs in MTBC, mycobacterial interspersed repetitive units (MIRUs). MIRUs are 40±100 bp DNA elements often found as tandem repeats and dispersed in intergenic regions of the MTBC genomes. Based on size, the MIRUs have been classified into three major types (Supply *et al.*, 1997). Type I sequences contain roughly 77 bp. Type II and type III MIRUs are characterized by a gap of 24bp and 15bp corresponding to the 30 and 50 portions of type I sequences, respectively. MIRUs are different from all other repetitive elements in that they do not contain dyad symmetries, but most MIRUs contain an open reading frame ORFs (Supply *et al.*, 1997), that overlaps the termination and initiation codons of their flanking genes and are oriented in the same direction as the ORFs. However, some MIRUs are also found within predicted coding regions. Within the MTBCs more than 40 different MIRU/VNTR loci have been identified and at least 24 of them are considered to be polymorphic (figure 4). Early findings also suggested that these interspersed bacterial minisatellite-like structures are stable and may evolve slowly in mycobacterial populations as analysis of 12 variable loci using three genealogically distant BCG substrains (*M. bovis* BCG Japan, Glaxo and Pasteur) found MIRU 4 as the only locus with variable repeats among the three. MIRU-VNTRs are remarkably stable and therefore adequate for tracking key events in epidemiological investigations. At the same time, MIRU-VNTRs provide a high resolution essential to differentiate unrelated strains. Two to eight alleles are at each of the 12 loci, yielding approximately 20 million possible combinations of alleles. The discriminatory power of MIRU genotyping is almost as great as that of IS*6110*-based genotyping (see below). MIRU analysis can be automated and can thus be used to evaluate large numbers of strains, yielding intrinsically digital results that can be easily catalogued on a computer database. A Website has been set up so that a worldwide database of MIRU patterns can be referenced (MIRU-VNTR*plus* (Allix-Beguec *et al*, 2008; Weniger *et al*, 2010).

4   Mobile Genetic Element (MGE)

The genomes of most organisms, from bacteria to mammals, have been found to contain Mobile Genetic Elements (MGEs). Mobile elements are involved in genomic rearrangements and virulence acquisition, and hence, are important elements in bacterial genome evolution. These elements are defined by their ability to remove themselves from one region of the genome and insert themselves into another region. MGEs were first identified by Barbara McClintock in the 1950s (McClintock, 1951), where they were found to alter the colour of maize kernels. However, they were originally dismissed as passive elements or 'junk DNA' and it is only in recent years that the major influence they play in genome evolution, particularly through their regulation of gene activity, has become appreciated.

MGEs are grouped according to their mechanism of transposition. Class I MGEs, or retrotransposons, move within the genome by being transcribed to RNA and then back to DNA by reverse transcriptase, while class II MGE's (often known as transposons) encode a transposase and move directly from one position to another within the genome using a 'cut and paste' or 'copy' mechanism. In bacteria, transposons are often referred to as insertion sequences (IS) and these are further classified according to structural similarities. Within the MTBCs a number of IS elements such as IS*986* and IS*987* have been identified as major cause of both genetic and phenotypic diversity within the members and among different strains of the same species but the most studied is the insertion sequence IS*6110* (Eisenach *et al.*, 1994; Miller *et al.*, 1994). Nevertheless, sequencing analysis has indicated that the three elements are basically identical, differing only in a few nucleotides and in their 3-bp terminal sequences. IS*6110* is 1,361 bp long and contains 28-bp, imperfect inverted repeats at its extremities with three mismatches and 3-bp direct repeats that probably result from repetition of the target sequence. Among the various mycobacterial species examined, IS*6110* was detected only in species belonging to the MTBC. A search in the EMBL data bank has revealed homologies with IS*3411*, an insertion element from *E. coli* (McAdam *et al*, 1990; Dale, 1995).

Most members of the MTBC, including MTB, MAF, contain multiple IS*6110* copies although *M. bovis* generally contains only one copy and limited transposition is observed. This insertion element is present in the DR region of almost all analysed MTBC species and strains, thus it is considered to be the site of the original insertion site into the MTBC early in its evolution. The number and position (insertion site) of IS*6110* copies in the genome of different MTBC strains is variable; the number ranges from none found in a few strains, to 25 different elements. Due to its great abundance and varied distribution in the genome, it has been suggested that the insertion sequence IS*6110* is an important contributor to the natural variation of the MTBCs. As has been indicated earlier, IS*6110* deletion and recombination are major mechanisms involved in the diversity in the MTBC's direct repeat region and hence evolution of the MTBCs.

Mapping of IS*6110* transpositional insertion points in MTB has demonstrated that no obvious insertion site sequence specificity exists, although more subtle sequence preferences may possibly occur. However, insertion sites are not random and integration of hot-spots exist (Sampson *et al.*, 1999). These may be defined as genomic regions that exhibit integration frequencies that are above the level expected if integration is assumed to be randomly distributed. They include the DR region (Hermans *et al.*, 1991), the phospholipase C gene region (Raynaud *et al.*, 2002), members of the PPE gene family (Chaitra *et al.*, 2005), and the intergenic region between the DnaA and DnaN genes (Rajagopalan *et al.*, 1995a; 1995b), as well as other ISs themselves, such as IS*1547* (also described as the ipl site) (Fang et al, 1997). One preferential intergenic insertion sites of IS*6110* appears to be the origin of chromosome replication (*oriC*) region, which is essential for the initiation of bacillary replication (Kurepina, 1998). Insertions of IS*6110* in the *oriC* region raise questions such as: do IS*6110* insertions in *oriC* alter the rate of DNA replication and therefore the growth rate? If so, are there consequences of this insertion on the bacillary morphology, growth and virulence? In one study, the authors tried to answer these questions, by studying two isogenic groups of MTB strains obtained from the sputa of two patients. The integration site of IS*6110* in *oriC*, the *in-vivo* and *in-vitro* duplication time as well as the bacillary size and morphology of the strains were determined. Isogenic strains containing the IS*6110* element in *oriC* exhibited a diminished growth rate and average dimensions of the bacilli were modified; moreover, they were less virulent in a mouse model (Casart *et al* 2008). When residing in transcriptionally silent genomic regions IS*6110* is inactive and rarely undergoes transposition. However, when inserted into a transcriptionally active region of the genome the transposition rate of IS*6110* is greatly increased, presumably due to an increase in transposase production (Craig, 1997). This finding suggests that a single transpositional event may generate a sudden burst of transpositional activity if the element is incorporated into a transcriptionally active site (Craig, 1997). With each additional duplication event the chance that an element will be integrated into an active genomic region and undergo increased transposition and duplication increases. Consequently, the copy number of IS*6110* may quickly increase, resulting in strains with an intermediate or high copy number. Insertion point mapping studies also detect genomic regions where IS integration is rare or absent (Seungtai *et al.*, 2009). This strongly suggests that integration into these regions is detrimental to the organism.

IS*6110* is suggested to be a major contributor to phenotypic variation within the MTBC and that it has influence on the evolution of the pathogen. IS*6110* has been shown to influence gene expression through integration into protein coding genomic regions, the ability to undergo recombination events resulting in gene deletion, and the upregulation of genes due to its intrinsic promoter activity and its spontaneous insertion has been associated with drug resistance (Kivi *et al.,* 2002). Recently, a statistically significant association was found between extrathoracic TB and insertion- and deletion- mutations in the *plcD* gene due to an IS*6110* insertion (Kong *et al.,* 2005). However, the effect of the genetic rearrangements mediated by IS*6110* transpositions on the course of the infection remains unclear. IS*6110* can upregulate downstream genes through an outward-directed promoter in its 3′ end. This activity has been demonstrated for upregulation of the two-component system PhoP/PhoR (Carlos *et al.,* 2004). Promoter activity was orientation dependent and was localized within 110-bp fragment adjacent to the right terminal inverted repeat (Alonso *et al.,* 2011). The Beijing lineage contains a larger number of IS*6110* copies than other lineages (Alonso *et al.,* 2011) and this could be related to the special characteristics of this family in terms of virulence and capacity for rapid dissemination.

The high degree of IS*6110* polymorphism, both in a numerical and positional sense, between different MTBC strains, has made it a useful marker for strain genotyping. Accordingly, the standardised IS*6110* fingerprinting method (Nicoletta, *et al.,* 2005) has become the most widely used genotyping method in molecular epidemiological studies of *M. tuberculosis*). This is because IS*6110* transposition events are generally common enough to allow differentiation between more distantly evolved strains but are still rare enough to show stability within more closely related strains. They are thus useful in distinguishing between recent epidemiological events (transmission) and distant epidemiological events (reactivation). In practice, two or more isolates with identical or near-identical (±1 band) IS6110 fingerprints (known as a cluster) are generally accepted as representing a recent transmission event (Figure 5). However, due to the technological demands of this technique and inter-laboratory differences in obtained results, PCR-based methods based on other repetitive markers such as VNTR are gradually replacing this method for epidemiological investigations.

5   Single Nucleotide Polymorphism

Allelic variation in the MTBC also arises from random nucleotide mutation, which can be deletion, insertion or substitutions (SNPs). Two classes of substitutions, referred to as synonymous and nonsynonymous single nucleotide polymorphisms (SNPs), can occur in genes that encode proteins (Kimura, 1983; Schork *et al.* 2000; Gut 2001). Nonsynonymous SNPs (nsSNPs) result in amino acid replacements and hence provide substrate for evolutionary selection. In contrast, synonymous SNPs (sSNPs) do not alter the structure of proteins and are evolutionarily neutral or nearly so (Kimura 1983; Schork *et al.* 2000; Gut, 2001). Numerous studies of 56 genes in several hundred MTBC strains suggested that there is about one synonymous nucleotide substitution per 10,000 nucleotide sites (Kapur *et al.* 1994; Sreevatsan *et al.* 1997a; Musser *et al.* 2000).

Some of the mutations are specific to distinct phylogentic groups of the MTBCs, and therefore, SNP analysis is currently being used for phylogenetic analysis (Streevatsan *et al;* Stucki *et al* 2012*).* SNPs are particularly useful for phylogenetic studies because they are less subject to selective pressure than are other genetic markers. The phylogenetic information obtained with SNP analysis have been found to correspond to that found with large deletion analysis, and in the case of MTBC, has an added advantage of devoid of [1]convergence evolution and hence lack [2]homoplasy (Comas *et al,* 2009). The isolates of the MTBC organisms were previously assigned to one of three principal genotypic groups (PGG) based on the combinations of polymorphisms at *katG* codon 463 and *gyrA* codon 95. Group 1 has the allelic combination *katG* codon 463 CTG (Leu) and *gyrA* codon 95 ACC (Thr); group 2 has *katG* 463 CGG (Arg) and *gyrA* codon 95 ACC (Thr), and group 3 organisms have *katG* 463 CGG (Arg) and *gyrA* codon 95 AGC (Ser). All isolates of *M. bovis*, *M. microti*, and MAF studied had the combination of polymorphisms characteristic of PGG 1. In contrast, MTB isolates fall into each of the three groups (Streevatsan *et al*, 1997). Some of the SNP assays that have been used of differentiation of the MTBCs include SNP in the narGHJI and oxyR genes for differentiating *M. bovis* from MTB; more are indicated in Table 4.

Lineage	SNP_Name	Primer	Primer Sequence	Probe	Probe_seq
Euro-American (red)	katG463	katG463_F	CCGAGATTGCCAGCCTTAAG	H37Rv_probe	6FAM-CAGATCCGGGCATC
		katG463_R	GAAACTAGCTGTGAGACAGTCAATCC	Mutant_probe	VIC-CCAGATCCTGGCATC
Blue (RD105)	Rv2952_0526n	Rv2952_F	CCTTCGATGTTGTGCTCAATGT	H37Rv_probe	6FAM-CCCAGGAGGGTAC
		Rv2952_R	CATGCGGCGATCTCATTGT	Mutant_probe	VIC-CCCAGGAAGGTACT
Pink (RV3221c)	Rv3221c_0085n	RV3221c_F	TGTCAACGAAGGCGATCAGA	H37Rv_probe	6FAM-ACAAGGGCGACGTC
		RV3221c_R	GACCGTTCCGGCAGCTT	Mutant_probe	VIC-ACAAGGGCGACATC
Purple (Rv3804c T-C)	Rv3804c_0012	Rv3804c_F	GCATGGATGCGTTGAGATGA	H37Rv_probe	6FAM-AAGAATGCAGCTTGTCGA
		Rv3804c_R	CGAGTCGACGCGACATACC	Mutant_probe	VIC-AAGAATGCAGCTTGTTGA

Table 4: List of Lineage, SNP, Primer and Probe for major Lineage typing. Stucki et al, 2001.

Homolka and colleagues analysed a set of 108 global collections of both human adapted and animal adapted MTBCs, strains (excluding *M. canetti*) representing five different ecotypes. Hershberg and colleagues sequenced 89 structural genes which together corresponded to 65,829 base pairs per strain, or 1.5% of the 4.4 Mbp genome of MTBC. SNP analysis of these 89 genes comprised housekeeping genes, antigens and additional genes such as that of putative drug targets, showed greater genetic diversity of the human-adapted organisms than previously thought. The phylogenetic analysis showed that all the animal-adapted members of MTBC form one group relative to the rest of the phylogeny, but more closer to the MAF West-Africa II lineage than the other MTBC lineages. This suggests that even though these animal strains belong to four distinct ecotypes adapted to distinct animal host species, they represent only a proportion of the genetic diversity found in all of the human MTBC

(Figure 2b, Hershberg *et al*, 2008). The genomes of the MTBCs are found to contain high proportion of dN/dS ratio (Homolka *et al.*, 2009; Comas *et al* 2010). The findings from the same study showed that unlike that reported earlier by Rocha, the high non-synonymous mutations may not be deleterious to the MTBCs, and may neither be the result of artefact due to the clonal genome butthe reduction in selective constrain.

> [1] Convergence Evolution: This describes the acquisition of the same biological trait in unrelated lineages/ organisms not closely related independently evolve similar traits
>
> [2] Homoplasy: The phenomenon of similarity in species/lineages of different ancestry that is the result of convergent evolution

Gutacker and collegues 2000, studying the genetic relationships among strains compared the 4.4-Mb genome sequences of *M. tuberculosis* strain H37Rv and CDC1551 and identified only ~900 SNPs located in open reading frames, which confirms the restricted allelic variation in MTBs. Approximately 65% of the SNPs were nsSNPs, an unanticipated result given that sSNPs are expected to outnumber nsSNPs except under situations involving positive selection (Kimura, 1983). Restricted allelic variation limits the utility of multilocus sequence analysis (Maiden *et al.* 1998) for estimating genetic relationships among MTBC strains and for studying relationships between strain genotype and patient phenotype, however there are other evidence suggesting this may not be true.

However, some SNPs have been identifiedin MTBC that alter activities of enzymes thought to be involved in pathogenesis and hence specific genes, and the finding of more functional genetic diversity than previously expected. For example, nitrate reduction is believed to be vital for the survival of tubercle bacteria under hypoxic/anaerobic conditions that are thought to prevail within granulomas. Nitrate reductase activity is rapidly induced in MTB under hypoxic conditions and is attributed to the induced expression of the nitrate/nitrite transporter gene, narK2. By contrast, *M. bovis* and *M. bovis* BCG (BCG) do not support the hypoxic induction of either nitrate reductase activity or narK2. The induction defect in the narK2X operon in *M. bovis* and BCG is caused by a -6T/C single nucleotide polymorphism (SNP) in the -10 promoter element essential for narK2X promoter activity. Keating *et al.*, 2005, identified that *M. bovis* is not able to grow in medium with only glycerol as carbon source but requires supplementation with pyruvate in glycerol medium. Thus *M. bovis* has a deficiency in central metabolism that has profound implications for in vivo growth and nutrition. Not only is *M. bovis* unable to use glycerol as a sole carbon source but the lack of a functioning pyruvate kinase (PK) means that carbohydrates cannot be used to generate energy. This disruption in sugar catabolism is caused by a single nucleotide polymorphism in *pykA*, the gene which encodes PK, that substitute's glutamic acid residue 220 with an aspartic acid residue. Substitution of this highly conserved amino acid residue renders PK inactive and thus blocks the ATP generating roles of glycolysis and the pentose phosphate pathway. This mutation has been also found to occur in other members of the MTBC, namely *M. microti* and at least in the West-African genotype II of MAF.

5.1   Adaptive Changes which Cause Drug Resistance

Several studies have demonstrated that mutations in drug target genes are associated with resistance to antituberculous drugs, however, most of the studies have been concentrated on MTB strains and limited data are available regarding *M. bovis* and MAF isolates. Several genes involved in resistance to isoniazid (*katG*, *ahpC*, *inhA*, and the *oxyR-ahpC* intergenic region), rifampin(RMP) (*rpoB*), streptomycin (*rrs*, *rpsL*), ethambutol (*embB*), and quinolones (*gyrA*) have been studied. These genes, or fragments of genes, usually amplified and sequenced. The mode of action of the key first-line drug RMP and the molecular mechanism of resistance have been explored in detail in previous studies (Homolka *et al.*, 2009). For example, several investigations showed that mutations in the 81-bp hot spot region (codon 426 to 452) of the *rpoB* gene are solely responsible for resistance in at least 90% of all RMP-resistant strains (Musser, 1995; Homolka *et al.*, 2009). SNP analysis is therefore very useful for the determination of drug resistance in human TB. Sequence analysis indicates that nucleotide substitutions in these genes cause a change in the encoded amino acid. However, other mutations have been described in different strains. A study by Romero et al sequencing of the *rpoB* gene revealed a substitution mutation in codon 531 (TCG□TTG, Ser□Leu) in the two human MDR isolates. In addition to these mutations, mutations in other regions have been associated with specific drug resistance. Wang *et al.*, 2007 demonstrated that Rv2629 A191C mutations were present in 99.1% of rifampin-resistant and 0% of rifampin-susceptible clinical MTB isolates and that over expression of the Rv2629 191C allele in *Mycobacterium smegmatis* produced an eightfold increase in rifampin resistance. However, further work involving phylogenetic analysis has proven that this allele is specifically associated with single nucleotide polymorphism cluster group 2 (SCG-2), a phylogenetic lineage that corresponds to the Beijing-W clade of MTB and that in contrast to the findings of *Wang et al.*, 2007 the over expression of either Rv2629 191 allele in *M. smegmatis* did not produce an increase in rifampin resistance. The findings therefore argue against Rv2629 191C allele association with rifampin resistance and that the allele cannot be used as a molecular target to detect rifampin resistance. The allele appears to be an excellent marker for the Beijing-W clade/SCG-2 phylogenetic group (Chakravorty *et al.*, 2008). Sequence analysis of 58 multidrug-resistant MTBC strains from Germany and 55 susceptible strains from a reference collection comprising major phylogenetic lineages confirmed that variations in Rv2629, 191A/C and 965C/T, are specific for genotypes Beijing and Ghana, respectively, but not involved in the development of rifampicin (Homolka *et al.*, 2009).

Streevatsan *et al.*, 1997 sequenced 26 structural genes of MTB, *M. bovis*, MAF and *M. microti*, found that allelic variation within these organisms is driven by drug resistance. Compilation of the two mega bases of sequence data for the 26 genes revealed that greater than 95% of nucleotide substitutions caused amino acid replacements or other mutations in gene regions linked to antibiotic resistance and driven to high frequency by direct drug selection. Over all 26 genes examined, only 32 polymorphic nucleotide sites were identified that have not been directly associated with antibiotic resistance.

6   The PE/PPE Multigene Family

Sequence analysis of the MTB reference strain H37Rv genome identified two large families of genes encoding glycine, rich proteins designated PE (Pro-Glu) and PPE (Pro Pro-Glu) (*Cole et al. 1998*). The H37Rv genome contains 99 members of the PE family and 68 members of the PPE family respectively and together account for around 10% of the organism's genomic coding potential and is encoded by 176 open reading frames (McEvoy, *et al.*, 2009). The PE genes are characterised by the presence of a proline-glutamic acid motif at positions 8 and 9 within a highly conserved N-terminal domain consisting of around 110 amino acids. Similarly, PPE genes contain a proline-proline-glutamic acid at positions 7–9 in a highly conserved N-terminal domain of approximately 180 amino acids. The C-terminal domains of both PE and PPE protein families are highly variable in both size and sequence and often contain repetitive DNA sequences that differ in copy number between genes. Indeed, several studies have revealed varying degrees of PE/PPE sequence polymorphism between MTB clinical isolates. While some analysis reported a high degree of polymorphism within the pe_pgrs33, pe_pgrs16, ppe18 and pe_pgrs26 genes, others who analysed other PE members did not find any polymorphisms but found these members to be very homogenous. Using comparative sequence analysis of 18 publicly available MTBC whole genome sequences, that aligned 33 pe and 66 ppe genes in order to detect the frequency and nature of genetic variation, it was shown that nsSNP's in pe (excluding pgrs) and ppe genes are 3.0 and 3.3 times higher than in non-pe/ppe genes respectively and that numerous other mutation types are also present at a high frequency.

Diversity was revealed by differences in size as revealed by PCR products and also by SNP analysis (Qi *et al.*, 2009). In addition to sequence variation, gene expression alterations may contribute to antigenic variation and these have also been noted in pe/ppe genes from different MTB strains.

Their genes have a conserved structure and repeat motifs that could be a potential source of antigenic variation in MTBCs. Pe/ppe genes are scattered throughout the genome and PE/PPE pairs are usually encoded in bicistronic operons although this is not universally so. This gene family has evolved by specific gene duplication events. PE/PPE proteins are either secreted or localized to the cell surface. The function of PE/PPE proteins remains enigmatic but studies suggest that they are secreted or cell surface associated and may be involved in bacterial virulence, and could participate in evasion of the host immune response.

6.1   Correlation of genetic Diversity and Clinical Presentation

The impact of strain variation for human disease has been well established for a number of bacterial pathogens such as *Escherichia coli*, *Neisseria menigitidis*, *Haemophylus influenzae*, *Bordetella* and *Streptococcus* species. In these bacterial species, some strains are more likely to cause invasive disease than others because such virulent phenotypes posses distinct virulent markers such as genes associated with the production of toxins. However, no such genetic marker has been identified for the MTBC. Infection with the MTBC results in a range of clinical phenotypes ranging from asymptomatic infection through localised diseased lungs to different forms of more invasive/disseminated disease. As has been outlined above, some SNPs, insertion elements and genomic deletions have been associated with clinical features of different strains and species (Vishnoi *et al.*, 2007; Vishnoi *et al.*, 2008); but if and how MTBC genomic diversity influences human disease in clinical settings remains an open question. A possible role for strain diversity in human tuberculosis (TB) is increasingly being suggested from work in various infection models (Davila *et al.*, 2010). For example, experimental studies using macrophage and animal models have shown that strains of human MTBC differ in virulence and immunogenicity (Coscolla and Gagneux, 2010; Levine, 2006). Beginning in the first half of the last century, numerous studies carried out in guinea pigs demonstrated that a significant proportion of MTBC strains isolated from TB patients in South India were less virulent compared to strains from the United Kingdom (Coscolla and Gagneux, 2010). However, no concrete conclusions have been made regarding strain genetic diversity and clinical presentation; for example while in Gambia it was concluded that MAF infects more HIV co-infected patients (de Jong *et al.*, 2010a), this findings were not concluded from a study in Ghana that involved more than two thousand cases (Meyer et al, 2008; de Jong *et al.*, 2010b). While many factors, including host and environmental factors like, nutritional aspects, as well as the extent of co-morbidities such as diabetes will affect the outcome of TB infection and disease, more systematic work needs to be conducted in this area to ascertain the role of strain diversity and outcome of infection in TB.

Acknowledgement

I am very grateful to Prof Sebastien Gagneux, Isaac Darko Otchere and Adwoa Asante-Poku for reviewing this Manuscript; I also thank Ms Agnes Baidoo for formatting the final document. I received funding from Ghana Government, Royal Society Leverhulme Trust African Award Scheme and Wellcome Trust Fellowship award **REF NO. 097134/Z/11/Z**

References

Achtman, M. (2008). Evolution, population structure, and phylogeography of genetically monomorphic bacterial pathogens. Annu Rev Microbiol 62: 53-70.

Achtman, M. (2011). Insights from genomic comparisons of genetically monomorphic bacterial pathogens. Phil Trans R Soc 367: 860–867. doi:10.1098/rstb.2011.0303.

Aga, R. S., Fair, E., Abemethy N. F., Hoynes, T., Woldemariam, M., et al.(2006). Microevolution of the direct repeat locus of Mycobacterium tuberculosis in a strain prevalent in San Francisco. J Clin Microbiol 44(4): 1558–1560.

Allix-Béguec, C., Harmsen, D., Weniger, T., Supply, P., Niemann, S. (2008). Evaluation and user-strategy of MIRU-VNTRplus, a multifunctional database for online analysis of genotyping data and phylogenetic identification of Mycobacterium tuberculosis complex isolates. J. Clin Microbiol 46(8): 2692-2699.

Aranaz, A., Cousins, D., Mateos, A., Dominguez, L. (2003). Elevation of Mycobacterium tuberculosis subsp. caprae Aranaz et al. 1999 to species rank as Mycobacterium caprae comb. nov., sp. Int J Syst Evol Microbiol 53: 1785–1789.

Alsaadi, A. I., Smith, D. W. (1973). Fate of virulent and attenuated Mycobacteria in guinea-pigs infected by respiratory route. Am Rev Respir Dis 107:1041–1046.

Alonso, H., Aguilo, J. I., Samper S., Antonio C. J., Campos-Herrero I. M., et al. (2011). Deciphering the role of IS6110 in a highly transmissible Mycobacterium tuberculosis Beijing strain, GC1237, Tuberculosis doi: 10.1016/j.tube.2010.12.007.

Arruda, S., Boom, G., Knights, R., Huima-Byron, T., Riley, L. W. (1993). Cloning of an M. tuberculosis DNA fragment associated with entry and survival inside cells. Science 261: 1454-1457.

Barnes, P.F. and Cave, M. D. (2003). Molecular Epidemiology of Tuberculosis. New Engl J Med 349:1149-1156.

Barrangou, R., Fremaux, C., Deveau, H., Richards, M., Boyaval, P., et al. (2007). CRISPR provides acquired resistance against viruses in prokaryotes. Science 315: 1709–1712.

Bart, M. J., van, G. M., Van der Heide, H. G., Boekhorst, J., Hermans, .P, et al. (2010). Comparative genomics of prevaccination and modern Bordetella pertussis strains. BMC Genomics 11: 627. (doi:10.1186/1471-2164-11-627).

Behr, M. A., Wilson, M. A., Gill, W.P., Salamon, H., Schoolnik G. K., Rane, S. and Small, .P M. (1999). Comparative genomics of BCG vaccines by whole-genome DNA microarray. Science 284: 1520-1523.

Brosch, R., Gordon, S. V., Pym, A., Eiglmeier, K., Garnier, T., et al. (2000). Comparative genomics of the mycobacteria. Int J. Med Microbial 290: 143-152.

Brosch, R., Gordon, S. V., Marmiesse, M., Brodin, P., Buchrieser, C., et al. (2002). A new evolutionary scenario for the Mycobacterium tuberculosis complex. Proc Natl Acad Sci 99(6): 3684–3689.

Brudey, K., Driscoll, J. R., Rigout, L., Prodinger, W. M., Gori, A., et al. (2006). Mycobacterium tuberculosis complex genetic diversity: mining the fourth international spoligotyping database (SpolDB4) for classification, population genetics and epidemiology. BMC Microbiol. 6: 23.

Carlos, Y., Menéndez, SC, Pérez, ME, Samper, S, Gómez, A. B., et al. (2004). IS6110 Mediates Increased Transcription of thephoP Virulence Gene in a Multidrug-Resistant Clinical Isolate Responsible for Tuberculosis Outbreaks J Clin Microbiol 42(1): 212-219.

Casart, Y, Turcios, L., Florez, I., Jaspe, R., Guerrero, E., et al. (2008). IS6110 in oriC affects the morphology and growth of Mycobacterium tuberculosis and attenuates virulence in mice. Tuberculosis (Edinb). 88(6):545-552.

Castets, M., Boisvert, H., Grumbach, F., Brunel, M., Rist, N. (1968). Tuberculosis bacilli of the African type: preliminary note. Rev Tuberc Pneumol 32: 179–184.

Chaitra, M. G., Hariharaputran, S., Chandra, N. R., Shaila, M. S., Nayak, R. (2005). Defining putative T cell epitopes from PE and PPE families of proteins of Mycobacterium tuberculosis with vaccine potential. Vaccine 23: 1265–1272.

Chakravorty, S. B., Aladegbami, A. S., Motiwala, Y., Dai, H., Safi, M., et al. (2008). Rifampin resistance, Beijing-W clade-single nucleotide polymorphism cluster group 2 phylogeny, and the Rv2629 191-C allele in Mycobacterium tuberculosis strains. J Clin Microbiol 46: 2555-2560.

Cole, S. T., Brosch, R., Parkhill. J., Garnier, T., Churcher, C., et al. (1998). Deciphering the biology of Mycobacterium tuberculosis from the complete genome sequence. Nature 393(6685): 537-544.

Comas, I., Homolka, S., Niemann, S., Gagneux, S. (2009). Genotyping of Genetically Monomorphic Bacteria: DNA Sequencing in Mycobacterium tuberculosis Highlights the Limitations of Current Methodologies. PLoS ONE 4(11): e7815. doi:10.1371/journal.pone.0007815.

Comas, I., Chakravartti, J., Small, P. M., Galagan, J., Niemann, S., et al. (2010). Human T cell epitopes of Mycobacterium tuberculosis are evolutionarily hyperconserved. Nat Genet 42: 498–503. (doi:10.1038/ng.590).

Coscolla, M., Gagneux, S. (2010.) Does Mycobacterium tuberculosis genomic diversity explain disease diversity? Drug Discov Today Dis Mech 7: e43–e59.

Cousins, D. V., Bastida, R., Cataldi, A., Quse, V., Redrobe, S., et al. (2003). Tuberculosis in seals caused by a novel member of the Mycobacterium tuberculosis complex: Mycobacterium pinnipedii sp. nov. Int J Syst Evol Microbiol 53: 1305–1314.

Craig, N. L. (1997). Target site selection in transposition. Annu Rev Biochem 66: 437–474. doi: 10.1146/annurev.biochem.66.1.437.

Dale, J. W. (1995). Mobile genetic elements in mycobacteria. Eur Respir J Suppl 20: 633s-648s.

Daniel, T. M. (1990). The rapid diagnosis of tuberculosis: a selective review. J Lab Clin Microbiol 116: 277-282.

Davila, J., Zhang L., Marrs C. F., Durmaz R., Yang Z. (2010). Assessment of the genetic diversity of Mycobacterium tuberculosis esxA, esxH, and fbpB genes among clinical isolates and its implication for the future immunization by new tuberculosis subunit vaccines Ag85B-ESAT-6 and Ag85B-TB10.4. J. Biomed Biotechnolol, doi:10.1155/2010/208371.

de Jong, B. C., Hill, P. C., Brookes, R. H., Otu, J. K., Peterson, K. L., et al. (2005). Mycobacterium africanum: a new opportunistic pathogen in HIV infection? AIDS 19(15): 1714-1715.

de Jong, B. C., Hill, P. C., Brookes, R. H., Gagneux, S., Jeffries, D. J., et al. (2006). Mycobacterium africanum elicits an attenuated T cell response to early secreted antigenic target, 6 kDa, in patients with tuberculosis and their household contacts. J Infect Dis 193(9): 1279-1286.

de Jong, B. C., Hill, P. C., Aiken, A., Awine, T., Antonio, M., et al. (2008). Progression to active tuberculosis, but not transmission, varies by Mycobacterium tuberculosis lineage in The Gambia. J Infect Dis. 198(7):1037-1043.

de Jong, B. C., Adedifa, I., Walther, B., Hill, P. C., Anthonio, M., et al. (2010a). Differences between TB cases infected with M. africanum, West-African type 2, relative to Euro-American M. tuberculosis-an update. FEMS Immunol Med Microbiol 58(1): 102-105.

de Jong, B. C., Antonio, M., Gagneux, S. (2010b). Mycobacterium africanum Review of an Important Cause of Human Tuberculosis in West Africa. PLoS Negl. Trop Dis 4, e744.

de la Cruz, F., Davies, J. (2000). *Horizontal gene transfer and the origin of species: lessons from bacteria.* Trends Microbiol 8: 128–133.

Demay, C., Liens, B., Burguière, T., Hill, V., Couvin, D., et al. (2012). *SITVITWEB-a publicly available international multimarker database for studying Mycobacterium tuberculosis genetic diversity and molecular epidemiology* Infect Genet Evol 12(4):755-766.

Eisenach, K. D., Sifford, M. D., Cave, M. D., Bates, J. H., Crawford, J. T. (1994). *Detection of Mycobacterium tuberculosis in sputum samples using a polymerase chain reaction.* Am Rev Respir Dis 144: 1160-1163.

Elhay, M. J., Oettinger, T., and Andersen, P. (1998). *Delayed type hypersensitivity responses to ESAT-6 and MPT64 from Mycobacterium tuberculosis in the guinea pig.* Infect Immun 66: 3454–3456.

Epplen, C., Epplen, J. T., Frank, G., Miterski, B., Santos, E. J., et al. (1997). *Differential stability of the (GAA)n tract in the Friedreich ataxia (STM7) gene.* Hum Genet 99: 834–836.

Fang, Z., Forbes, K. J. (1997). *A Mycobacterium tuberculosis IS6110 preferential locus (ipl) for insertion into the genome.* J Clin Microbiol 35: 479–481.

Fang, Z., Morrison, N., Watt, B., Doig, C., Forbes, K. J. (1998). *IS6110 transposition and evolutionary scenario of the direct repeat locus in a group of closely related Mycobacterium tuberculosis strains.* J Bacteriol 180: 2102–2109.

Ferdinand, S., Valetudie, G., Sola, C., Rastogi, N. (2004). *Data mining of Mycobacterium tuberculosis complex genotyping results using mycobacterial interspersed repetitive units validates the clonal structure of spoligotyping-defined families.* Res Microbiol 155: 647–654.

Frota, C. C., Hunt, D. M., Buxton, R. S., Rickman, L., Hinds, J., et al. (2004). *Genome structure in the vole bacillus, Mycobacterium microti, a member of the Mycobacterium tuberculosis complex with a low virulence for humans.* Microbiol 150: 1519–1527.

Gagneux, S., DeRiemer, K., Vanb, T., Kato-Maedab, M., de Jong, B. C., et al. (2006). *Variable host-pathogen compatibility in Mycobacterium tuberculosis.* Proc Natl Acad Sci 103: 2869-2873.

Gagneux, S. (2012). *Host-pathogen coevolution in human tuberculosis.* Phil Trans R Soc 367: 850-859.

Gandhi, N. R., Moll, A., Sturm, A. W., Pawinski, R., Govender, T., et al. (2006). *Extensively drug-resistant tuberculosis as a cause of death in patients co-infected with tuberculosis and HIV in a rural area of South Africa.* Lancet 368(9547): 1575-1580.

Garnier, T., Eiglmeier, K., Camus, J. C., Medina, N., Mansoor, H., et al. (2003). *The complete genome sequence of Mycobacterium bovis.* Proc Natl Acad Sci USA 100: 7877–7882.

Gilson, E., Clement, J. M., Brutlag, D., Hofnung, M. (1984). *A family of dispersed repetitive extragenic palindromic DNA sequences in E. coli.* EMBO J. 3: 1417-1421.

Gilson, E., Perrin, D., Clement, J. M., Szmelcman, S., Dassa ,E., et al. (1986). *Palindromic units from E. coli as binding sites for a chromoid-associated protein.* FEBS Lett 206(2): 323–328.

Gordon, S. V., Brosch, R., Billault, A., Garnier, T., Eiglmeier, K., et al (1999). *Identification of variable regions in the genomes of tubercle bacilli using bacterial rtificial chromosome arrays.* Mol Microbiol 32: 643–656.

Groenen, P. M. A., Bunschoten, A. E., van Soolingen, D., van Embden, J. D. A. (1993). *Nature of DNA polymorphism in the direct repeat cluster of Mycobacterium tuberculosis: application for strain differentiation by a novel typing method.* Mol Microbiol 10: 1057–1085.

Groenheit, R., Ghebremichael, S., Svensson, J., Rabna, P., Colombatti, R., et al. (2011). *The Guinea-Bissau Family of Mycobacterium tuberculosis Complex Revisited.* PLoS ONE 6(4): e18601. doi:10.1371/journal.pone.0018601.

Gut, I. G. (2001). *Automation in genotyping of single nucleotide polymorphisms.* Hum Mutat 17(6): 475-492.

Gutacker, M., Valsangiacomo, C., Piffaretti, J. C. (2000). *Identification of two genetic groups in Bacteroides fragilis by multilocus enzyme electrophoresis: distribution of antibiotic resistance (cfiA, cepA) and enterotoxin (bft) encoding genes.* Microbiol 146: 1241–1254.

Hermans, P. W., van Soolingen, D., Bik, E. M., de Haas, P. E., Dale, J. W., et al. (1991). Insertion element IS987 from Mycobacterium bovis BCG is located in a hot-spot integration region for insertion elements in Mycobacterium tuberculosis comlex strains. Infect Immun 59: 2695-2709.

Hershberg, R., Lipatov, M., Small, P. M., Sheffer, H.., Niemann, S., et al (2008). High Functional Diversity in Mycobacterium tuberculosis Driven by Genetic Drift and Human Demography. PLoS Biol 6(12): e311. doi:10.1371/journal.pbio.0060311.

Holt, K. E., Parkhill, J., Mazzoni, C. J., Roumagnac, P., Weill, F-X, et al. (2008). High-throughput sequencing provides insights into genome variation and evolution in Salmonella typhi. Nat Genet 40: 987–993. (doi:10. 1038/ng.195).

Homolka, S., Post, E., Oberhauser, B., Garawani, A. G., Westman, L., et al. (2008). High genetic diversity among Mycobacterium tuberculosis complex strains from Sierra Leone BMC Microbiology 8:103 doi:10.1186/1471-2180-8-103.

Horwitz, M. A., Lee, B. W., Dillon, B. J., Harth, G. (1995). Protective immunity against tuberculosis induced by vaccination with major extracellular proteins of Mycobacterium tuberculosis . Proc Natl Acad Sci USA 92: 1530–1534.

Homolka, S., Köser, C. A., Rüsch-Gerdes J. S., Niemann, S. (2009). Single-Nucleotide Polymorphisms in Rv2629 Are Specific for Mycobacterium tuberculosis Genotypes Beijing and Ghana but Not Associated with Rifampin Resistance. J Clin Microbiol 47(1): 223–226.

Huard, R. C., Fabre, M., de Haas, P. L. C. O., van Soolingen, D., Cousins, D., et al. (2006). Novel Genetic Polymorphisms That Further Delineate the Phylogeny of the Mycobacterium tuberculosis Complex. J Bacteriol 188(12): 4271-4287.

Kamerbeek, J., Schouls, L., Kolk, A., van Agterveld, M., van Soolingen, D, et al. (1997). Simultaneous detection and strain differentiation of Mycobacterium tuberculosis for diagnosis and epidemiology. J Clin Microbiol 35(4): 907–914.

Kapur, V., Whittam, T. S., Musser , J. M. (1994). Is Mycobacterium tuberculosis 15,000 years old? J Infect Dis 170: 1348–1349.

Keating, L. A., Wheeler, P. R., Mansoor, H., Inwald, J. K., Dale, J., et al. (2005). The pyruvate requirement of some members of the Mycobacterium tuberculosis complex is due to an inactive pyruvate kinase: implications for in vivo growth. Mol Microbiol 56(1): 163–174.

Kent, P. T., Kubica, G. P. (1985). Public health Mycobacteriology: A guide for the level 111 laboratory. US Department of Health and Human Services. (CDC) 86-21654; 6: 57-68.

Kimura, M. (1983). The Neutral Theory of Molecular Evolution. Cambridge University Press, Cambridge.

Kong, Y., Cave, M. D., Yang, D., Zhang, L., Marrs, C. F., et al. (2005). Distribution of insertion and deletion-associated genetic polymorphisms among four Mycobacterium tuberculosis phospholipase C genes and associations with extrathoracic tuberculosis: a population-based study. J Clin Microbiol 43: 6048-6053.

Kurepina, N. E., Sreevatsan, S., Plikaytis, B. B., Bifani, P. J., Connell, N. D., et al. (1998). Characterization of the phylogenetic distribution and chromosomal insertion sites of five IS6110 elements in Mycobacterium tuberculosis: non-random integration in the dnaA-dnaN region. Tuber Lung Dis 79: 31-42.

Kuroda, M., Serizawa, M., Okutani, A., Sekizuka, T., Banno, et al. (2010). Genome-wide single nucleotide polymorphism typing method for identification of Bacillus anthracis species and strains among B. Cereus group species. J Clin Microbiol 48: 2821–2829. (doi:10.1128/JCM.00137-10).

Lari, N., Rindi, L., Sola, C., Bonanni, D., Rastogi, N., et al. (2005). Genetic Diversity, Determined of the basis of katG463 and gyrA95 Polymorphisms, Spoligotyping, and IS6110 Typing, of Mycobacterium tuberculosis Complex Isolates from Italy. J Clin Microbiol 43: 1617-1624.

Levin, B. R. (1996). The evolution and maintenance of virulence in microparasites. Emerg. Infect Dis 2: 93–102. (doi:10.3201/eid0202.960203).

Lewis, N. K., Liao, R., Guinn, K. M., Hickey, M. J., Smith, S., et al. (2003). Deletion of RD1 from Mycobacterium tuberculosis Mimics Bacille Calmette-Guérin Attenuation. J Infect Dis 187(1): 117–123.

Losada, L., Ronning, C. M., DeShazer, D., Woods, D., Fedorova, N., et al. (2010). *Continuing evolution of Burkholderia mallei through genome reduction and large-scale rearrangements. Genome Biol Evol 2: 102–116. (doi:10.1093/gbe/evq003).*

Mahairas, G. G., Sabo, P. J., Hickey, M. J., Singh, D. C., Stover, C. K . (1996). *Molecular analysis of genetic differences between Mycobacterium bovis BCG and virulent M. bovis J Bacteriol 178: 1274–1282.*

Maiden, M. C., Bygraves, J. A., Feil, E., Morelli, G., Russell, J. E., et al. (1998). *Multi-locus sequence typing: a portable approach to the identification of clones within populations of pathogenic microorganisms. Proc Natl Acad Sci 95(6): 3140-3145.*

Malik, A. N., Godfrey-Faussett, P. (2005). *Effects of genetic variability of Mycobacterium tuberculosis strains on the presentation of disease. Lancet Infect Dis 5: 174–183.*

Manca, C., Tsenova, L., Barry III, C. E., Bergtold, A., Freeman, S., et al. (1999). *Mycobacterium tuberculosis CDC1551 induces a more vigorous host response in vivo and in vitro, but is not more virulent than other clinical isolates. J Immunol 162: 6740-6746.*

Manca, C., Tsenova, L., Bergtold, A., Freeman, S., Tovey, M., et al. (2001). *Virulence of a Mycobacterium tuberculosis clinical isolate in mice is determined by failure to induce Th1 type immunity and is associated with induction of IFN-alpha /beta. Proc Natl Acad Sci USA 98: 5752-5757.*

Manca, C., Tsenova, L., Freeman, S., et al. (2005). *Hypervirulent M. tuberculosis W/Beijing Strains Upregulate Type I IFNs and Increase Expression of Negative Regulators of the Jak-Stat Pathway. J Interferon Cytokine Res 25: 694-701.*

Marten, K. M., Liu, X., Raychaudhuri, S., Altman, R. B., Small, P. M. (2002). *Determining the Genomic Locations of Repetitive DNA Sequences with a Whole-Genome Microarray: IS6110 in Mycobacterium tuberculosis. J Clin Microbiol 40(6): 2192–2198.*

McAdam, R. A., Hermans, P. W., van Soolingen, D., Zainuddin, Z. F., Catty, D., et al. (1990). *Characterization of a Mycobacterium tuberculosis insertion sequence belonging to the IS3 family. Mol Microbiol 4(9):1607-1613.*

McEvoy, C. R., van Helden, P. D., Warren, R. M., Van Pittius, N. C. G. (2009). *"Evidence for a rapid rate of molecular evolution at the hypervariable and immunogenic PPE38 gene region," Evolutionary Biology 9(1): 237.*

McClintock, B. (1951). *Cold Spring Harbor Symp. Quant Biol 16: 13-47.*

Meyer, C. G., Scarisbrick, G., Niemann, S., Browne, E. N., Chinbuah, M. A., et al. (2008). *Pulmonary tuberculosis: virulence of Mycobacterium africanum and relevance in HIV co-infection. Tubercul (Edinb). 88(5):482-489.*

Miller, N., Hernandez, S. G., Cleary, T. J. (1994). *Evaluation of Gen-Probe Amplified Mycobacterium Tuberculosis Direct Test and PCR for direct detection of Mycobacterium tuberculosis in clinical specimens. J Clin Microbiol 32: 393-397.*

Mitchison, D. A, Wallace, J. G., Bhatia, A. L., Selkon, J. B., Subbaiah, T. V., et al. (1960). *A comparison of the virulence in guinea-pigs of South Indian and British tubercle bacilli. Tubercle 41:1–22. [PubMed: 14423002].*

Monot, M., Honore, N., Garnier, T., Zidane, N., Sherafi, D., et al. (2009). *Comparative genomic and phylogeographic analysis of Mycobacterium leprae. Nat Genet 41: 1282–1289.*

Morelli, G., Song, Y., Mazzoni, C. J., Eppinger, M., Roumagnac, P., et al. (2010). *Yersinia pestis genome sequencing identifies patterns of global phylogenetic diversity. Nat Genet 42: 1140–1143. (doi:10.1038/ng.705).*

Mostowy, S., Cousins, D., Brinkman, J., Aranaz, A., Behr, M. A. (2002). *Genomic deletions suggest a phylogeny for the Mycobacterium tuberculosis complex. J Infect Dis 186: 74–80.*

Musser, J. M. (1995). *Antimicrobial agent resistance in Mycobacteria: molecular genetic insights. Clin Microbiol Rev 8: 496–514.*

Nakamura, Y., Leppert, M., O'Connell, P., Wolff, R., Holm, T., et al. (1987). *Variable Number of Tandem Repeat (VNTR) Markers for Human Gene Mapping Science', Science 235: 1616-1622.*

Nakamura, Y., Carlson, M., Krapcho, K., Kanamori, M., White, R. (1988). `New Approach for Isolation of VNTR markers', Amer J of Hum Genet 43: 854-859.

Namouchi, A., Didelot, X., Schöck, U., Gicquel, B., Rocha, E. P. (2012). After the bottleneck: Genome-wide diversification of the Mycobacterium tuberculosis complex by mutation, recombination, and natural selection. Genome Res 22(4):721-34.

Niemann, S., Rusch-Gerdes, .S, Joloba, M. L., Whalen, C. C., Guwatudde, D., et al. (2002). Mycobacterium africanum subtype II is associated with two distinct genotypes and is a major cause of human tuberculosis in Kampala, Uganda. J Clin Microbiol 40(9) 3398-3405.

Ozcaglar, C., Shabbeer, A., Vandenberg, S., Yerner, B., Bennett, K. P. (2011). Sublineage structure analysis of Mycobacterium tuberculosis complex strains using multiple-biomarker tensors. BMC Genomics 12(suppl 2).S1

Parwati, I., van Crevel, R., van Soolingen, D. (2010). Possible underlying mechanisms for successful emergence of the Mycobacterium tuberculosis Beijing genotype strains. Lancet Infect Dis 10: 103-111.

Perkins, M. D., Cunningham, J. (2007). Facing the Crisis: Improving the Diagnosis of Tuberculosis in the HIV Era. J Inf Dis 196(S1): S15-S27.

Philipp, W. J. , Nair, S. , Guglielmi, G., Lagranderie, M., Gicquel, B., et al. (1996.) Physical mapping of Mycobacterium bovis BCG Pasteur reveals differences from the genome map of Mycobacterium tuberculosis H37Rv and from M. bovis Microbiol 142: 3135–3145.

Portevin, D., Gagneux, S., Comas, I., Young, D. (2011). Human Macrophage Responses to Clinical Isolates from the Mycobacterium tuberculosis Complex Discriminate between Ancient and Modern Lineages. PLoS Pathog 7(3): e1001307. doi:10.1371/journal.ppat.1001307.

Qi, W., Käser, M., Röltgen, K., Yeboah-Manu, D., Pluschke, G. (2009). Genomic Diversity and Evolution of Mycobacterium ulcerans Revealed by Next-Generation Sequencing. PLoS Pathog 5(9): e1000580. doi:10.1371/journal.ppat.1000580.

Raynaud, C., Guilhot, C., Rauzier, J., Bordat, Y., Pelicic, V., et al. (2002). Phospholipases C are involved in the virulence of Mycobacterium tuberculosis. Molecular Microbiol 45: 203–217.

Reed, M. B., Gagneux, S., Deriemer, K., Small, P. M., Barry III, C. E., et al.(2004). A glycolipid of hypervirulent tuberculosis strains that inhibits the innate immune response. Nature 431: 84-87.

Rodriguez-Campos, S., Romero, B., Aranaz, A., Bezos, J., de Juan, L., et al. (2011). Limitations of Spoligotyping and Variable-Number Tandem-Repeat Typing for Molecular Tracing of Mycobacterium bovis in a High-Diversity Setting. J Clin Microbiol 49(9): 3361–3364.

Rajagopalan, M., Qin, M. H., Steingrube, V. A., Nash, D. R., Wallace, J. R. J., Madiraju, MVVS (1995a). Amplification and cloning of the Mycobacterium tuberculosis dnaA gene. Gene 163: 75–79.

Rajagopalan, M., Qin, M. H., Nash, D. R., Madiraju, M. V. V. S. (1995b). Mycobacterium smegmatis dnaA region and autonomous replication activity. J Bacteriol 177: 6527–6535.

Richards, R. I., Sutherland, G. R. (1992). Dynamic mutations: A new class of mutations causing human disease. Cell 70: 709–712.

Rosenkrands, I. P. B., Rasmussen, M., Carnio, S., Jacobsen ,M., Theisen, et al. (1998). Identification and characterization of a 29- kilodalton protein from Mycobacterium tuberculosis culture filtrate recognized by mouse memory effector cells. Infect Immun 66: 2728–2735.

Sampson, S. L., Warren, R. M., Richardson, M. G., van Der Spuy, D., van Helden, P. D. (1999). Disruption of coding regions by IS 6110 insertion in Mycobacterium tuberculosis. Tuberc Lung Dis 79: 349–359.

Schork, N. J., Fallin, D., Lanchbury, J. S. (2000). Single nucleotide polymorphism and the future of genetic epidemiology. Clin Genet 58: 250–264.

Sharples, G. J., Lloyd, R. G. (1990). A novel repeated DNA sequence located in the intergenic regions of bacterial chromosomes. Nucleic Acids Res 18: 6503-6508.

Smith, T. (1898). A comparative study of bovine tubercle bacilli and of human bacilli from sputum. J Exp Med 3: 451–511.

Sola, C., Rastogi, N., Gutierrez, M. C., Vincent, V., Brosch, R., et al. (2003). Is Mycobacterium africanum subtype of the Mycobacterium tuberculosis complex? J Clin Microbiol 41: 1345-1346.

Sreevatsan, S., Pan, X., Stockbauer, K. E., Connell, N. D., Kreiswirth, B. N., et al. (1997). Restricted structural gene polymorphism in the Mycobacterium tuberculosis complex indicates evolutionarily recent global dissemination. Proc Natl Acad Sci 94: 9869–9874.

Stucki, D., Malla, B., Hostettler, S., Huna, T., Feldmann, J., et al. (2012.) Two New Rapid SNP-Typing Methods for Classifying Mycobacterium tuberculosis Complex into the Main Phylogenetic Lineages. PLoS One. 7(7): e41253.

Supply, P., Magdalena, J., Himpens, S., Locli, C. (1997). Identification of novel intergenic repetitive units in a Mycobacterial two- Component system operon. Mol. Microbiol. 26: 991-1003.

Supply, P., Mazars, E., Lesjean, S., Vincent, V., Gicquel, B. B., et al. (2002). Variable human minisatellite-like regions in the Mycobacterium tuberculosis genome. J Mol Biol 36(3): 762-771.

Supply, P., Warren, R. M., Banuls, A-L, Lesjean, S., van der Spuy, G. D., et al. (2003). Linkage disequilibrium between minisatellite loci supports clonal evolution of Mycobacterium tuberculosis in a high tuberculosis incidence area. Mol. Microbiol. 47: 529–538 (2003).

Tekaia, F., Gordon, S. V., Garnier, T., Brosch, R., Barrell, B. G., et al. (1999). Analysis of the proteome of Mycobacterium tuberculosis in silico. Tuber Lung Dis 79: 329–342.

Toure, I. M. (1982). [The status of Mycobacterium africanum in West Africa]. Bull Int Union Tuberc 57: 241–249.

Truman, R. W., Singh, P., Sharma, R., Busso, P., Rougemont, J., et al. (2011). Probable zoonotic leprosy in the southern United States. N Engl J Med 364: 1626–1633. (doi:10.1056/NEJMoa1010536).

Tsenova, L., Ellison, E., Harbacheuski, R., Moreira, A. L., Kurepina, N., et al. (2005). Virulence of Selected Mycobacterium tuberculosis Clinical Isolates in the Rabbit Model of Meningitis Is Dependent on Phenolic Glycolipid Produced by the Bacilli. J Infect Dis 192: 98-106.

Udwadia, Z. (2009). "Emergence of New Forms of Totally Drug-Resistant Tuberculosis Bacilli", Chest, April 6 2009 http://chestjournal.chestpubs.org

van Embden, J. D. A., van Gorkom, T., Kremer, K., Jansen, T., van der Zeijst, B. A. M., et al. (2000). Genetic variation and evolutionary origin of the direct repeat locus of Mycobacterium tuberculosis complex bacteria. J. Bacteriol 182: 2393–2401.

Velayati, A. A., Masjedi, M. R., Farnia, P., Tabarsi, P., Ghanavi, J., et al. (2009). Emergence of new forms of totally drug-resistant tuberculosis bacilli: super extensively drug-resistant tuberculosis of totally drug-resistant strain in Iran. Chest 136: 420-425.

Vishnoi, A., Roy, R., Bhattacharya, A. (2007). Comparative analysis of bacterial genomes: identification of divergent regions in mycobacterial genomes using an anchor based approach. Nucl Aci Res 35(11): 3654-3667.

Vishnoi, A., Srivastava A., Roy, R., Bhattacharya, A. (2008). MGDD: Mycobacterium tuberculosis genome divergence database. BMC Genom 9:1–4.

Wang, Q., Yue, J., Zhang, L., Xu ,Y., Chen, J., et al. (2007). A newly identified 191A/C mutation in the Rv2629 gene that was significantly associated with rifampin resistance in Mycobacterium tuberculosis. J Proteome Res 6: 4564-4571.

Warren, D., Johnson, J. R., Johnson, C. W., Franklin, C., Lowe, F. C. (2002). Genitourinary Tuberculosis Campbell's Urology. 8th ed. Saunders. WHO report.Treatment of tuberculosis: Guidelines for National Programmes, 3rd ed. WHO, Geneva, 2003 ttp://www.who.int/docstore/gtb/publications.

Warren, R. M., Streicher, E. M., Sampson, L., van der Spuy, D., Richardson, M., et al. (2002). Microevolution of the direct repeat region of Mycobacterium tuberculosis: implications for interpretation of spoligotyping data. J Clin Microbiol 40: 4457–4465.

Warren, R. M., G. D. van der Spuy, M, Richardson, N., Beyers, M. W., Borgdorff, M. A., et al. (2002). Calculation of the stability of the IS6110 banding pattern in patients with persistent Mycobacterium tuberculosis disease. J Clin Microbiol 40: 1705–1708.

Weniger, T., Krawczyk, J., Supply, P., Niemann, S., Harmsen, D. (2010). MIRU-VNTRplus: a web tool for polyphasic genotyping of Mycobacterium tuberculosis complex bacteria. Nucleic Acids Res 38: W326-331.

World Health Organization (2008). Global tuberculosis control: surveillance, planning, financing. Geneva: (WHO/HTM/TB/2008.393).

World Health Organization (2006). Extensively drug-resistant tuberculosis (XDR.TB): recommendations for prevention and control. Weekly Epidemiol Record 81: 430-432.

World Health Organization (2010). WHO Guidelines for the programmatic management of drug-resistant tuberculosis. Fact Sheet No.104.

World Health Organization (2012). 'Totally Drug Resistant' tuberculosis: a WHO consultation on the diagnostic definition and treatment options", WHO, Geneva, 2012 www.who.int/tb/challenges/xdr.

Yeboah-Manu, D., Asante-Poku, A., Bodmer, T., Stucki, D., Koram, K., et al. (2011). Genotypic Diversity and Drug Susceptibility Patterns among M. tuberculosis Complex Isolates from South-Western Ghana. PLoS ONE 6(7): e21906. doi:10.1371/journal.pone.0021906.

Yoon, S., Xuan, Z., Makarov, V., Ye, K., Sebat, J. (2009). Sensitive and accurate detection of copy number variants using read depth of coverage. Genome Res 19(9): 1586–1592.

Zhang, M., Gong, J., Yang, Z., Samten, B., Cave, M. D., et al. (1999). Enhanced capacity of a widespread strain of Mycobacterium tuberculosis to grow in human macrophages. J Infect Dis 179, 1213-1217.

Negative Influence on Human Organism both *M. tuberculosis* and Anti-tuberculous Therapy: How to Find Balance?

Ekaterina Kulchavenya
Urogenital Department, Novosibirsk TB Research Institute
Novosibirsk Medical University, Russia

1   Introduction

Tuberculosis (TB) and HIV/AIDS have reached such proportions worldwide that the development of civil societies is seriously endangered. According to the World Health Organization (WHO) report 2008, the worldwide estimated incidence of new cases of TB increased in 2006 to 9.2 million (139 per 100 000 on average). Large proportions of cases occur in Asia and Africa; 55% and 31%, respectively (WHO reports, 2008). There were an estimated 8.8 million incident cases of TB globally in 2010, 1.1 million deaths (range, 0.9 million–1.2 million) among HIV-negative cases of TB and an additional 0.35 million deaths (range, 0.32 million–0.39 million) among people who were HIV-positive (WHO reports, 2010 -2011; Raviglione, M., 2003).

One-third of the world's population is currently infected with Mycobacterium tuberculosis (Mtb).TB kills more youths and adults than any other infectious disease. Every four seconds someone falls ill with TB and every 10 seconds someone dies from TB. Left untreated, a person with active TB can infect between 10 and 15 people every year. TB accounts for 9% of deaths among women between 15 and 44 years of ages compared with wars, which accounts for 4%, HIV for 3% and heart diseases for 3% of deaths. Of all causes of death TB holds the eighth place, of all infectious diseases the fourth place and of infectious diseases in adults the first place (WHO reports, 2008).

Extrapulmonary TB (EPTB) is not well-known, so it is often overlooked, but it is dangerous too. WHO recognized TB as a global problem, but meant TB as a whole, mostly pulmonary TB (PTB). Urogenital TB (UGTB) is not involved in attention of WHO, although UGTB is the second most common form of TB in countries with a severe epidemic situation and the third most common form in regions with low incidence of TB. 70% of men who died from tuberculosis of all localizations had prostate tuberculosis which had mostly been overlooked during their life time. In actual figures, this means about 12,000 men yearly in Russia. Prostate TB has an importance due to: 1). It is a sexually transmitted disease; 2). It leads to infertility; 3). It results, like any prostatitis, in chronic pelvic pain, that significantly reduces a quality of life; 4). It decreased a sexual function, that reduces a quality of life again. Bacillum Calmette Guerin (BCG) vaccine is used for the therapy of bladder cancer and may play a role in the incidence of urogenital tuberculosis as well as a kidney transplantation (Kul'chavenia, E.V. & and Muzyko, L.V., 2007).

Mycobacterium tuberculosis has been found in the bones of ancient bison, which lived 17000 years ago, and seems to have existed on Earth as long as the history of man. For ages mankind has paid fatal tribute to tuberculosis, which now accounts for about 5000 human deaths daily. Many well-known people were victims of TB throughout history. TB killed: Pharaoh Tutankhamun, Napoleon II of France, Cardinal Richelieu, Baruch Spinoza, Jean-Jacques Rousseau, Robert Burns, Amedeo Modigliani, Vivien Leigh and many, many others.

TB is a disease caused by **Mycobacterium tuberculosis,** first revealed by Robert Koch in 1882. Before this time TB was considered as a kind of cold and as a congenital disease. There are no reports about clinical features of TB in persons who lived before 18th century, like Baruch de Spinoza or Cardinal Richelieu. However, we can learn from the history of Anton Chekhov, a famous Russian writer who was also a doctor. He reports having pulmonary TB with hemoptysis, bone TB with skeletal deformation, intestinal TB with melena and urogenital TB with gross-haematuria. Common symptoms of TB have been: coughing, weight loss, loss of appetite, night sweats, pain, fever, dysuria, weakness, anemia and bleeding.

2   Innate Human Resistance to Tuberculosis

Tuberculosis, again, is a leading cause worldwide of human mortality attributable to a single infectious agent (WHO report, 2012); nevertheless, the infection of human organism with Mycobacterium tuberculosis doesn't lead to disease obligatory, by all means. Recent studies have revealed numerous polymorphisms implicated in host susceptibility to TB. Human organism may have an innate resistance to Mtb. Demonstrative lesson of this fact was "Lubeck disaster". Between 10 December 1929 and 30 April 1930, 251 infants born in the old Hanseatic town of Lubeck received three doses of BCG vaccine by the mouth during the first ten days of life. Of these 251, 72 died of TB, most of them in two to five months and all but one before the end of the first year. In addition, 135 suffered from clinical TB but eventually recovered; and 44 became tuberculin-positive but remained well. The vaccine used was later found to have been contaminated with a human tuberculosis strain being studied in same lab (Wilson, 1931). All children were equally infected by Mtb – and some of them died, some of them – got sick with clinical TB, and 17.5% remained healthy, because they had good innate resistance to TB.

A hallmark of Mtb infection is the ability of most (90-95%) healthy adults to control infection through acquired immunity, in which antigen specific T cells and macrophages arrest growth of Mtb bacilli and maintain control over persistent bacilli. In addition to CD4+ T cells, other T cell subsets such as, gammadelta, CD8+ and CD1-restricted T cells have roles in the immune response to Mtb. A diverse T cell response allows the host to recognize a wider range of mycobacterial antigens presented by different families of antigen-presenting molecules, and thus greater ability to detect the pathogen (Boom et al., 2003).

3   Mtb Induced Response on TB

Mtb induces vigorous immune responses, yet evades host immunity, persisting within phagosomes of the infected macrophages. Toll-like receptors (TLRs) play an essential role in the recognition of Mtb components by macrophages and dendritic cells, resulting in not only activation of innate immunity but also development of antigen-specific adaptive immunity (Fratazzi et al., 1999). Induction of early death of the infected cells may be one of the strategies of host defense against Mtb because macrophages go into apoptosis upon infection with Mtb, resulting in suppression of the intracellular replication (Danelishvili et al., 2003). Inerferon-gamma (IFN-gamma) also plays an important role in protection. The cytokine that is produced from natural killer (NK) cells and dendritic cells at the early period of infection strongly induces not only macrophage activation but also development of antigen-specific IFN-gamma-producing CD4+T cells. Since antigen-specific CD8+ T cells and CD1-restricted T cells are also reported to contribute to the protective immunity, cooperation of these T cells is essential for the host resistance (Kawamura, 2006). This phenomenon lied in the basis of the therapy for bladder cancer with BCG vaccine. Zbar B. et al. (1970) discovered, that intradermal inoculation of mixtures containing living tumor cells and living Mycobacterium bovis (strain BCG) into unimmunized syngeneic guinea pigs resulted in an inflammatory reaction to the BCG, and there was no progressive tumor growth. In 1976 first patients with recurrent superficial bladder tumors have been treated by vesical and intradermal administration of Bacillus Calmette-Guerin (BCG). The pattern of recurrence in 9 patients has been altered favorably (Morales et al., 1976). These preliminary results lied in the base of concept on BCG therapy for bladder cancer. Intravesical BCG significantly reduces the risk of progression after transurethral resection in patients with superficial bladder cancer who receive maintenance treatment. Thus, it is the agent of choice for patients with intermediate and high risk papillary tumors and those with carcinoma in situ (Bohle & Bock, 2004; Sylvester *et al.*, 2002). Nevertheless alongside with positive results many complications of BCG therapy, including lethal, were noted (Gupta *et al.*, 1998; Foster, 1997).

3.1   History Case

Below the case of severe complications of BCG therapy, treated in our Clinic, is shown.

Patient B.A.I., 50 years. In 2003 superficial urothelial carcinoma of a bladder was diagnosed, transurethral resection was performed without any adjuvant therapy. Control cystoscopy in 2004 presented relapse of the tumor in 4 sites. Transurethral resection was repeated and pathomorphologically urothelial carcinoma without invasion of lamina propria was found. After this operation the patient left the city and didn't address to a doctor during 6 years. In March 2010 he was admitted in urological clinic because of gross-haematuria. Cystoscopy presented multitude (more than 10) tumors of 5 – 20 mm in diameter. Transurethral resection was repeated again; pathomorphologically – low grade urothelial carcinoma T1 was found. In one month BCG-therapy in dose 100 mg weekly was started. After 3rd instillation dysuria, fever appeared. Levofloxacin 500 mg was prescribed, and in one week temperature became normal, but dysuria was the same, bladder capacity decreased till 50 ml intervals between urination were about 30 minutes. In august, 2010 control cystoscopy revealed a solitary ulcer, tubercles. This picture was estimated as bladder TB and anti-TB therapy was recommended. But the patient got sick in myocardial infarction, underwent cardio-surgery and only 07.09.2010 he was admitted in urogenital clinic of TB Institute.

The patient complained of frequent painful urination both at day and at night. Complex examination revealed pyuria, haematuria, soft anemia. Functions of kidneys and a liver were normal, PSA - 0,3 ng/ml. X-ray examination showed a stone 15 x 10 mm in the right kidney with hydronephrosis. Left kidney was normal. Retrograde cystogramm showed left vesico-uretral reflux, bladder capacity was 50 ml. Mycobacteriuria was not found by any method (microscopy, PCR, culture). Atypical cells in urine were not found too.

Diagnosis was: bladder cancer T1N0M0G1, urolithiasis, the stone in the right kidney. Hydronephrosis of right kidney. Bladder tuberculosis grade 4. Vesico-uretral reflux on right. MBT-.

The patients took rifampicin, isoniazid, pyrazinamid and cicloserin for 4 months that resulted in disappearance of the pain but frequency was the same, bladder volume was 50 ml. He was operated on 24.01.2011. Simultaneously pyelolithototomy, cystprostatectomy, appendectomy and ileocystoplastic by Studer were performed. Figures 1-4 demonstrate operation material and hystology.

Pathohistology: bladder urothelium with focal thinning down to 1-2 epithelial cells. Lamina propria is obviously edematous, hyperemic, contains petechia. Diffuse lymphocytic and neutrophilic infiltrates in mucosa, some lymphoid follicles occur. Papillary lesion is identical of other mucosa by structure. Bladder wall is significantly desorganized by sclerotic expansion, smooth muscle fascicles are thin and fragmented. Prostate: nonspecific chronic inflammatory infiltrate with significant focal neutrofilic component, especially intra- and periductular. Stromal fibrosis in prostate, atrophic and cystic ductal changes. Appendix contain few epithelioid- and giant (Langhans') cell granulomas, including one within follicular germinal center. Thus, BCG therapy provoked local TB as well as generalized TB. Nevertheless histological signs of neither TB nor cancer were not found.

On control examination in 2 months the capacity of an artificial bladder was 400 ml, urination free, but sometimes there was night incontinence.

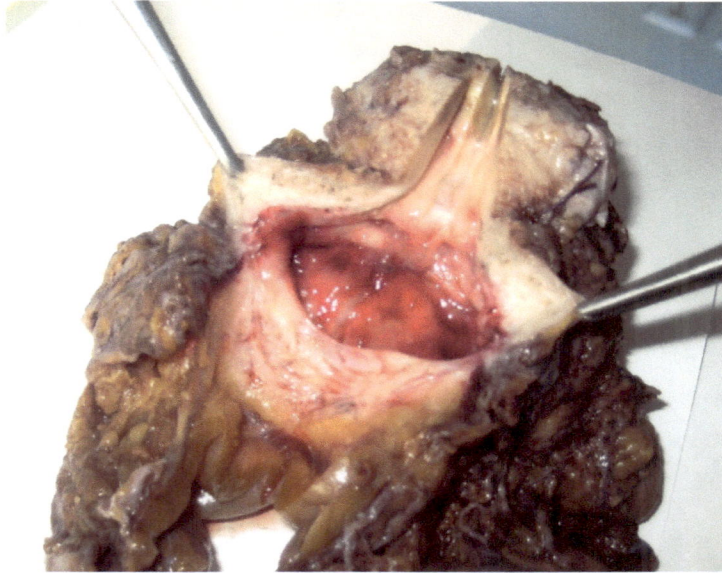

Figure 1: Removed bladder and prostate of B.A.I. on sagittal section. The diameter 4.5 cm, thick walls. Mucous membrane is reddish with hemorrhages. Prostate is grey, dense, at a glance without pathology

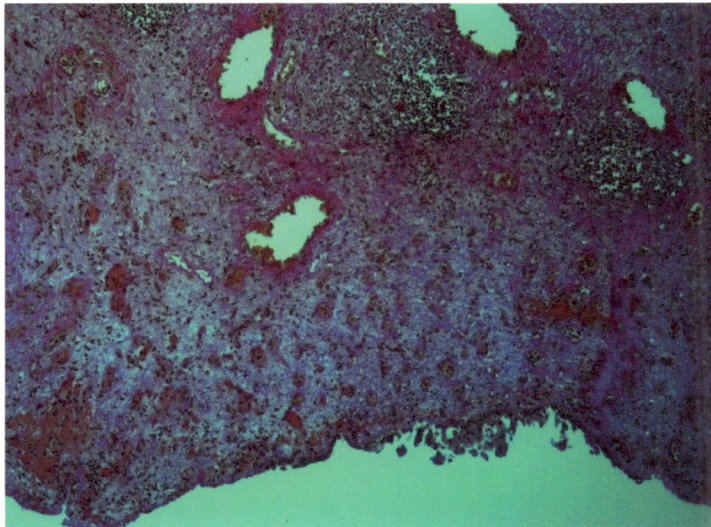

Figure 2: Chronic erosive cystitis. Wide erosion of bladder epithelium (bottom). Lamina propria shows neoangiogenesis (granulation tissue), edema and early collagenic fibrosis. Focal mononuclear inflammatory infiltration, formation of lymphoid follicles, and more mature fibrosis (top). van Gieson, x120.

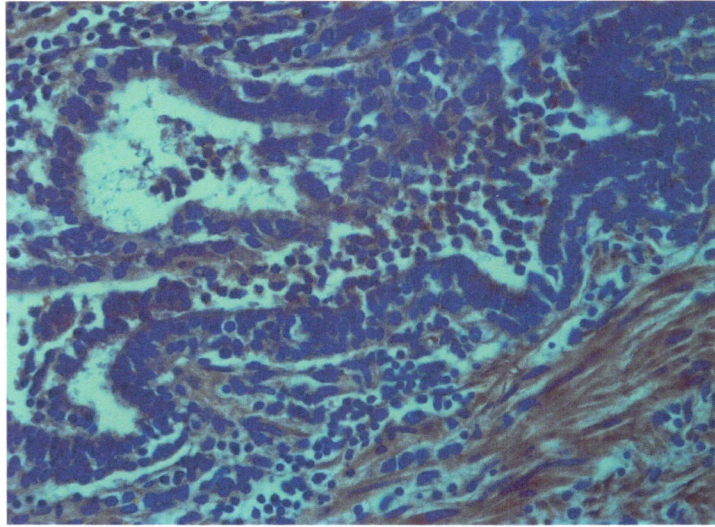

Figure 3: Prostate. Polymorphocellular interstitial infiltration, granulocytes fill dilated ductular lumens. Hematoxylin and eosin. x600.

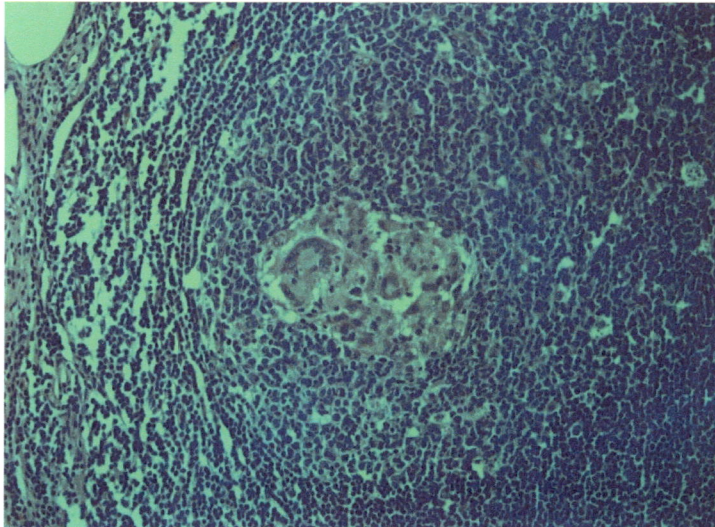

Figure 4: Appendix. Granuloma is located within germinal center of lymphoid follicle and consist of epithelioid and giant multinucleated Langhans cells. Hematoxylin and eosin. x300.

4   Genetic Control of Acquired Response on Tuberculosis

Each stage of the host response to Mtb is under genetic control, including the initial encounter with Mtb by macrophages, epithelial cells and dendritic cells in the lung, induction of the inductive T cell response, and killing by activated macrophages within granulomas. Although environmental factors are important determinants of progression to disease, there is a genetic component underlying susceptibility to TB, the basis of which may vary in different populations (Yim & Selvaraj, 2010). Activation of the P2X7 receptor, an ATP-gated Ca2+ channel, leads to the activation of phospholipase D, and the induction of apoptosis with death of the infecting Mtb. Macrophages from subjects who are heterozygote, homozygote or compound heterozygote for these polymorphisms fail to undergo apoptosis and show partial or complete inhibition of mycobacterial killing. One of these non-functioning polymorphisms was significantly associated with increased susceptibility to TB disease, particularly extrapulmonary disease (Britton *et al.*, 2007).

Thuong *et al.* (2008) hypothesized that macrophages from individuals with different clinical manifestations of TB would have distinct gene expression profiles and that polymorphisms in these genes may also be associated with susceptibility to TB. Gene expression profiles in Mtb-stimulated and unstimulated macrophages was compared and identified 1,608 and 199 genes that were differentially expressed by >2- and >5-fold, respectively. These results suggest that genome-wide studies can provide an unbiased method to identify critical macrophage response genes that are associated with different clinical outcomes and that variation in innate immune response genes regulate susceptibility to TB.

5   Cellular and Proteins Immune Response on TB

Phagocytosed Mtb either multiply inside the endocytic compartment of mononuclear phagocytes or they are destroyed by the host cell, so TB is controlled by the cellular immune response. Protection against Mtb depends on alpha/beta T-cells expressing the CD4 or CD8 phenotype. T-cell-mediated immunity amplifies macrophage capacities to kill and digest the bacilli (Peng *et al.*, 2011). Specific alpha/beta T-cells produce several cytokines that attract and activate macrophages and additional lymphocytes, such as: interferon-gamma (IFN-gamma) which has the capacity to activate several antimicrobial properties of macrophages; tumour necrosis factor-alpha (TNF-alpha) a key cytokine involved in granuloma formation; interleukins 2, 6 and 8 (IL-2; IL-6 and IL-8); and interleukin 12 (IL-12), a candidate cytokine for the induction of Th1 cells (Munk & Emoto, 1995). Furthermore, CD4+ and CD8+ T-cells display cytotoxic activity, which permits them to control mycobacterial growth through destruction of the infected cells. Escaping bacteria are subsequently ingested and destroyed by surrounding macrophages activated by T-cells. There is evidence to associate gamma/delta T-cells with antimycobacterial immunity, such as their preferential accumulation in inflammatory lesions, in necrotic areas of tuberculous lymphadenitis, and potent in vitro stimulation by Mtb components. In addition, Mtb activated gamma/delta T-cells are cytolytic and secrete several cytokines. Hence, clinical tuberculosis is associated with T-cell reactivity which controls the local concentrations of tubercle bacilli (Pinheiro *et al.*, 2012).

In TB-induced response participate several types of proteins: macrophage receptors, such as the mannose receptor (MR, CD206), dendritic cell-specific ICAM-3-grabbing nonintegrin (DC-SIGN, CD209), Dectin-1, Toll-like receptors (TLRs), complement receptor 3 (CR3, CD11b/CD18), nucleotide oligomerization domain 1 (NOD1) and NOD2, CD14, P2X7, and the vitamin D nuclear receptor; soluble C-type lectins, such as surfactant proteins and mannose-binding lectin; phagocyte cytokines, such as tumor necrosis factor (TNF), interleukin-1β (IL-1β), IL-6, IL-10, IL-12, and IL-18; chemokines, such as IL-8, monocyte chemoattractant protein, RANTES, and CXCL10; and other important innate immune molecules, such as inducible nitric oxide synthase and solute carrier protein 11A1 (Rojasm *et al.*, 1999). Polymorphisms in these genes have been variably associated with susceptibility to TB among different populations (Azad *et al.*, 2012; Wu *et al.*, 2012). In most of the clinical cases of TB, the production of IL-

12, IL-18 and IFN-gamma is increased, however, the group of relatively lower cytokine production did not respond well to the treatment. In addition, the plasma level of one of the chemokines, IP-10, was shown to be an indicator for the severity of the disease (Mitsuyama *et al.*, 2003; Volpe *et al.*, 2006).

6   Pathogenesis of TB Infection

Most common route of transmissions of Mtb is respiratory one, when infectious can be spread by coughing, sneezing, laughing, singing, or just talking. Also are possible alimentary transmission – usually through milk from ill cows; direct and indirect physical contact, including sexual; iatrogenic transmission with BCG instillation for bladder cancer therapy; transplacental transmission (unusual); blood transmission through a mosquito bite (extremely rarely) (Kulchavenya, 2009). Independent of the route of infection Mtb are spread by bloodstream and lymphatic system throughout the body (so-called primary dissemination). Of course, direct contact more often leads to the skin TB, alimentary route – to intestinal TB, prostate TB may be a cause of a genital TB in sexual partner etc. But after respiratory contamination lungs may by intact, and kidney or lymphonodal TB develops, as well as TB meningitis after alimentary contamination is possible (McDonough & Kress, 1995; Kulchavenya *et al.*, 2007).

Since the main route of entry of the causative agent is the respiratory route, alveolar macrophages are the important cell types, which combat the pathogen. There are various aspects of macrophage-mycobacterium interactions. The role of macrophage in host response such as binding of Mtb to macrophages via surface receptors, phagosome-lysosome fusion, mycobacterial growth inhibition/killing through free radical based mechanisms such as reactive oxygen and nitrogen intermediates; cytokine-mediated mechanisms; recruitment of accessory immune cells for local inflammatory response and presentation of antigens to T cells for development of acquired immunity is very important (Kee *at al.*, 2012). The macrophage apoptosis in containing the growth of the bacilli as well as other components of innate immune response such as natural resistance associated macrophage protein, neutrophils, and natural killer cells play the role too (Esin *et al.*, 2008). The specific acquired immune response through CD4 T cells, mainly responsible for protective Th1 cytokines and through CD8 cells bringing about cytotoxicity, also has been described. Humoral immune response is seen though not implicated in protection (Portevin & Young, 2013). Mtbs are endowed with mechanisms through which they can evade the onslaught of host defense response: diminishing the ability of antigen presenting cells to present antigens to CD4(+) T cells; production of suppressive cytokines; escape from fused phagosomes and inducing T cell apoptosis (Raja, 2004).

7   The Role of Macrophages and Apoptosis

Alveolar macrophages (AMs) are exposed to frequent challenges from inhaled particulates and microbes and function as a first line of defense with a highly regulated immune response because of their unique biology as prototypic alternatively activated macrophages. Lung collectins, particularly surfactant protein A (SP-A), contribute to this activation state by fine-tuning the macrophage inflammatory response. Pienaar & Lerm (2013) created the mathematical model of the initial interaction between Mtb and macrophages, which considers the interplay between bacterial killing and the pathogen's interference with macrophage function. Their results revealed an oscillating balance between host and pathogen, but the balance was transient and varies in length, indicating that stochasticity in the bacterial population or host response could contribute to the diverse incubation periods observed in exposed individuals.

Nguyen *et al.* (2012) have found, that during short-term (10 min-2 h) exposure, SP-A's regulation of human macrophage responses occurs through decreased activity of kinases required for proinflammatory cytokine production. Exposure of human macrophages to SP-A for 6-24 h upregulates expression of IL-1 receptor-associated kinase M (IRAK-M), a negative regulator of TLR-mediated NF-κB activation. In contrast to TNF-α and IL-6, the surfactant components upregulate LPS-mediated immunoregulatory IL-10 production, an effect reversed by IRAK-M knockdown.

Microarray analysis of infected human alveolar macrophages found serine protease inhibitor 9 (PI-9) to be the most prominently expressed of a cluster of apoptosis-associated genes induced by virulent Mtb. Inhibition of PI-9 by small inhibitory RNA decreased Mtb-induced expression of the antiapoptotic molecule Bcl-2 and resulted in a corresponding increase in production of caspase 3, a terminal effector molecule of apoptosis. Thus PI-9 induction within human mononuclear phagocytes by virulent Mtb serves to protect these primary targets of infection from elimination by apoptosis and thereby promotes intracellular survival of the organism (Toossi *et al.*, 2012).

Mtb interacts with macrophages and epithelial cells in the alveolar space of the lung, where it is able to invade and replicate in both cell types (Schaale *et al.*, 2013). Both virulent and attenuated Mtb induce apoptosis in macrophages; however, the attenuated strain – H37Ra resulted in significantly more apoptosis than the virulent strain H37Rv after 5 days of infection. In contrast, cytotoxicity of alveolar cells was the result of necrosis, but not apoptosis (Danelishvili, 2003). Although infection with Mtb strains resulted in apoptosis of 14% of the cells on the monolayer, cell death associated with necrosis was observed in 59% of alveolar epithelial cells after 5 days of infection (Danelishvili, 2003). Anti-apoptotic Bcl-2, Mcl-1, Bfl-1 and Bcl-xL in the cells were significantly upregulated following infection with K-strain (belongs to the Beijing family, is the most frequently isolated clinical strain of Mtb in Korea) compared with H37Rv, whereas Bax was slightly upregulated in response to infection with both H37Rv and K-strain. The highly virulent K-strain keeps cellular apoptosis as a host defense mechanism to a minimum and induces necrosis in macrophages (Sohn *et al.*, 2009).

M. avium as well as Mtb replicate in human macrophages and induce apoptosis. Incubation of freshly added uninfected autologous macrophages with apoptotic M. avium-infected macrophages results in 90% inhibition of bacterial growth. Apoptosis also prevents the release of intracellular components and the spread of mycobacterial infection by sequestering the pathogens within apoptotic bodies (Fratazzi *et al.*, 1999). Authors believe, that consistent with the model that host cell apoptosis is a defense mechanism against mycobacteria is the finding that the virulent Mtb strain H37Rv induces substantially less macrophage apoptosis than the attenuated strain H37Ra.

8   The Role of the Lung Epithelium during TB

Lung epithelial cells (A549) were used as a model in which to examine cytotoxicity during infection with either virulent or avirulent mycobacteria in order to further establish the role of the lung epithelium during TB. Infection of A549 cells with Mtb strains Erdman and CDC1551 demonstrated significant cell monolayer clearing, whereas infection with either Mycobacterium bovis BCG or Mycobacterium smegmatis LR222 did not. Clearing of Mtb-infected A549 cells correlated to necrosis, not apoptosis. Treatment of MBT-infected A549 cells with streptomycin demonstrated a significant reduction in the necrosis of A549 cell monolayers (Dobos *et al.*, 2000).

Coculture of infected sputum from TB patients with neutralizing antibodies to TGF-beta or TNF-alpha decreased spontaneous (P < or = 0.05) and Mtb-induced (P < or = 0.02) T-cell apoptosis by 50-90%, but effects were not additive. During TB, predisposition of CD4 T-cells to apoptosis may involve both low expression of Bcl-2, and excessive expression of TGF-beta TNF-alpha and FasL (Hirsch *et al.*, 2005).

9   Other Factors of Acquired Response on TB

Granulysin is an important defensive molecule expressed by human T cells and NK cells and has a cytolytic activity against microbes including Mtb and tumors. Expression of 15kD (15K) granulysin protein and mRNA in CD8 positive T cells in the patients infected with drug sensitive TB or MDR-TB M. tuberculosis were lower than that in the healthy volunteers, suggesting that granulysin treatment might improve the TB disease in human (Kita *et al.* 2011).

Chemokines (CK) are potent leukocyte activators and chemoattractants and participate in granuloma formation, functions critical for the immune response to Mtb. It was hypothesized by Saukkonen (2002) that infection of AM with different strains of Mtb elicits distinct profiles of CK, which could be altered by human immunodeficiency virus (HIV) infection. Macrophage inflammatory protein-1 alpha (MIP-1 alpha), and MIP-1 beta were the major beta-CK produced in response to Mtb infection. Virulent Mtb (H37Rv) induced significantly less MIP-1 alpha than did the avirulent strain (H37Ra), while MIP-1 beta production was comparable for both strains. MIP-1 alpha and MIP-1 beta were induced by the membrane, but not cytosolic, fraction of Mtb. Mtb-induced CK secretion was partly dependent on tumor necrosis factor alpha (TNF-alpha). MIP-1 beta suppressed intracellular growth of Mtb two- to threefold. Thus, beta-CK contribute to the innate immune response to Mtb infection (Saukkonen, 2002).

The pathophysiology of Mtb infection is linked to the ability of the organism to grow within macrophages. Lung myeloid dendritic cells are a newly recognized reservoir of Mtb during infection. Iron acquisition is critical for Mtb growth. Access of Mtb to Fe may influence its growth in macrophages and dendritic cells (Olakanmi *et al.*, 2013). Infection with Mtb is accompanied by an intense local inflammatory response which may be critical to the pathogenesis of TB. Activation of components of the innate immune response, such as recruitment of polymorphonuclear (PMN) and mononuclear phagocytes and induction of pro-inflammatory cytokines, such as tumor necrosis factor alpha (TNF-alpha), by Mtb occurs early after Mtb infection, however, may persist as the organism establishes itself within granulomas. Mtb and its protein and non-protein components are potent in induction of cytokines and chemokines from PMN and monocytes (Toossi, 2000).

Mtb survive inside macrophages by manipulating microbicidal functions such as phago-lysosome fusion, production of reactive oxygen species and nitric oxide, and by rendering macrophages non-responsive to IFN-gamma (Alemán *et al.*, 2007). Mtb-infected lung tissue does however not only contain macrophages, but also significant numbers of infiltrating polymorphonuclear neutrophils (PMN). These are able to phagocytose and kill ingested Mtb, but are short-lived cells that constantly need to be removed from tissues to avoid tissue damage (Hedlund *et al.*, 2010). Engulfment of Mtb-induced apoptotic PMN by macrophages initiates secretion of TNF-alpha from the macrophages, reflecting a pro-inflammatory response. Moreover, Mtb-induced apoptotic PMN up-regulate heat shock proteins 60 and 72 (Hsp60,

Hsp72) intracellularly and also release Hsp72 extracellularly. Both recombinant Hsp72 and released Hsp72 enhanced the pro-inflammatory response to both Mtb-induced apoptotic PMN and Mtb. This stimulatory effect of the supernatant was abrogated by depleting the Hsp72 with immunoprecipitation (Persson *et al.*, 2008).

In addition to direct bactericidal activities, such as phagocytosis and generation of reactive oxygen species (ROS), neutrophils can regulate the inflammatory response by undergoing apoptosis. Infection of human neutrophils with Mtb induces rapid cell death displaying the characteristic features of apoptosis such as morphologic changes, phosphatidylserine exposure, and DNA fragmentation. Both a virulent (H37Rv) and an attenuated (H37Ra) strain of Mtb were equally effective in inducing apoptosis. Pretreatment of neutrophils with antioxidants or an inhibitor of NADPH oxidase markedly blocked Mtb-induced apoptosis but did not affect spontaneos apoptosis (Perskvist *et al.*, 2002). The Mtb-induced apoptosis was associated with a speedy and transient increase in expression of Bax protein, a proapoptotic member of the Bcl-2 family, and a more prominent reduction in expression of the antiapoptotic protein Bcl-x(L). Phagocytosis of Mtb-induced apoptotic neutrophils markedly increases the production of proinflammatory cytokine TNF-alpha by human macrophages (Gagliardi *et al.*, 2005; Maianski *et al.*, 2003).

Nitric oxide (NO), synthesized from l-arginine by NO synthases, is a small, diffusible, highly reactive molecule with dichotomous regulatory roles under physiological and pathological conditions. NO can promote apoptosis (proapoptosis) in some cells, whereas it inhibits apoptosis (antiapoptosis) in other cells. This complexity is a consequence of the rate of NO production and the interaction with biological molecules such as iron, thiols, proteins, and reactive oxygen species. Long-lasting production of NO acts as a proapoptotic modulator. However, low or physiological concentrations of NO prevent cells from apoptosis induced by trophic factor withdrawal, Fas, TNFalpha, and lipopolysaccharide (Chung *et al.*, 2001).

The slow growth and chronic nature of Mtb infection result in prolonged exposure to antigens, and hence further T cell sensitization. To survive in macrophages, Mtb has evolved mechanisms to block immune responses (Rojas *et al.*, 1999). These include modulation of phagosomes, neutralization of macrophage effector molecules, stimulating the secretion of inhibitory cytokines, and interfering with processing of antigens for T cells. The relative importance of these blocking mechanisms likely depends on the stage of Mtb infection: primary infection, persistence, reactivation or active tuberculosis. The balance of the host-pathogen interaction in Mtb infection is determined by the interaction of T cells and infected macrophages. The outcome of this interaction results either in control of Mtb infection or active disease (Boom *et al.*, 2003).

10   Acquired Response on TB in Co-morbid Patients

Any co-morbidity makes worse the response on TB. The association of Mtb with monocytes was significantly lower in diabetics than non-diabetics (p = 0.02). Poorly-controlled type 2 diabetes mellitus was significantly associated with the lower interaction of Mtb with monocytes (Jeon & Murray, 2008; Gomez *et al.*, 2013).

Human macrophages represent the first line of defense for the containment of Mtb infection. After phagocytosis, macrophages express activation surface markers and produce proinflammatory cytokines and chemokines whose main role is to control pathogen spreading by recruiting peripheral lymphocytes and monocytes at the site of inflammation. However, in the case of a concomitant human immunodeficiency virus (HIV) infection, these signals strongly enhance the susceptibility to viral infection both at the viral entry and replication levels (Patel *et al.*, 2007). Under these conditions, viral expansion extends beyond tissue macrophages to T cells and vice-versa, according to the emerging viral phenotype. In absence of an efficient immune response, Mtb can replicate in macrophages in an uncontrolled fashion culminating in macrophage death by apoptosis. As a consequence, a more severe form of immunedepression, involving both innate and specific immune responses, could be responsible for both ematogenous mycobacterial dissemination and extrapulmonary form of TB in HIV-infected patients (Mariani *et al.*, 2001). During HIV/TB, systemic immune activation is dissociated from microbial translocation. Changes in circulating sCD14 and LPS are dependent on CD4 T-cell count (Toossi *et al.*, 2013). Expression of CycT1 in response to Mtb was assessed in mononuclear cells from pleural fluid (PFMC) and blood (PBMC) from HIV/TB patients with pleural TB, and in blood monocytes (MN) from singly infected HIV-1-seropositive subjects. Higher expression of CycT1 mRNA in PFMCs as compared to PBMCs from HIV/TB-coinfected subjects was found (Toossi *et al.*, 2012).

Concomitant intestinal helminth infection in TB patients had a negative impact (P < 0.05) on absolute frequencies of CD3(+), CD4(+), CD8(+), natural killer (NK) T and CD4(+) CD25(high) T cell subsets when compared to either TB patients or healthy controls. In addition to a depressed anti-Mtb immunity, TB + Helm patients also presented with more severe radiological pulmonary disease, with a significant difference (P = 0.013) in the number of involved lung zones at the end of TB treatment (Resende *et al.*, 2007).

11   Vaccines Against TB Infection

To improve an acquired response on TB a special vaccine were created (Anderson & Doherty, 2005). Aronson et al. (2004) estimated the efficacy of BCG vaccine, calculated for each 10-year interval using a Cox regression model with time-dependent variables based on tuberculosis events. The overall incidence of tuberculosis was 66 and 138 cases per 100 000 person-years in the BCG vaccine and placebo groups, respectively, for an estimate of vaccine efficacy of 52% (95% confidence interval, 27%-69%).

Infection of human monocytes with M. bovis BCG induced macrophage inflammatory protein (MIP)-1alpha and MIP-1beta secretion in a dose-dependent manner. The ability of M. bovis BCG to produce CC-chemokines might lead to protection in the acquired immune response of mycobacterial infection (Méndez-Samperio *et al.*, 2003). The BCG was initially administered as a live oral vaccine. This route of administration was stopped in 1930 following the Lübeck (Germany) disaster. The intradermal route of administration was later found to be safe for mass vaccination, through studies conducted in the 1930s (Boom *et al.*, 2003). Okada has developed a novel TB vaccine; a combination of the DNA vaccines expressing mycobacterial heat shock protein 65 (HSP65) and interleukin 12 (IL-12) delivered by the hemagglutinating virus of Japan (HVJ)-liposome or-envelope (HSP65+IL-12/HVJ). This vaccine provided remarkable protective efficacy in mouse and guinea pig models compared to the BCG vaccine, on the basis of an induction of the CD8 positive CTL activity against TB antigens and improvement of the histopathological tuberculosis lesions, respectively. The Elispot assay showed that HSP65+IL-12 DNA/HVJ vaccine induced a greater number of IFN-gamma producing T cells than BCG in the mouse model (Okada, 2008). This vaccine also provided therapeutic efficacy against multidrug resistant TB (MDR-TB) and extremely drug resistant TB (XDR-TB) in murine models (Okada, 2006; Okada & Kita, 2010; Okada *et al.*, 2011).

Also recombinant virus-vectored TB vaccine was developed. A recombinant replication-deficient adenoviral (Ad) vector was engineered to express Mtb Ag85A. Single administration of this Ad vaccine via the intranasal route provided potent immune protection from pulmonary Mtb challenge. Respiratory mucosal boosting immunization with Ad vaccine was effective in enhancing T-cell activation and immune protection following parenteral DNA or BCG prime immunization (Wang *et al.*, 2004; Xing & Lichty, 2006; Abalos *et al.*, 2011).

Guinea pigs immunized with extracellular proteins (EP) and then challenged with aerosolized Mtb exhibit protective immunity: they were consistently protected against clinical illness, including weight loss. Actively growing Mtb release immunoprotective molecules extracellularly, that a subunit vaccine against TB is feasible; extracellular molecules of Mtb are potential candidates for a subunit vaccine (Pal & Horwitz, 1992).

Blazevic *et al.* (2013) developed a murine aerosol challenge model to investigate responses capable of protecting against mucosal infection. Mice received vaccinations intranasally with CpG-adjuvanted antigen 85B (Ag85B/CpG) and/or Bacillus Calmette-Guerin (BCG). Protection against aerosol challenge with a recombinant GFP-expressing BCG was assessed. Mucosal prime/boost vaccinations with Ag85B/CpG and BCG were protective, but did not prevent lung infection (Blazevic *et al.* 2013). Indicating more efficacious mucosal vaccines are needed

Bacille Calmette-Guérin (BCG) is the only vaccine available today and has been used for more than 90 years with astonishing safety records. However, its efficacy remains controversial. No universal BCG vaccination policy exists, with some countries merely recommending its use and others that have implemented immunization programs (Luca & Mihaescu, 2013). Despite the fact that mechanisms underlying the lack of pulmonary protection provided by the BCG remain poorly understood, it remains the "Gold Standard" for vaccine-mediated protection against Mtb and will continue to be used for the foreseeable future. The only approved TB vaccine is the Bacille Calmette-Guerin (BCG), which provides protection against childhood miliary tuberculosis and has been administered intradermally in humans for almost a century (Horvath & Xing, 2013). There is no any evidence of sufficient novel vaccines against TB in human, and none special vaccine against TB+HIV has been developed.

12   Risk and Benefit of Antituberculous Therapy

Humankind's fight against TB dramatically changed after 1945, after creation first of anti-TB drug – streptomycin. For this discovery *Selman Abraham Waksman* was awarded with Nobel Prize in 1952.

Nearly all of the following drugs were discovered between 1945 and 1970 years: streptomycin, PAS, isoniazid, thiacetazone, pyrazinamide, kanamycin, amykacin, viomycin, capreomycin, ethionamide, cycloserine, clofazimine, rifampicin and ethambutol. Anti-TB dugs made most cases curable. Unfortunately, every medal has its reverse. Euphoria, caused by success of chemotherapy of TB, decreased soon – mostly due to development of drug resistance and poor tolerance of the therapy. Both these facts enforced each other. As Mtb may have natural resistance, it is necessary to combine a minimum of three different drugs. The more drugs take the patient – the more risk of development of side effects. Many side effects limit chemotherapy and provoke drug resistance (Didilescu & Craiova, 2011; Wada *et al.*, 1999).

After several decades without any notable progress, there are encouraging results in research and development of anti-TB drugs, the result of a large number of projects now in competition. Along with developing new drugs to treat tuberculosis (TMC207, SQ109, LL3858) are being reassessed others to optimize their effectiveness in order to shorten and simplify therapy (rifampin and rifapentine) and three other drugs, currently used for other indications, were forwarded towards TB (gatifloxacin and moxiflox-acin, linezolid). Moxifloxacin, a fluoroquinolone, improved the activity of the standard drug regimen when substituted for ethambutol (Wada, 2001).

High incidence of liver toxicity induced by pyrazinamide, rifampicin, isonoazid was revealed. The risk factors of drug-induced hepatitis so far reported included elderly, positive hepatitis C virus antibody, low serum albumin and so on (Grosset *et al.*, 2012). Liver injury was characterized as being mild and moderate and the type of injury associated was represented by pure cholestasis and hepatocanalicular le-sions. Probably, rifampicin is the drug responsible for this kind of evolution aggravating the hepatotoxici-ty induces by isoniazid and pyrazinamide (Mitchison & Davies, 2012). Liver injury was characterized as being mild and moderate and the type of injury associated was represented by pure cholestasis and hepa-tocanalicular lesions (Kolpakova *et al.*, 2001). Probably, rifampicin is the drug responsible for this kind of evolution aggravating the hepatotoxicity induces by isoniazid and pyrazinamide. Isoniazid and pyra-zinamide are both well-known hepatotoxic drugs. When isoniazid is used, the hepatic lesion appears be-fore than when pyrazinamide is used (de Souza *et al*, 1996).

Drug intolerance was noted in 40.1% of patients with renal TB. Pyrazinamide, streptomycin, and ethambutol were most toxic to these patients. There was a higher likelihood of drug intolerance in fe-males with bilateral nephrotuberculosis complicated by chronic renal failure (Kul'chavenia & Kuz-netsov,1998; Shutskaia *et al.*, 1991).

The profile of patients treated by DOTS scheme and presenting with adverse reactions showed that majority of the patients (53%) had gastrointestinal reactions, the commonest presenting complaint being nausea and vomiting. General aches and pains were complained by about 35% and giddiness was the pre-senting complaint in 27% irrespective of the use of streptomycin. Skin rash and itching was complained by about 17% of patients and 11% complained of arthralgia, while only 1% had hepatotoxicity during treatment. Majority of the adverse reactions (67%) were observed within the first four weeks of treatment (Pereira *et al.*, 2000; Dhingra *et al.*, 2004; Zierski & Bek, 1980).

Layer & Engelhardm (1986) described a case lupus erythematosus (SLE) and concomitant pulmo-nary tuberculosis in a 46-year-old female patient. In the course of the tuberculostatic therapy, there oc-curred six episodes of exacerbation of drug-induced SLE signs and symptoms including fever, myalgia, swelling of joints, butterfly rash and high titers of antinuclear antibodies. These exacerbations were in-duced by single-agent or combination therapy with ethambutol, pyrazinamide, streptomycin and/or prothionamide and resolved readily after discontinuation of the drug(s).

Isoniazid-induced lupus erythematosus affects either sex equally and the most common presenting feature is arthralgia or arthritis with anemia. Fever and pleuritis occur in approximately half of the cases, and pericarditis in approximately 30% of cases.

Siddiqui & Khan (2002) reported a case of isoniazid-induced lupus erythematosus presenting with cardiac tamponade. A 73-year-old man was treated with isoniazid for 8 months at a dose of 300 mg a day. The patient responded to the withdrawal of the isoniazid therapy and placement of a pericardial window. It was described drug-induced heart failure in advanced pulmonary tuberculosis (Daynes,1974), hyperu-ricaemia induced by ethambutol (Narang *et al.*, 1983) and pyrazinamide (Solangi *et al.*, 2004).

13   Sexual dysfunction in male patients with pulmonary tuberculosis

TB patients have to take many medicines for a long time; anti-TB therapy negatively influences not only on mycobacterium tuberculosis, but also on human organism. A comparative study of 105 newly diagnosed patients with PTB and 37 volunteers aged 18 to 39 years has been carried out to estimate their sexual function. Patients with pulmonary tuberculosis showed deterioration of all components of copulatory act, from sexual desire to orgasm, in spite of absence of any related diseases of urogenital system. The degree of disorders in the group of patients with cavernous PTB was significantly higher than in patients with infiltrative PTB and it was correlated with a severity of intoxication syndrome.

Adequate anti-TB therapy could improve sexual function of a man with pulmonary tuberculosis by arresting the inflammatory TB process and reducing intoxication. Nevertheless even after 6 months of the therapy there was still significant difference in subjective assessment of copulative functions in both TB groups compared to the healthy volunteers. After 3 months of combined chemotherapy ejaculatory disorders developed, mostly – delayed ejaculation. We explained it by toxicity effect of anti-TB drugs (Kulchavenya *et al.*, 2012).

Thus, tuberculosis worsened a male sexual function, and etiotropic anti-TB therapy improved it, but only in first three months, then dynamic slowed. Anti-TB drugs are aggressive not for Mycobacteria tuberculosis only, but for human organism too.

14   Conclusion

Thus there is an innate resistance of the human organism to Mtb – and it is a main reason why TB, potentially lethal disease, doesn't destroy all humankind. Mtb itself stimulates acquired response on TB that improves the resistance of the human organism. Special vaccine increases this resistance too – but actually BCG only is approved, others are experimental. Efficiency of BCG is not satisfied, complication of BCG is possible, nevertheless BCG is a "Gold standard" and now we have no alternative. Medical science may help to reinforce both innate and acquired response on TB, nevertheless, genetical predisposition plays important role. Inadequate chemotherapy for tuberculosis leads to development of drug resistance of Mbt and adverse effects, forming circulus vituosus. There was noted specific negative side effect – delayed ejaculation. To avoid adverse effects of anti-TB chemotherapy address drug delivery by lymphotropic introduction was recommended, laser therapy, optimal pathogenetic therapy (phytotherapy, antioxidant etc) (Kulchavenya, 2009; Kulchavenya & Krasnov, 2010).

Acknowledgement

I would like to thank my friend and assistant Denis Kholtobin.

References

Abalos, R.M., Burgos, J.A., Saunderson, P., & Sakatani, M. (2011). Development of therapeutic and prophylactic vaccine against Tuberculosis using monkey and transgenic mice models. Hum Vaccin. Jan-Feb;7 Suppl:108-14. Epub 2011 Jan 1.

Alemán, M., de la Barrera, S., Schierloh, P., Yokobori, N., Baldini, M., Musella, R., Abbate, E. & Sasiain, M. (2007). Spontaneous or Mycobacterium tuberculosis-induced apoptotic neutrophils exert opposite effects on the dendritic cell-mediated immune response. Eur J Immunol. Jun;37(6):1524-37.

Anderson, P. & Doherty, T.M. (2005). The success and failure of BCG–implications for a novel tuberculosis vaccine. Nat Rev Microbiol.;3(8):656-662.

Aronson, N.E., Santosham, M., Comstock, G.W., Howard, R.S., Moulton, L.H., Rhoades, E.R. &Harrison. L.H. (2004). Long-term efficacy of BCG vaccine in American Indians and Alaska Natives: A 60-year follow-up study. JAMA. May 5;291(17):2086-91.

Azad, A.K., Sadee, W., & Schlesinger, L.S. (2012). Innate immune gene polymorphisms in tuberculosis. Infect Immun. Oct;80(10):3343-59. doi: 10.1128/IAI.00443-12. Epub 2012 Jul 23.

Blazevic, A., Eickhoff, C.S., Stanley, J., Buller, M.R., Schriewer, J., Kettelson, E.M. & Hoft, D.F. (2013). Investigations of TB vaccine-induced mucosal protection in mice. Microbes Infect. Oct 8. pii: S1286-4579(13)00192-5. doi: 10.1016/j.micinf.2013.09.006. [Epub ahead of print]

Bohle, A. & Bock, P.R. (2004). Intravesical bacillus Calmette-Guerin versus mitomycin C in superficial bladder cancer: formal meta-analysis of comparative studies on tumor progression. Urology Apr; 3(4) : 682-7. http://www.ncbi.nlm.nih.gov/pubmed/15072879

Boom, W.H., Canaday, D.H., Fulton, S.A., Gehring, A.J., Rojas, R.E., & Torres, M. (2003). Human immunity to M. tuberculosis: T cell subsets and antigen processing. Tuberculosis (Edinb). 83(1-3):98-106.

Britton, W.J., Fernando, S.L., Saunders, B.M., Sluyter, R., & Wiley, J.S. (2007). The genetic control of susceptibility to Mycobacterium tuberculosis. Novartis Found Symp. 281:79-89; discussion 89-92, 208-9.

Chung, H.T., Pae, H.O., Choi, B.M., Billiar, T.R, & Kim, Y.M. (2001). Nitric oxide as a bioregulator of apoptosis. Biochem Biophys Res Commun. Apr 20;282(5):1075-9.

Danelishvili, L., McGarvey, J., Li, Y.J., & Bermudez, L.E. (2003). Mycobacterium tuberculosis infection causes different levels of apoptosis and necrosis in human macrophages and alveolar epithelial cells. Cell Microbiol. Sep;5(9):649-60.

Daynes, G. (1974). Drug-induced heart failure in advanced pulmonary tuberculosis. S Afr Med J. Nov 23;48(57):2352-3.

Dhingra, V.K., Rajpal, S., Aggarwal, N., Aggarwaln, J.K., Shadab, K. & Jain, S.K. (2004). Adverse drug reactions observed during DOTS. J Commun Dis. Dec;36(4):251-9.

Didilescu, C. & Craiova, U.M. (2011). Present and future in the use of anti-tubercular drugs. Pneumologia. Oct-Dec;60(4):198-201.

Dobos, K.M., Spotts, E.A., Quinn, F.D., & King, C.H. (2000). Necrosis of lung epithelial cells during infection with Mycobacterium tuberculosis is preceded by cell permeation. Infect Immun. Nov;68(11):6300-10.

Esin, S., Batoni, G., Counoupas, C., Stringaro, A., Brancatisano, F.L., Colone, M., Maisetta, G., Florio, W., Arancia, G. & Campa, M. (2008). Direct binding of human NK cell natural cytotoxicity receptor NKp44 to the surfaces of mycobacteria and other bacteria. Infect Immun. Apr;76(4):1719-27. doi: 10.1128/IAI.00870-07. Epub 2008 Jan 22.

Fratazzi, C., Arbeit, R.D., Carini, C., Balcewicz-Sablinska, M.K., Keane, J., Kornfeld, H., & Remold, H.G. (1999). Macrophage apoptosis in mycobacterial infections. J Leukoc Biol. Nov;66(5):763-4.

Foster, D.R. (1997). Miliary tuberculosis following intravesical BCG treatment Br J Radiol. Apr;70(832):429.

Gagliardi, M.C., Teloni, R., Giannoni, F., Pardini, M., Sargentini, V., Brunori, L., Fattorini, L. & Nisini, R. (2005). Mycobacterium bovis Bacillus Calmette-Guerin infects DC-SIGN- dendritic cell and causes the inhibition of IL-12 and the enhancement of IL-10 production. J Leukoc Biol. Jul;78(1):106-13. Epub 2005 Apr 21.

Global tuberculosis control: WHO report 2011. Available from: http://www.who.int/tb/publications/global_report/2008/pdf/report_without_annexes.pdf. http://www.who.int/tb/publications/global_report/2011/gtbr11_full.pdf

Gomez, D.I., Twahirwa, M., Schlesinger, L.S., & Restrepo, B.I. (2013). Reduced Mycobacterium tuberculosis association with monocytes from diabetes patients that have poor glucose control. Tuberculosis (Edinb). Mar;93(2):192-7. doi: 10.1016/j.tube.2012.10.003. Epub 2012 Nov 3.

Grosset, J.H., Singer, T.G. & Bishai, W.R. (2012). New drugs for the treatment of tuberculosis: hope and reality. Int J Tuberc Lung Dis. Aug;16(8):1005-14. doi: 10.5588/ijtld.12.0277.

Gupta, R.C., Lavengood, R. Jr., & Smith, J.P. (1988). Miliary tuberculosis due to intravesical bacillus Calmette- Guerin therapy Chest. Dec;94(6):1296-8.

Jeon, C.Y & Murray, M.B. (2008). Diabetes mellitus increases the risk of active tuberculosis: a systematic review of 13 observational studies. PLoS Med. Jul 15;5(7):e152. doi: 10.1371/journal.pmed.0050152.

Hedlund, S., Persson, A., Vujic, A., Che, K.F., Stendahl. O. & Larsson, M. (2010). Dendritic cell activation by sensing Mycobacterium tuberculosis-induced apoptotic neutrophils via DC-SIGN. Hum Immunol. Jun;71(6):535-40. doi: 10.1016/j.humimm.2010.02.022. Epub 2010 Mar 11.

Hirsch, C.S. Johnson, J.L., Okwera, A., Kanost, R.A., Wu, M., Peters, P., Muhumuza, M., Mayanja-Kizza, H., Mugerwa, R.D. Mugyenyi, P., Ellner, J.J., & Toossi, Z. (2005). Mechanisms of apoptosis of T-cells in human tuberculosis. J Clin Immunol. Jul;25(4):353-64.

Horvath, C.N. & Xing, Z. (2013). Immunization strategies against pulmonary tuberculosis: considerations of T cell geography. Adv Exp Med Biol. 2013;783:267-78. doi: 10.1007/978-1-4614-6111-1_14.

Kita, Y., Okada, M., Nakajima, T., Kanamaru, N., Hashimoto, S., Nagasawa, T., Kaneda, Y., Yoshida, S., Nishida, Y., Nakatani, H., Takao, K., Kishigami, C., Nishimatsu, S., Sekine, Y., Takamori, Y., McMurray, D.N., De la Cruz, E.C., Tan, E.V., Kawamura, I. (2006). Protective immunity against Mycobacterium tuberculosis. Kekkaku. Nov;81(11):687-91.

Kee, S.J., Kwon, Y.S., Park, Y.W., Cho, Y.N., Lee, S.J., Kim, T.J., Lee, S.S., Jang, H.C., Shin, M.G., Shin, J.H., Suh, S.P. & Ryang, D.W. (2012). Dysfunction of natural killer T cells in patients with active Mycobacterium tuberculosis infection. Infect Immun. Jun;80(6):2100-8. doi: 10.1128/IAI.06018-11. Epub 2012 Mar 12.

Kolpakova, T.A., Kolpakov, M.A, Bashkirova, Iu.V., Rachkovskaia, L.N., Burylin, S.Iu. & Liubarskiĭ, M.S. (2001). Effects of the enterosorbent SUMS-1 on isoniazid pharmacokinetics and lipid peroxidation in patients with pulmonary tuberculosis and drug-induced hepatic lesions. Probl Tuberk.;(3):34-6.

Kul'chavenia, E.V. & Kuznetsov, P.V. (1998). Complications of polychemotherapy for renal tuberculosis. Probl Tuberk.;(1):28-30.

Kulchavenya, E., Filimonov, P., & Shvetsova, O. (2007). An Atlas of a Urogenital tuberculosis and other extrapulmonary localizations (monograph). Novosibirsk: «Tirazh-Sibir».

Kulchavenia, E.V. & Muzyko, L.V. (2007). [Two cases of tuberculosis after transplantation of the kidney]. Urologiia, (6): 80-2.

Kulchavenya, E. (2009).Tuberculosis of urogenital system in Urology: National Manual Lopatkin N, Editor. Geotar-Media: Moscow. p. p.584-601.

Kulchavenya, E. & Krasnov, V. (2010). Selected questions of TB-urology(monograph). Novosibirsk: «Nauka».

Layer, P. & Engelhardm M. (1986). Tuberculostatics-induced systemic lupus erythematosus. Dtsch Med Wochenschr. Oct 17;111(42):1603-5.

Luca, S. & Mihaescu, T. (2013). History of BCG Vaccine. Maedica (Buchar). Mar;8(1):53-8.

Maianski, N.A., Roos, D. & Kuijpers, T.W. (2003). Tumor necrosis factor alpha induces a caspase-independent death pathway in human neutrophils. Blood. Mar 1;101(5):1987-95. Epub 2002 Oct 10.

Mariani, F., Goletti, D., Ciaramella, A., Martino, A., Colizzi, V., & Fraziano M. (2001). Macrophage response to Mycobacterium tuberculosis during HIV infection: relationships between macrophage activation and apoptosis. Curr Mol Med. May;1(2):209-16.

Méndez-Samperio, P., Vázquez, A., & Ayala, H. (2003). Infection of human monocytes with Mycobacterium bovis BCG induces production of CC-chemokines. J Infect. Aug;47(2):139-47.

Mitchison, D. & Davies, G. (2012). The chemotherapy of tuberculosis: past, present and future. Int J Tuberc Lung Dis. Jun;16(6):724-32. doi: 10.5588/ijtld.12.0083.

Mitsuyama, M., Akagawa, K., Kobayashi, K., Sugawara, I., Kawakami, K., Yamamoto, S., & Okada, Z. (2003). Up-to-date understanding of tuberculosis immunity. Kekkaku. Jan;78(1):51-5.

Morales, A., Eidinger, D., & Bruce, A.W. (1976). Intracavitary Bacillus Calmette-Guerin in the treatment of superficial bladder tumors J Urol. Aug;116(2):180-3.

Munk, M.E. & Emoto, M. (1995). Functions of T-cell subsets and cytokines in mycobacterial infections. Eur Respir J Suppl. Sep;20:668s-675s.

McDonough, K.A. & Kress, Y. (1995). Cytotoxicity for lung epithelial cells is a virulence-associated phenotype of Mycobacterium tuberculosis. – Infect Immun. Dec;63(12):4802-11.

Narang, R.K., Agarwal, M.C., Raina, A.K., Singh, S.N., Bihari, K. & Sharma, S.N. (1983). Hyperuricaemia induced by ethambutol. Br J Dis Chest. Oct;77(4):403-6.

Nguyen, H.A., Rajaram, M.V., Meyer, D.A., & Schlesinger, L.S. (2012). Pulmonary surfactant protein A and surfactant lipids upregulate IRAK-M, a negative regulator of TLR-mediated inflammation in human macrophages. Am J Physiol Lung Cell Mol Physiol. Oct 1;303(7):L608-16. doi: 10.1152/ajplung.00067.2012. Epub 2012 Aug 10.

Okada, M. (2008). The development of novel vaccines against tuberculosis. Nihon Rinsho Meneki Gakkai Kaishi. Oct;31(5):356-68.

*Okada, M., & Kita, Y. (2010). Anti-tuberculosis immunity by cytotoxic T cells * granulysin and the development of novel vaccines (HSP-65 DNA+IL-12 DNA). Kekkaku. Jun;85(6):531-8.*

Okada, M., Kita, Y., Nakajima, T., Kanamaru, N., Hashimoto, S., Nagasawa, T., Kaneda, Y., Yoshida, S., Nishida, Y., Nakatani, H., Takao, K., Kishigami, C., Nishimatsu, S., Sekine, Y., Inoue, Y., McMurray, D.N., & Sakatani, M. (2011). Novel prophylactic vaccine using a prime-boost method and hemagglutinating virus of Japan-envelope against tuberculosis. Clin Dev Immunol. 2011:549281. doi: 10.1155/2011/549281. Epub 2011 Mar 7.

Okada, M. (2006). Novel vaccines against M. tuberculosis. Kekkaku. Dec;81(12):745-51.

Olakanmi, O., Kesavalu, B., Abdalla, M.Y. & Britigan, B.E. (2013) Iron acquisition by Mycobacterium tuberculosis residing within myeloid dendritic cells. Microb Pathog. Sep 22;65C:21-28. doi: 10.1016/j.micpath.2013.09.002. [Epub ahead of print].

Pal, P.G. & Horwitz, M.A. (1992). Immunization with extracellular proteins of Mycobacterium tuberculosis induces cell-mediated immune responses and substantial protective immunity in a guinea pig model of pulmonary tuberculosis. Infect Immun. Nov;60(11):4781-92.

Patel, N.R., Zhu, J., Tachado, S.D., Zhang, J., Wan, Z., Saukkonen, J. & Koziel, H. (2007). HIV impairs TNF-alpha mediated macrophage apoptotic response to Mycobacterium tuberculosis. J Immunol. Nov 15;179(10):6973-80.

Peng, H., Wang, X., Barnes, P.F., Tang, H., Townsend, J.C. & Samten, B. (2011). The Mycobacterium tuberculosis early secreted antigenic target of 6 kDa inhibits T cell interferon-γ production through the p38 mitogen-activated protein kinase pathway. J Biol Chem. Jul 8;286(27):24508-18. doi: 10.1074/jbc.M111.234062. Epub 2011 May 17.

Pereira, R.M., Tresoldi, A.T. & Hessel, G. (2000). Isoniazid-induced hepatic failure. Report of a case. Arq Gastroenterol. Jan-Mar;37(1):72-5.

Pienaar, E. & Lerm, M. (2013). A mathematical model of the initial interaction between Mycobacterium tuberculosis and macrophages. J Theor Biol. Oct 7. pii: S0022-5193(13)00465-7. doi: 10.1016/j.jtbi.2013.09.029. [Epub ahead of print]

Pinheiro, M.B., Antonelli, L.R., Sathler-Avelar, R., Vitelli-Avelar, D.M., Spindola-de-Miranda, S., Guimarães, T.M., Teixeira-Carvalho, A., Martins-Filho, O.A. & Toledo V.P. (2012). CD4-CD8-αβ and γδ T cells display inflammatory and regulatory potentials during human tuberculosis. PLoS One;7(12):e50923. doi: 10.1371/journal.pone.0050923. Epub 2012 Dec 11.

Persson, Y.A., Blomgran-Julinder, R., Rahman, S., Zheng, L., & Stendahl, O. (2008). Mycobacterium tuberculosis-induced apoptotic neutrophils trigger a pro-inflammatory response in macrophages through release of heat shock protein 72, acting in synergy with the bacteria. Microbes Infect. Mar;10(3):233-40. doi: 10.1016/j.micinf.2007.11.007. Epub 2007 Nov 29.

Perskvist, N., Long, M., Stendahl, O., & Zheng, L. (2002). Mycobacterium tuberculosis promotes apoptosis in human neutrophils by activating caspase-3 and altering expression of Bax/Bcl-xL via an oxygen-dependent pathway. J Immunol. Jun 15;168(12):6358-65.

Portevin, D. & Young, D. (2013). Natural killer cell cytokine response to M. bovis BCG Is associated with inhibited proliferation, increased apoptosis and ultimate depletion of NKp44(+)CD56(bright) cells. PLoS One. Jul 15;8(7):e68864. doi: 10.1371/journal.pone.0068864. Print 2013.

Raja, A. (2004). Immunology of tuberculosis. Indian J Med Res. 2004 Oct;120(4):213-32.

Raviglione, M., 2003 The TB epidemic from 1992 to 2002.- Tuberculosis. - 2003. – Vol. 83.:P.4–14.

Resende, C.T., Hirsch, C.S., Toossi, Z., Dietze, R., & Ribeiro-Rodrigues, R. (2007). Intestinal helminth co-infection has a negative impact on both anti-Mycobacterium tuberculosis immunity and clinical response to tuberculosis therapy. Clin Exp Immunol. Jan;147(1):45-52.

Rojas, R.E., Balaji, K.N., Subramanian, A. & Boom, W.H. (1999). Regulation of human CD4(+) alphabeta T-cell-receptor-positive (TCR(+)) and gammadelta TCR(+) T-cell responses to Mycobacterium tuberculosis by interleukin-10 and transforming growth factor beta. Infect Immun. 1999 Dec;67(12):6461-72.

Saukkonen, J.J., Bazydlo, B., Thomas, M., Strieter, R.M., Keane, J., & Kornfeld, H. (2002). Beta-chemokines are induced by Mycobacterium tuberculosis and inhibit its growth. Infect Immun. Apr;70(4):1684-93.

Schaale, K., Brandenburg, J., Kispert, A., Leitges, M., Ehlers, S. & Reiling, N. (2013) Wnt6 Is Expressed in Granulomatous Lesions of Mycobacterium tuberculosis-Infected Mice and Is Involved in Macrophage Differentiation and Proliferation. J Immunol. Oct 11. [Epub ahead of print]

Shutskaia, E.I., Priakhina, V.N., Kolpakova, T.A., & Kurilovich, G.M. (1991). Drug-induced nephropathy in patients with tuberculosis of the lungs. Probl Tuberk.;(4):48-9.

Siddiqui, M.A. & Khan, I.A. (2002). Isoniazid-induced lupus erythematosus presenting with cardiac tamponade. Am J Ther. Mar-Apr;9(2):163-5.

Solangi, G.A., Zuberi, B.F., Shaikh, S. & Shaikh, W.M. (2004). Pyrazinamide induced hyperuricemia in patients taking anti-tuberculous therapy. J Coll Physicians Surg Pak. Mar;14(3):136-8.

Sohn, H., Lee, K.S., Kim, S.Y., Shin, D.M., Shin, S.J., Jo, E.K., Park, J.K., & Kim, H.J. (2009). Induction of cell death in human macrophages by a highly virulent Korean Isolate of Mycobacterium tuberculosis and the virulent strain H37Rv. Scand J Immunol. Jan;69(1):43-50. doi: 10.1111/j.1365-3083.2008.02188.x.

de Souza, A.F., de Oliveira, e Silva. A., Baldi, J., de Souza, T.N. & Rizzo, P.M. (1996). Hepatic functional changes induced by the combined use of isoniazid, pyrazinamide and rifampicin in the treatment of pulmonary tuberculosis. Arq Gastroenterol. Oct-Dec;33(4):194-200.

Sylvester, R.J., van der Meijden, A.P., & Lamm, D.L. (2002) Intravesical bacillus Calmette-Guerin reduces the risk of progression in patients with superficial bladder cancer: a meta-analysis of the published results of randomized clinical trials. J Urol Nov;168(5):1964-70. http://www.ncbi.nlm.nih.gov/pubmed/12394686

The Global Plan to Stop TB, 2011–2015. Geneva, World Health Organization, 2010 (WHO/HTM/STB/2010. 2)

Thuong, N.T., Dunstan, S.J., Chau, T.T., Thorsson, V., Simmons, C.P., Quyen, N.T., Thwaites, G.E., Thi Ngoc Lan, N., Hibberd, M., Teo, Y.Y., Seielstad, M., Aderem, A., Farrar, J.J., & Hawn, T.R. (2008). Identification of tuberculosis susceptibility genes with human macrophage gene expression profiles. PLoS Pathog. Dec;4(12):e1000229. doi: 10.1371/journal.ppat.1000229. Epub 2008 Dec 5.

Toossi, Z., Funderburg, N.T., Sirdeshmuk, S., Whalen, C.C., Nanteza, M.W., Johnson, D.F., Mayanja-Kizza, H., & Hirsch, C.S. (2013). Systemic Immune Activation and Microbial Translocation in Dual HIV/Tuberculosis-Infected Subjects. J Infect Dis. Apr 2. [Epub ahead of print]

Toossi, Z., Wu, M., Hirsch, C.S. Mayanja-Kizza, H., Baseke, J., Aung, H., Canaday, D.H., & Fujinaga, K. (2012). Activation of P-TEFb at sites of dual HIV/TB infection, and inhibition of MTB-induced HIV transcriptional activation by the inhibitor of CDK9, Indirubin-3'-monoxime. AIDS Res Hum Retroviruses. Feb;28(2):182-7. doi: 10.1089/AID.2010.0211. Epub 2011 May 6.

Toossi, Z., Wu, M., Rojas, R., Kalsdorf, B., Aung, H., Hirsch, C.S., Walrath, J., Wolbink, A., van Ham, M., & Silver, R.F. (2012). Induction of serine protease inhibitor 9 by Mycobacterium tuberculosis inhibits apoptosis and promotes survival of infected macrophages. J Infect Dis. Jan 1;205(1):144-51. doi: 10.1093/infdis/jir697. Epub 2011 Nov 16.

Toossi, Z. (2000). The inflammatory response in Mycobacterium tuberculosis infection. Arch Immunol Ther Exp (Warsz). 48(6):513-9.

Volpe, E., Cappelli, G., Grassi, M., Martino, A., Serafino, A., Colizzi, V., Sanarico, N., & Mariani, F. (2006). Gene expression profiling of human macrophages at late time of infection with Mycobacterium tuberculosis. Immunology. 2006 Aug;118(4):449-60.

Wada, M., Yoshiyama, T., Ogata, H., Ito, K., Mizutani, S. & Sugita, H. (1999). Six-months chemotherapy (2HRZS or E/4HRE) of new cases of pulmonary tuberculosis-six year experiences on its effectiveness, toxicity, and acceptability. Kekkaku. Apr;74(4):353-60.

Wada M. (2001). Effectiveness and problems of PZA-containing 6-month regimen for the treatment of new pulmonary tuberculosis patients. Kekkaku. Jan;76(1):33-43.

Wang, J., Thorson, L., Stokes, R.W., Santosuosso, M., Huygen, K., Zganiacz, A., Hitt, M., & Xing, Z. (2004). Single mucosal, but not parenteral, immunization with recombinant adenoviral-based vaccine provides potent protection from pulmonary tuberculosis. J Immunol. Nov 15;173(10):6357-65.

WHO. Global tuberculosis report 2012. Geneva: World Health Organization, 2012. http://www.who.int/tb/publications/global_report/en/index.html (accessed Dec 27, 2012).

Wilson, G. (1931). The Lubeck disaster. Am J Public Health Nations Health. March; 21(3): 282.

World Health Organization. Global Tuberculosis Control, Surveillance, Planning, Financing. 2008; Available from: http://www.who.int/tb/publications/global_report/2008/pdf/report_without_annexes.pdf.

Wu, M., Aung, H., Hirsch, C.S., & Toossi, Z. (2012). Inhibition of Mycobacterium tuberculosis-induced signalling by transforming growth factor-β in human mononuclear phagocytes. Scand J Immunol. Mar;75(3):301-4. doi: 10.1111/j.1365-3083.2011.02668.x.

Xing, Z. & Lichty, B.D. (2006). Use of recombinant virus-vectored tuberculosis vaccines for respiratory mucosal immunization. Tuberculosis (Edinb). May-Jul;86(3-4):211-7. Epub 2006 Feb 28.

Yim, J.J. & Selvaraj, P. (2010). Genetic susceptibility in tuberculosis. Respirology. Feb;15(2):241-56. doi: 10.1111/j.1440-1843.2009.01690.x.

Zbar, B., Bernstein, I., Tanaka, T., & Rapp, H.J. (1970) Tumor immunity produced by the intradermal inoculation of living tumor cells and living Mycobacterium bovis (strain BCG) Science. Dec 11;170(963):1217-8.

Zierski, M. & Bek, E. (1980). Side effects of various combinations of rifampin and isoniazid with ethambutol or streptomycin and pyrazinamide in short-term chemotherapy of newly-detected pulmonary tuberculosis. Pneumonol Pol. Jul;48(7):469-79.

Urogenital Tuberculosis as a Part of Extrapulmonary Tuberculosis: Epidemiology and Some Aspects of Diagnosis and Therapy

Ekaterina Kulchavenya

Urogenital Department, Novosibirsk TB Research Institute
Novosibirsk Medical University, Russia

1   Introduction

Tuberculosis (TB) is a current public health problem, remaining the most common worldwide cause of mortality from infectious disease. Tuberculosis (both pulmonary and extrapulmonary) leads to male and female infertility (Khanna & Agrawal, 2011; Kulshrestha *et al.*, 2011; Wise & Marella, 2003; Tzvetkov & Tzvetkova, 2006; Lenk & Schroeder, 2001; Scherban *et al.*, 2010; Wise & Shteynshlyuger, 2008), it is a sexually transmitted disease (Scherban & Kulchavenya, 2008) that explains why TB is not only a medical, but also a big social problem.

Urogenital tuberculosis (UGTB) is ancient but still now an unsolved problem. Clinical features are flexible and variable, UGTB mimics numerous other diseases that results in delayed diagnosis. Despite of about 7000 articles with key words "urogenital / genitourinary tuberculosis", there is none good multicenter study with high level of evidence on this problem. UGTB is an embodiment of contradictions – from terms and classification till therapy and management. Nevertheless we have to overcome this quagmire for best understanding this eternal enigmatic and potentially fatal dangerous disease.

2   Terminology and Classification

There are no unique classifications of extrapulmonary tuberculosis (EPTB) or urogenital tuberculosis. Some authors consider EPTB as TB of any organ, excluding exactly broncho-pulmonary lesion, so pleural TB they relate to the one of the form of EPTB too. Others think that division of lung and its cover pleura on two separate organs is incorrect, and ascribe both organs to pulmonary tuberculosis (PTB) and instead of EPTB use a term Extrathoracal Tuberculosis (ETTB), or extrarespiratory tuberculosis, which merge TB of all organs out of thorax. This is a reason for confusion with proportion of EPTB/ETTB forms.

The first note of urogenital TB was made by Porter (1894). Later Wildbolz (1937) suggested the term genitourinary TB. The term "Urogenital TB" is more logical, because kidney TB, which is usually primary, is diagnosed more often than genital TB (Singh *et al.*, 2013). Only 53% of patients with kidney TB had genital lesions, but in 61.9% patients with epididymorchitis and in 79.3% patients with TB of the prostate a renal lesion could be diagnosed (Kulchavenya, 2009; Gómez García *et al.*, 2010). In UGTB, the kidneys are the most common sites of infection and are infected through hematogenous spread of the bacilli, which then spread through the renal and genital tract (Abbara & Davidson, 2011). Although some authors believe that tuberculosis often affects the lower genitourinary system rather than the kidney. They found that tuberculosis of the lower genitourinary tract most commonly affects the epididymis and the testis, followed by bladder, ureter, prostate, and penis (Wise & Shteynshlyuger, 2008).

Actually the term UGTB is incorrect too, because it includes kidney TB, male genital tuberculosis (MGTB) and sometimes even female genital tuberculosis (FGTB) – but all these forms of the disease have their own clinical features and require their own approaches to diagnosis and management. Although there is an opinion, that, as TB is an infection disease caused by M. tuberculosis (Mtb), it should be diagnosed by identification of the infection agent only and therapy should be directed on elimination of Mtb only – without separation on particular forms with individual approach to the diagnosis and treatment.

3   Epidemiology

In 1984 EPTB remained a major health problem in Australia, where 24.3% of all new TB notifications were extrapulmonary origin. The commonest sites of disease were the lymph nodes, urogenital tract, pleura and bone (Dwyer *et al.*, 1987). By the 1980s, the availability of antituberculous chemotherapy reduced the incidence and prevalence of tuberculosis. Changing patterns of population emigration and the development of large pools of immune-compromised individuals reversed the downward trend of tuberculosis (Wise & Marella, 2003).

In past century in Oklahoma a greater proportion of newly diagnosed cases of extrapulmonary tuberculosis occurred in nonwhites. This was especially true to TB meningitis, TB lymphadenitis, and miliary tuberculosis (Snider, 1975). These days EPTB was frequent in Africa and had a great severity due to delayed diagnosis and multifocal forms (Aubry *et al.*, 1979). At Boston city in 80-ies of last century EPTB represented 4.5% of all new cases of active tuberculosis and tended to occur in older patients. Sites of involvement included lymph nodes, genitourinary tract, bone and articular sites, the meninges, peritoneum, adrenal glands, pericardium, and miscellaneous sites, in this order (Alvarez & McCabe, 1984).

In Spain from 1991 to 2008 among the 2,161 cases diagnosed, 1,186 were PTB and 705 EPTB. The number of EPTB cases decreased more slowly than PTB. EPTB increased from 30.6% of cases in 1991-1996 to 37.6% in 2003-2008 (lymphatic site increased 27%) (García-Rodríguez *et al.*, 2011). Authors concluded, that whilst there has been a reduction in the overall incidence of TB, the proportion of EPTB increased that could be explained by an increase in life expectancy and the predominance of women in the population, and by a decline in BCG vaccinated patients (García-Rodríguez *et al.*, 2011). In Nepal common sites for EPTB were lymph nodes (42.6 %) and peritoneum and/or intestines (14.8%) (Sreeramareddy *et al.*, 2008).

Within the last decade the spectrum of EPTB in Siberia has changed significantly (Kulchavenya, 2013). TB of the central nervous system almost doubled from 4.9% to 8.7%, mostly due to co-morbidity with HIV. Bone and joints TB increased by about half from 20.3% to 34.5%, and among this group TB spondylitis with neurological disorders predominated, the most debilitating form of the disease. The proportion of UGTB decreased from 42.9% to 31.7%. In contrary, there was a decrease of peripheral lymph nodes TB from 16.7% in 1999 to 11.2% in 2011, with fistulous disease still frequent. At the end of the last century ocular TB accounted for 7.4% and in 2008 (in 2009 listed in "others") for 4.4% of the patients with EPTB. Accordingly, in 1999 other form of TB accounted for 7.8% and in 2009 for 15.8% (in 2011 – 13.9%). The increase is partly due to inclusion of patients with ocular TB in this group, and partly due to better diagnosis of TB of the skin, abdominal organs, breast etc (Kulchavenya, 2013).

EPTB had an increasing rate in Turkey in 2001-2007. The reason remains largely unknown (Gunal *et al.*, 2011). The most commonly seen two types of EPTB were genitourinary TB (27.2%) and meningeal TB (19.4%). TB of bone/joints, pleura, lymph nodes, skin, and peritoneal TB occurred at a frequency ranging from 9.7% to 10.7% (Gunal *et al.*, 2011). In 2009 almost one-fifth of United States TB cases were extrapulmonary; unexplained slower annual case count decreases have occurred in EPTB, compared with annual case count decreases in pulmonary tuberculosis (PTB) cases. From 1993 to 2006 among 253,299 cases, 73.6% were PTB and 18.7% were EPTB, including lymphatic (40.4%), pleural (19.8%), bone and/or joint (11.3%), genitourinary (6.5%), meningeal (5.4%), peritoneal (4.9%), and unclassified EPTB (11.8%) cases (Peto *et al.*, 2009). In France in 2012 the most frequent clinical presentations of EPTB were lymphadenitis, pleuritis and osteoarticular TB. Peritoneal, urogenital or meningeal TB was less frequent, and their diagnosis was often difficult due to the wide differential diagnosis and the low sensitivity of diagnostic tests including cultures and genetic amplification tests (Mazza-Stalder *et al.*, 2012). In some countries the rate of growth of bone & joint TB reached the leading position among EPTB (Kulchavenya, 2013). Location of TB on the spine remains the most common form of skeletal TB, representing 62.2% of all osteo-articulary locations (Didilescu, C. & Tănăsescu, M., 2012; Wiler *et al.*, 2010). The skeletal form was responsible for 3% of the total number of cases, with 50% of these due to spinal tuberculosis (Vilar *et al.*, 2006).

UGTB usually results from the reactivation of old, dormant tuberculous diseases by pathogens of the Mycobacterium tuberculosis complex (Lenk, 2011). It was the second most common form of EPTB in countries with severe epidemic situation and the third most common form in regions with low incidence of TB (Colbert *et al.*, 2012; Kulchavenya *et al.*, 2012; Lima *et al.*, 2012), with more than 90% of cases occurring in developing countries (Abbara *et al.*, 2011). EPTB comprises 20-25% total burden of the disease in which UGTB is 4% by opinion of Singh *et al.*, 2013. It has been well described that the urogenital system is a common site of EPTB in adults, but the true incidence of UGTB is less clear, and reports have varied from 4% to 73% (Zarrabi & Heyns, 2009). It was found that UGTB represented 27% of extrapulmonary cases. Renal involvement in TB can be part of a disseminated infection or a localized genitourinary disease. Renal involvement by TB infection is underdiagnosed in most health care centers (Daher *et al.*, 2913). In nowadays UGTB is not commonly encountered in general urological practice in Australia and New Zealand. However, this infection is easily overlooked unless clinicians maintain a strong awareness of its possibility (Patterson *et al.*, 2012). In Japan because of the progress in anti-TB chemotherapy, it has become quite rare to diagnose patients with UGTB, however, the incidence of tuberculosis remains comparatively high, particularly in elder patients, among advanced countries (Miyake & Fujisawa).

Lin *et al.* (2009) in retrospective study compared patients with EPTB and PTB in southern Taiwan. They found, that among total of 766 TB patients in 102 (13.3%) EPTB was diagnosed, and in 664 (86.7%) – PTB, and 19.6% of EPTB patients also had PTB. The most frequently involved EPTB site was the bone and joints (24.5%). The incidence of EPTB vs. PTB decreased significantly for each decade increase in patient age. Multivariate logistic regression analysis showed that being female, not being diabetic, having end-stage renal disease and not smoking were independent risk factors for EPTB (Lin *et al.*, 2009).

131 history cases of UGTB patients, who were revealed in 2009 – 2011 years in Siberia, were analyzed (Kulchavenya, 2013). The most common form was kidney tuberculosis (74.8%). Isolated kidney tuberculosis (KTB) more often has met in women – 56.8%. Patients of middle and old age more often were revealed in stage of cavernous KTB; young patients had small forms. Among all UGTB patients asymptomatic course was in 12.2%, among KTB - in 15.9%. Every third patient complained of flank pain and dysuria (accordingly 35.2% and 39.8%), 17% presented toxicity symptoms, 9.1% - renal colic, 7.9% - gross-hematuria. M.tuberculosis in urine was found in 31.8% in all levels of isolated KTB as whole. UGTB has no any specific symptom, even sterile pyuria meets only in 25% only. The acute onset of tuberculous orchiepididydmitis was in 35.7% of patients, hemospermia was in 7.1%, dysuria - in 35.7%. The most common complaints for prostate tuberculosis were perineal pain (31.6%), dysuria (also 31.6%), and hemospermia (26.3%). Mtb in prostate secretion / ejaculate was revealed in this group in 10.5%. Authors concluded that all urogenital tract infections should be suspected on UGTB in patients living in the region with high incidence rate, who had contact with tuberculosis infection, who has recurrent course of the disease, resistant to standard therapy.

Isolated epididymo-orchitis is an unusual presentation of tuberculosis (Shenoy et al., 2012). In study of Singh at al. (2013), in UGTB kidney was the most affected organ (64.9%) following ureter (27.35%), urinary bladder (17.09%), prostate (3.4%) and epididymis (5.19%). In this study, none case of testicular and penile tuberculosis was encountered. Tuberculous epididymo-orchitis should be considered in the patients who present with a scrotal mass. The preoperative differentiation of tuberculous epididymoorchitis from non-tuberculous epididymo-orchitis and testicular tumor is difficult. In patients who have epididymal and testicular lesions, surgical excision provides the diagnosis (Suankwan et al., 2012). In Spain of the 371 male TB patients 34 (9.2%) had orchiepididymitis. Mean age was 52.7 years and the presenting symptom was scrotal swelling and/or pain. Over 50% of cases involved the right testis. MGTB associated renal tuberculosis and active disease in extraurological organs presented in 64% and 19.2% of cases, respectively. Diagnosis was established by culture of Mycobacterium tuberculosis recovery from urine and/or purulent scrotal exudates (Gómez García et al., 2010).

Some authors have found that UGTB affects more men than women (Benchekroun et al., 1998; Figueiredo & Lucon, 2008; el Khader et al, 2001 Tanthanuch et al., 2010; Nurkić, M., 2006); others – exactly the contrary (Aubry et al.,1979; García-Rodríguez et al., 2011; Mazza-Stalder et al., 2012; Singh et al., 2011; Singh et al., 2013). It have been seem UGTB, as any other kidney disease, should be more often in female patients, because menses, gravidity, inflammation of genitals may hinder the urine passage. Urinary stasis makes the possibility for fixation Mtb to urothelium, and, so, for developing renal TB.

As whole a proportion male:female among EPTB patients depends on form of the disease. Concerning UGTB superiority of female patients is when UGTB includes both urological and gynecological TB, but in some regions there were female superiority among urological TB too. Actually, for better estimation of epidemic situation UGTB should me divided on urological TB (including male genital TB), and female genital TB.

In eastern Sudan of the 2778 women presenting with various gynecologic symptoms, 44 suspected cases of FGTB were identified. Granulomatous tissue reactions were observed in 25 of the suspected FGTB cases, yielding an incidence of 0.9%. The majority (80%) of these patients presented with chronic pelvic and lower abdominal pain; however, 68.0% presented with pelvic mass, cyst and/or abscess; 48.0% had dyspareunia; 40.0% were infertile; 28% had menstrual dysfunction; 20.0% had dysmenorrhea; and 4.0% experienced postmenopausal bleeding. Body mass index, residence, and educational level were significantly different between women diagnosed with FGTB and those where FGTB was excluded (P values=0.02, 0.03, and 0.01, respectively). However, no significant differences were found in age and Bacillus Calmette-Guérin vaccination status (Ali & Abdallah, 2012).

Over a period of 30 months (July 1986 - December 1988) 57 cases of genital tuberculosis were diagnosed at Tygerberg Hospital (Margolis et al., 1998). Forty of these cases were diagnosed as a result of routine screening in 650 patients who presented with infertility and the other 17 were diagnosed in patients admitted to the gynaecological wards. The prevalence in patients presenting with infertility was 6.15%. The commonest gynaecological presenting symptom was infertility (73.7%). Dysmenorrhoea in 29.8% and deep dyspareunia in 12.3% were the only other frequently occurring gynaecological symptoms. Menstruation was normal in 50 patients (87.7%) (Margolis et al., 1998). In another study FGTB patients presented with infertility (70%), pelvic/abdominal pain (55%), and menstrual disturbances (25%). Tuberculosis involved the endometrium in 55.88%, tubes in 23.53%, ovaries in 14.71% and cervix in 5.88% of the 68 cases (Mondal & Dutta, 2009). In fifteen-year retrospective study of 110 cases in eastern India a total number of 110 cases of FGTB from 92 patients were included. Patients presented with infertility (70%), pelvic/ abdominal pain (55%) and menstrual disturbances (25%). Female genital tuberculosis involved the vulva (2), vagina (1), cervix (5), endometrium (66), fallopian tube (24) and in 12 patients - ovaries (Mondal, 2013).

A total of 85 women of genital TB, who underwent diagnostic laparoscopy for infertility or chronic pelvic pain were enrolled in the retrospective study in India. Most women were from poor socioeconomic status (68.1%). Past history of TB was seen in 34.1% women with PTB in 22.35% women with EPTB. Most women presented with infertility (90.6%: primary 72.9%; secondary 17.6%) while the rest had chronic pelvic pain (9.4%). Diagnosis of genital TB was made by histopathological evidence of TB granuloma in 18.8%, positive polymerase chain reaction (PCR) in 64.7% and laparoscopic findings of genital TB in 47.1%. The various findings on laparoscopy were tubercles on peritoneum (12.9%) or ovary (1.2%), tubovarian masses (7.1%), caseous nodules (5.8%), encysted ascitis in 7.1% women. Various grades of pelvic adhesions were seen in 65.8% women (Sharma et al., 2008).

A retrospective clinicopathological study of 1,548 cases of FGTB between 1940 and 2011 was conducted in Turkey. The mean age of the cases was 29.49 years. Involvement of the endometrium was noted in 1,073, fallopian tubes in 164, cervix in 157, and 154 had multiple organ involvement. Clinically, 115 cases (7.4%) were diagnosed as having primary infertility and 12 cases (0.8%) as having secondary infertility. There was a coexistent carcinoma in 1.5% of the cases. Peritoneal tuberculosis in 21 cases and tuberculous lymphadenitis in 7 cases were seen as well (Türkmen et al., 2012).

4   Predisposition

About 2 billion people are infected with Mycobacterium tuberculosis; they are carriers of latent infection, forming a large reservoir for reactivation of tuberculosis (Barry et al., 2009). Thus any contemporary person has a risk to be infected with Mycobacterium tuberculosis (Mtb) and, in unfavorable conditions, to get sick with TB. Nevertheless, the infection of human organism with Mtb doesn't lead to disease obligatory, by all means. Recent studies have revealed numerous polymorphisms implicated in host susceptibility to TB. Human organism may have an innate resistance to Mtb. Object lesson of this fact was "Lubeck disaster". Between 10 December 1929 and 30 April 1930, 251 infants born in the old Hanseatic town of Lubeck received three doses of BCG vaccine by the mouth during the first ten days of life. Of these 251, 72 died of TB, most of them in two to five months and all but one before the end of the first year. In addition, 135 suffered from clinical TB but eventually recovered; and 44 became tuberculin-positive but remained well. The vaccine used was later found to have been contaminated with a human tuberculosis strain being studied in same lab (Wilson G., 1931). All children were equally infected by Mtb – and some of them died, some of them – got sick with clinical TB, and 17.5% remained healthy, because they had good innate resistance to TB.

Factors leading to the increased incidence of tuberculosis include the high incidence of tuberculosis among the AIDS population, and the emergence of drug-resistant strains of tuberculosis (Gusmão et al., 1998; Fekak et al., 2003) TB with AIDS tends to occur in a younger population, is often extrapulmonary or with atypical lung involvement. Drug resistance is similar in patients with and without AIDS (Cremades Romero et al., 1998).

A cross-sectional study on extra pulmonary tuberculosis suspected patients was conducted at University of Gondar Hospital from January 2012 to April, 2012. The overall prevalence of smear positive EPTB was 34 (9.9%), and half of them (52.9%) were positive for human immunodeficiency virus. Of these cases of EPTB, lymph node tuberculosis constituted the largest proportion (82.4%). Previous history of tuberculosis (OR = 4.77, 95% CI 1.86-12.24), contact to a known tuberculosis cases (OR = 6.67 95% CI 2.78-16.90), history of underlying diseases (OR = 2.79 95% CI 1.15-6.78) and income (OR = 12.9 95% CI 2.25-68.02) were significantly associated with extra pulmonary tuberculosis infection (Zenebe *et al.*, 2013).

For UGTB poor prognostic factors included age over 65 years (HR = 4.03; 95%; CI: 1.27-12.76), cardiovascular disease (HR = 5.96; 95% CI: 1.98-17.92), receiving steroids (HR = 10.16; 95% CI: 2.27-45.47), not being treated (HR 4.81; 95% CI 1.12-20.67) (Hsu *et al.*, 2011).

Furthermore, infectious adverse events associated with intravesical instillation therapy with bacille Calmette-Guérin (BCG), which is one of the most useful agents against non-muscle invasive bladder cancer, are frequently developed (Wise & Marella, 2003; Drechsler & Kirch, 2010; Miyake & Fujisawa, 2011; Kulchavenya *et al.*, 2012). Congenital anomalies of urogenital tract, renal cysts, kidney transplantation and urolithiasis significantly increase a risk of development UGTB. The incidence of tuberculosis has been estimated to be as much as 10-fold higher among renal failure patients than among the general population (Chan *et al.*, 1996; Gusmão *et al.*, 1998; Kulchavenya & Muzyko, 2007; Korzeniewska A *et al.*, 2009; Rabbani *et al.*, 2011; Takeshita *et al.*, 2012).

5 Pathogenesis of TB infection

Most common route of transmissions of Mtb is respiratory one, when infectious can be spread by coughing, sneezing, laughing, singing, or just talking. Also alimentary transmission is possible – usually through milk from ill cows; direct and indirect physical contact, including sexual; iatrogenic transmission with BCG instillation for bladder cancer therapy; transplacental transmission (unusual); blood transmission through a mosquito bite - extremely rarely (Kulchavenya, 2009).

Independent of the route of infection Mtb are spread by bloodstream and lymphatic system throughout the body (so-called primary dissemination). Of course, direct contact more often leads to the skin TB, alimentary route – to intestinal TB, prostate TB may be a cause of a genital TB in sexual partner etc. But after respiratory contamination lungs may by intact, and kidney or lymphonodal TB develops, as well as TB meningitis after alimentary contamination is possible (Brühl & Walpert, 1989; Türkmen *et al.*, 2012). Very rare case of TB of placenta is shown below.

Case: Women 24 year, married, was examined in time of pregnancy by standard volume, was estimated as healthy. She had never any contact with TB infection. Delivery was in time, normal, physiological with healthy girl (weight 3200 g, length 51 sm). As in Russian Federation in big clinics placenta is investigated by histology normally in any case, placenta of our patient was investigated too. Patohistology revealed TB inflammation with cells of Pirogov-Langhans, and Mtb in the specimen, colored by Ziehl-Neelsen technique. Figures 1-2 demonstrate TB of placenta. In 3 month ultrasound investigation shown a calcified focus in the right ovarium. Baby remained well.

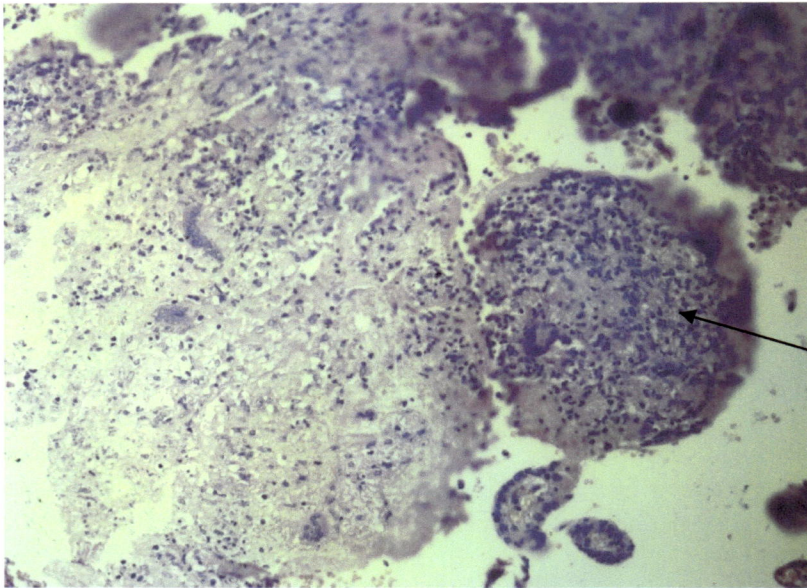

Figure 1: A large epithelioid-cell granuloma with caseous necrosis in the center (is shown by arrow). x100. Hematoxylin and eosin.

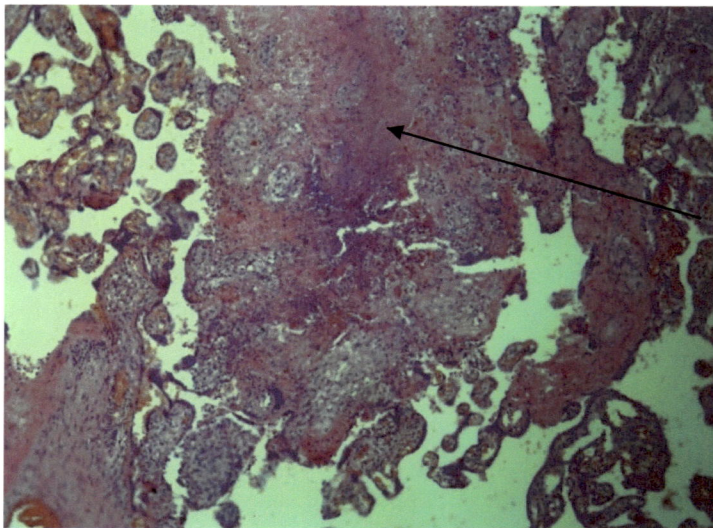

Figure 2: TB caseous necrosis masses (is shown by arrow). x100. Hematoxylin and eosin.

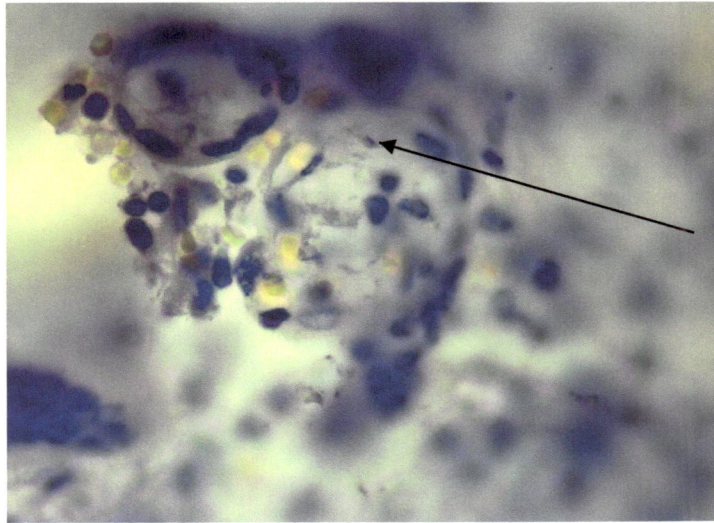

Figure 3: Numerous acid-fast bacilli within inflammed area (is shown by arrow). x1000. Ziehl-Neelsen.

6   Classification

For real estimation of epidemic level the disease should be in-time diagnosed and well classified. UGBT is an infectious disease of kidneys, urinary tract and male genitals, caused by M. tuberculosis. Clear definition and classification are necessary for correct therapy. Classification of any disease includes dispersion on forms and stages and exact definition for each stage. Each stage implies different approach to the management, so accurate classification is a base for good results of the therapy.

We proposed a following classification (Kulchavenya, 2004) of UGTB:

I. Kidney TB (KTB);

II. Male genital tuberculosis (MGTB);

III. Female genital tuberculosis (FGTB);

IV. Generalized UGTB when both kidneys and genitals are involved.

6.1   Kidney TB is divided on:

1 stage – non-destructive form, TB of parenchyma.

Tuberculosis of the renal parenchyma – minimal initial form of nondestructive nephrotuberculosis, when it is possible not only clinical, but also anatomic recovery. Urinalysis in children may be normal, although in adults may be found moderate leucocyturia. Radiographic signs of renal disease are absent. The structure of pelviocalyceal system is normal, destruction or retention are not assigned.

2 stage – small-destructive form, TB papillitis.

Tubercular papillitis may be one-and two-sided, single and multiple. M. tuberculosis in urine is not found always; usually is complicated by urinary tract tuberculosis. Should be cured by chemotherapy; with inadequate etiopathogenetic therapy ureteral strictures may form that require surgical correction. The prognosis is favorable.

3 stage – destructive form with one or two caverns (cavernous kidney TB).

Cavernous renal tuberculosis pathogenically develops by two ways - from tuberculosis of parenchyma or from papillitis. In the first case a subcortical cavity is forming, not associated with the CPS, the clinical picture is similar to renal carbuncle. Mostly such cavern is diagnosed after surgery. Cavernous nephrotuberculosis can be mono- and bilateral. If in one kidney tubercular papillitis is diagnosed, and in another - a cavern revealed, the case is classified as cavernous nephrotuberculosis, by more severe form of disease. The complications develop in more than a half of the patients. Usually cavernous nephrotuberculosis requires surgery (partial nephrectomy, plastic of ureter)

4 stage – widespread destructive form with more than 2 caverns (policavernous kidney TB).

Polycavernous renal tuberculosis presupposes occurrence of several cavities, which may lead to decreasing of renal function. As an extreme case, pyonephrosis may develop with the formation of the fistula. At the same time the self-recovery is possible, the so-called «kidney's autoamputation» - imbibition of caverns with calcium salts and complete obliteration of the ureter. Complications develop almost always, the contralateral kidney is often involved too. Usually is cured by radical operation.

5 stage – urinary tract tuberculosis (UTB) – secondary for KTB, includes TB of ureter, bladder TB of 1-4 grades, urethral TB. Bladder TB is divided on following grades:

- 1 *stage* – Infiltrative form - tubercles;

- 2 *stage* – Ulcerous form – erosive;

- 3 *stage* – spastic cystitis (false microcystis) actually overactive bladders;

- 4 *stage* - true microcystis, up to full shrinkage of the bladder.

Complications of KTB/UTB: strictures, fistula, renal failure, arterial hypertension.

6.2   Male Genital Tuberculosis (MGTB) is divided on:

- Orchiepidydimitis (mono- and bilateral)

- Prostate TB (infiltrative or cavernous forms)

- TB of seminal vesicles

- TB of penis

Complications of MGTB: strictures, fistula, infertility, sexual dysfunction.

Clinical features and symptoms significantly varied between different forms of UGTB. The approach to the therapy and management of UGTB should be differential. KTB 1-2 levels should be treated with chemotherapy, KTB 3 level may require partial nephrectomy, KTB 4 level is indicated for nephrectomy – by open surgery or laparoscopically. Stricture of ureter is indicated for reconstructive surgery only in KTB 1- 3 levels, KTB 4 level with stricture of ureter is indicated for nephrureterectomy. Bladder TB 1-2 grades should be treated by chemotherapy, bladder TB 3 grade requires additional prescription of trospium chloride, bladder TB grade 4 is indicated for cystectomy and reconstructive enteroplactic operation.

MGTB should be treated with chemotherapy; fistula, discharge sinus are indicated for surgery. Generalized UGTB is managed depending on forms of KTB and MGTB.

Chemotherapy for any form of UGTB includes initial intensive phase and continuation phase, which should be different accordingly clinical classification as well as drug sensibility of M.tuberculosis. For un-complicated KTB 1 level 6-month's standard chemotherapy with 4 anti-TB drugs (isoniazide (H), rifampicin (R), pyrazinamide (Z), streptomycin (S)) may be enough; KTB 2 level requires 8 months of the therapy, KTB 3-4 levels – more then 8, and S should me excluding from the scheme, but fluoroquinolones and PAS, cycloserin should be added as well as pathogenetic therapy.

Thus, UGTB is multivariant disease, and standard unified approach to it is impossible. Join term "UGTB" has insufficient information in order to estimate therapy, surgery and prognosis – as well as to evaluate the epidemiology. Uniform approach to the therapy and management of UGTB independently of clinical forms leads to poorer results, then individual one. Using clinical classification will improve the efficiency of the therapy of UGTB. Diagnosis "UGTB" as whole has a little information, it is insufficiently both for estimation of epidemiology and choosing of approach of the therapy. The clinical classification is simple and clear, it is enough for estimation of the form and stage of disease and for definition of correct optimal treatment.

7   Clinical Features

UGTB usually results from the reactivation of old, dormant tuberculous diseases by pathogens of the Mycobacterium tuberculosis complex. The diagnosis of tuberculosis of the urinary tract is based on the case history, the finding of pyuria in the absence of infection as judged by culture on routine media and by radiological imaging (Lenk, 2011). In the study of el Khader *et al.* (2001) the most frequent clinical symptoms were irritative symptoms (47.3%). Fever, anorexia and weight loss were rare (11%). 16% of patients had an isolated genital lesion. 14% presented with renal failure (mean serum creatinine: 18 mg/l). Only 5.2% presented with bacilluria. Urography showed abnormalities in 80% of cases. The most frequent abnormality was a non-functioning silent kidney in 40.3%. The clinical presentations of tuberculous epididymo-orchitis included scrotal mass (80%), scrotal pain (44%), micturition syndrome (8%), urethral discharge (4%), and scrotal fistula (4%). One third of the patients had pulmonary tuberculosis. Sixteen percents of the patients had underlying human immunodeficiency virus infection (Suankwan *et al.*, 2012). Benchekroun *et al.* (1998) analyzed 80 patients with UGTB between 1985 and 1995. These patients consisted of 50 males (62.5%) and 30 females (37.5%) with a mean age of 38 years (range: 20 to 50 years). Intravenous urography revealed silent kidney in 26% of cases, ureterohydronephrosis in 36% of cases, small bladder in 17% of cases, and was normal in only 5% of cases. Renal function was impaired in 32% of patients. The diagnosis was confirmed by a positive smear in the urine in 64% of cases, bladder biopsy in 20% of cases and pathological examination of the operative specimen in 20% of cases.

Urogenital tuberculosis raises major diagnostic problems due to the frequently atypical and misleading clinical features. It is a serious disease as the lesions are often multifocal and extensive, requiring major surgical resection and urinary tract reconstruction (Benchekroun *et al.*,1998). Diagnosis is often difficult because TB has a variety of clinical findings. It can mimic numerous other disease entities. A high level of clinical suspicion allows early diagnosis and timely initiation of proper management (Teo & Wee, 2011; Muttarak *et al.*, 2005). The nonspecific clinical features of UGTB make the early and accurate diagnosis of the disease difficult. Hematuria, lower urinary tract symptoms, flank pain, and scrotal swelling are the most common presenting features. Chronic epididymitis associated with a draining scrotal sinus is often associated with UGTB (Zarrabi & Heyns, 2009). The most presenting symptoms were polyuria, dysuria and acidic urinary pH with pyuria. 80% of the patients had abnormal imaging studies of the urinary system, with hydronephrosis being the most frequently found condition (Tanthanuch *et al.*, 2010). In review of 8961 cases from the world literature there was shown great difference between clinical features of UGTB in different regions depending on epidemic situation, advancing of country etc (Figueiredo & Lucon, 2008).

Patients usually exhibit local symptoms. Fever, weight loss and anorexia are uncommon. Eighty-nine percent of the patients had abnormal urinalysis: hematuria and/or pyuria (Kao *et al.*, 1996). Patients can present with unusual complaints not immediately suspicious for tuberculosis (Colbert *et al.*, 2012); this infection is easily overlooked unless clinicians maintain a strong awareness of its possibility (Patterson *et al.*, 2012). In Moscow UGTB manifested with chronic cystitis in 13.1%, subacute orchoepidydimitis in 13.1%, anatomofunctional alterations of the kidneys (hydronephrotic transformation, non-functioning kidney, ureteritis, etc.) in 28.5% of patients (Batyrov *et al.*, 2004). The diagnosis of renal TB can be hypothesized in a non-specific bacterial cystitis associated with a therapeutic failure or a urinalysis with a persistent leukocyturia in the absence of bacteriuria (Lima *et al.*, 2012). Non-optimal empiric therapy for urogenital tract infections (UTI) resulted in high level of co-morbidity UGTB and UTI, and old symptom "sterile pyuria" now lost its significance (Kulchavenya, 2010).

8   Laboratory Diagnosis

A delay in diagnosing UGTB is common and results in significant morbidity. Patients who are diagnosed at a late stage often have complications such as ureteral stricture with hydronephrosis, a shrunken bladder, autonephrectomy, or destruction of the testis by a cold abscess. This is unfortunate, because effective medical therapy is readily available (Zarrabi & Heyns, 2009).

Diagnostic of UGTB stays on 4 columns: bacteriology, pathohistology, radiology and provocative test with therapy ex juvantibus, but some simple and cheap tests may be useful too.

8.1   Urinalysis in the Diagnostic of UGTB

Urinalysis is the least invasive method of diagnosing UGTB. The classically described "sterile pyuria" is not very sensitive or specific for UGTB, but persisting sterile pyuria in an individual at risk should increase the clinician's index of suspicion (Zarrabi & Heyns, 2009).

The introduction of the 4-glass test according to Meares and Stamey (1968) was a great step forward to diagnose chronic prostatitis not only by symptoms, but also by investigation of segmented urine and prostatic secretion specimens to localize the inflammation/infection to the urethra, bladder or prostate (or any of these combinations). Thus, for many generations the Meares and Stamey 4-glass test was considered as "gold standard" and recommended not only for research but also for the general practicing urologist as routine test for diagnosing chronic prostatitis (Nickel, 2003). Unfortunately, one had to realize that these recommendations were not followed by several reasons, because the test is i) time consuming; ii) difficult to perform; iii) costly; and iv) bothersome for the patient (McNauhgton-Collins *et al.*, 2000).

This was mainly the reason why the pre-massage and post-massage 2-glass test (PPMT) was developed to facilitate the M&S 4-glass test (Nickel & Weidner, 2000; Nickel *et al.*, 2006). However, by the PPMT 2-glass test only the laboratory burden (cost) is reduced by reducing the number of specimens, but the discomfort for the patient remains the same, because the patient has to produce a midstream urine, interrupt micturition not to empty the bladder completely, because after the following prostatic massage by digital rectal examination (DRE) he is supposed to produce another urine specimen again during the same visit. First, not every patient can interrupt micturition before the bladder becomes empty. Second, voluntary stop of micturition converts laminar flow of urine in a turbulent one and thus provokes reflux of urine into the prostatic ducts, which is fraught with the risk to develop chemical burns, inflammation and prostatolithiasis. Another aspect using the M&S 4-glass test is probably even more serious. Patients assigned to the M&S 4-glass test are usually not informed that between VB1 and VB2 and thereafter continuous urination without interruption is necessary to produce a true midstream urine specimen which is necessary to i) diagnose concomitant cystitis and ii) serve also as basic comparative parameter by which localization of inflammation/infection to the urethra or prostate can be made possible. Interruption of urine flow between VB1 and VB2 and at the end of VB2 will lead to contraction of the prostate and thus contamination of urine with prostatic secretion.

We (Kulchavenya *et al*, 2011, 2012) developed a 3-glass test for screening of patients with clinical signs and symptoms of chronic prostatitis with the option of further tests for final diagnosis only in those patients where additional investigations are needed. This KE 3-glass test comprises three urine samples taken from only one continuous urine stream: VB1 comprises the first 10 ml, VB2 the midstream portion of a non interrupted stream, and VB3 the final portion at the very last end of the stream. As the prostate is a part of the external sphincter of the bladder, it contracts at the end of a micturition. Therefore the urine sample at the end of the micturition (VB3) corresponds practically to the urine sample after prostatic massage. However, the discomfort of prostatic massage by DRE can be avoided. Leucocyturia in the first portion (VB1) indicates an inflammation in the urethra, in the second portion (VB2) a general inflammation in the urinary bladder and/or upper urinary tract, and in the third portion (VB3) an inflammation in the prostate. Leucocyturia in all three portions may mirror inflammation of the total urinary system.

Therefore 3-glass test (i) allowed avoiding DRE for diagnosis of chronic prostatitis, and (ii) total leucocyturia is highly suspected on UGTB. Non-specific bacterial prostatitis as well as non-specific epididymitis very rare is accompanied by pyelonephritis. On contrary, MGTB combines with kidney TB in up to 80%. So patient with epididymitis and/or prostatitis, having pyuria in all 3 portions of urine is high suspicious on UGTB – if it is real pyuria, not contamination of urine by prostatic secretion, as inevitably in 4-glass test. In our study UGTB was revealed in patients with chronic prostatitis by 3-glass test in 1.8% (Kulchavenya *et al*, 2011).

8.2   Bacteriology

At least six specimens of urine, expressed prostatic secretion and ejaculate should be cultured, each onto at least three slants (Lowenstein - Jensen, Finn – II, Middlebrook 7H9-12) (Lenk, 2011). Nevertheless standard technique is positive in 36-57% of UGTB patients only (Kulchavenya, 2009; Batyrov *et al.*, 2004; Joo Yong Lee *et al.*, 2011; Tanthanuch *et al.*,2010). Positive cultures were by 15% higher, if sowing performed three times in one day (Zhuravlev *et al.*, 2012). 22,654 samples of urine were investigated by method of concentration and homogenization by Petroff and inoculated on Loewenstein culture media. All urine samples were taken from 4,192 patients. Positive culture was found in 358 urine samples (1.58%), in 173 patients (4.13%) (Nurkić, M., 2006). For MGTB diagnosis investigation in one day prostatic secretion, than post-massage urine, then ejaculate and post-ejaculate urine – by microscopy, culture and real-time polymerase chain reaction (PCR) each probe is recommended. Very important thing is the shortest time between collection of urine, prostatic secretion, and ejaculate and its sowing; optimal time should not be more than 40 min. (Kulchavenya, 2010). In order to identify mycobacteria and to perform antituberculous susceptibility tests, direct preparations stained with Ziehl – Nielsen (ZN) method to evaluate a smear microscopically or PCR method are insufficient; cultivation of mycobacteria is necessary (Aslan *et al.*, 2007). PCR was found to be useful in diagnosing early disease as well as confirming diagnosis in clinically suspected cases. False negative PCR was an important limitation in this technique (Thangappah *et al.*, 2011).

TB is an anthropozoonotic disease; it is a reason for possible cross-contamination human-animal and opposite (Dumonceaux *et al.*, 2011). Presence of Mycobacterium bovis in urine accounted for 4.2% - 12.5% of all UGTB cases (Blagodarnyĭ *et al.*, 1990; Berta *et al.*, 2011; Singh *et al.*, 2011).

To overcome the limitations of current urine-based diagnostic assays of UGTB, isothermal microcalorimetry was used to detect the metabolic activity of Mtb and other commonly neglected pathogenic mycobacteria in urine and accurately determine their growth parameters (Kumar *et al.*, 2012).

8.3   Pathohistology

One more problem of diagnosis of UGTB is loss of pathomorphological signs of TB, especially in co-morbidity with HIV-infection. For identification of Mtb biopsies and operation tissue should be investigated also by ZN method. Seventy eight tissue specimens (renal, prostate, epididymis, penile and soft tissue) from patients with clinically suspected UGTB were processed for both PCR and histopathological examination (HPE). In 87.1% samples, results for both PCR and HPE were coinciding. False positivity and false negativity was observed in 5.1% and 7.6% samples, respectively. With HPE as the gold standard, PCR has shown sensitivity of 87.5% and specificity of 86.7% and positive agreement between two tests was observed as significant. PCR results were obtained within a mean period of 3.4 days while those of HPE were obtained in 7.2 days. Authors concluded that tissue PCR is a sensitive and specific method for obtaining early and timely diagnosis of UGTB. Application of tissue PCR can augment the diagnostic accuracy in pathologically labelled granulomatous inflammations (Chawla *et al.*, 2012). In another study the possibility of the early rapid diagnosis of renal tuberculosis by PCR of renal biopsy specimens was estimated. It was found, that the sensitivity and specificity of real-time PCR were respectively 93.3% and 56.7%. The sensitivity and specificity of the urine M. tuberculosis culture were respectively 23.3% and 100% (Sun *et al.*, 2010).

There was no correlation between the histological findings and the mycobacteriological investigations. The investigation of tissue specimens on the presence of mycobacteria also from other organs of the urogenital tract is suitable method of the bacteriological proof of tuberculosis, especially in the absence or positive bacteriological findings from the urine or accessory gland secretion for the estimation of species and resistance of these bacteria (Lenk *et al.*, 1986).

It is necessary to keep in mind that biopsy for confirming UGTB by histology may have serious complications (Kulchavenya, 2010; Silva *et al.*, 2011) till generalization of TB in un-treated patient. Miliary TB was diagnosed in the patient resulting from the hematogenous spread following TRUS-guided prostate biopsy (Chul, 2011). Although sometimes biopsy may be useful in diagnostic UGTB (Shenoy *et al.*, 2012), and histologic follow-up was estimated as a good method for monitoring the efficacy of treatment. Transrectal prostate biopsy may be an important tool for the diagnosis and follow-up of prostatic tuberculosis (Lee *et al.*, 2011).

8.4   Radiology

Radiology is good method for diagnosis of UGTB – both prostate and kidney TB. Unfortunately this method is useful only for late cavernous forms, but our aim is early diagnosis. Pyelograms disclosed abnormalities in 94% and most revealed late changes (Kao *et al.*, 1996). Caverns of prostate and/or kidney are absolutely pathognomonic symptom, but caverns mean late-diagnosed complicated form, cavernous UGTB can't be cured by chemotherapy (Kulchavenya, 2010).

8.5   Provocation Test

In many cases provocation test with injection of 20-50-100 units of tuberculin subcutaneously may be useful. All laboratory investigations including body temperature are repeated 24 and 48 hours after tuberculin injection. The test is positive if leucocytosis, lymphocytopenia, leucocyturia, leucocytospermia and body temperature have increased by more than one degree. Also local reaction (hyperemia, induration in place of injection tuberculin) is to be taken into account. After provocative subcutaneous tuberculin test identification of MBT by culture or PCR increased by 16%. On the whole, this test improved the diagnosis of UGTB, especially the obscure, latent forms, to 63% (Kulchavenya & Kim, 2010).

8.6   Therapy ex Juvantibus

Therapy ex juvantibus may be 1st type, when patient receives antibiotic which doesn't inhibit Mtb, and 2nd type, when patient receives antibiotics which inhibit only Mtb (Kulchavenya, 2009). For therapy ex juvantibus 1st type fosfomycin, cefalosporins, and nitrofurantoin are suitable. For therapy ex juvantibus 2nd type we can use isoniazide, PAS, protionamide, etionamid, ethambutol, pyrazinamide. For good results of the therapy ex juvantibus pathognomonic therapy also is indicated: phytotherapy with canefron, non-steroid anti-inflammatory drugs etc (Kulchavenya and Kim, 2010).

9   Therapy

Drugs that can cure most TB patients have been available since the 1950s, yet TB remains the world's second most important cause of death by infectious diseases. Unfortunately, during about half a century none new drug was developed. In the same time resistance of Mtb has increased enormously. Mono-, poly, and multi-drug resistant Mtb to the basic antituberculous drugs was found in up to 52.2% of extrapulmonary TB patients and up to 78.7% in pulmonary TB patients (Kao *et al.*, 1996). Antituberculous drug treatment is based on an initial 2 month intensive phase with three or four drugs daily followed by a 4 month continuation phase with only two drugs (Lenk, 2011).

Medical treatment of genital TB is somewhat different from that of other TB, because prostatotropic drugs have to be preferred. In countries with low incidence of TB three antituberculous drugs with bactericidal activity may be sufficient for bacterial eradication and prevention of resistance. In epidemic regions patients with MGTB should be treated with four or five antituberculous drugs: isoniazid 10 mg/kg + rifampicin 10 mg/kg + pyrazinamid 20 mg/kg + streptomycin 15 mg/kg + PAS 150 mg/kg (or ofloxacin 800 mg or levofloxacin 500 mg daily) simultaneously for two to four months, followed by six to eight months of chemotherapy with isoniazid and rifampicin only (Kulchavenya, 2010).

WHO recommended reducing the treatment time to nine or six months with 4 drugs (isoniazid, rifampicin, pyrazinamid and streptomycin or ethambutol); in complicated or combined cases the length of the therapy may be 12-14 months. In cases of re-treatment, immunosuppression and HIV/AIDS the treatment time increases to nine or 12 months (World Health Organization, 2004; World Health Organization, 2008).

Chemotherapy for late-diagnosed complicated forms of UGTB is not enough effective, so surgery is indicated (Viswaroop et al., 2006). The organ-removing operations were conducted in 73% of patients (Batyrov et al., 2004). Surgery, whether in the acute setting (orchiectomy, nephrostomy) or after medical treatment (nephrectomy, cystoplasty), still plays an important role in the treatment of patients with UGTB (Zarrabi & Heyns, 2009).

To improve the chemotherapy for complicated form of UGTB with bladder involvement modified scheme was developed (Kulchavenya, 2010). "Modified" tetrad included isoniazid 10 mg/kg + rifampicin 10 mg/kg + pyrazinamid 20 mg/kg + ofloxacin 800 mg during 2 months. This was followed by a 6-10 months treatment with isoniazid and rifampicin only. In addition from the first day of the therapy all patients received trospium chloride 15 mg b.i.d during three months as pathogenetic treatment. The efficiency of modified tetrad was compared with results of the standard chemotherapy (isoniazid 10 mg/kg + rifampicin 10 mg/kg + pyrazinamid 20 mg/kg + streptomycin 15 mg/kg). The outcome analysis showed, that standard therapy was insufficient in more than a half of the cases: only 42.1% could be cured, 57.9% developed complications such as posttuberculous cystalgia (36.8%) and microcystis (21.1%). Patients treated by modified tetrad responded in a favourable manner: urinary frequency reduced about 75%, bladder capacity increased an average of 4.7 fold. Recovery was reached in 84.3%. Posttuberculous cystalgia developed in 15.7% only. None of the patients developed microcystis after the combined treatment. Tolerance to the treatment was good: only one patient had light side effect (mouth dryness).

10   Surgery

As UGTB is infection of the urogenital system, it should be cured by medicines, like any other UTI. And it may be cured – if it is diagnosed in-time, before development of destruction and caverns. Unfortunately, mostly due to late diagnostic, medical treatment may not result in resolution of symptoms. Surgical intervention and reconstruction of the urinary tract are frequently indicated (Viswaroop et al., 2006; Wise & Shteynshlyuger, 2008). The organ-removing operations were conducted in 73% of UGTB patients. Preoperative tuberculostatic therapy reduced frequency of postoperative complications. In early diagnosis, the organ was saved in operations in 9.4% only (Batyrov et al., 2004). It was found that such eradicative techniques as nephrectomy and nephruretherectomy still prevail. Early drainage of the kidney for its decompression allows preservation of the kidney and following reconstructive surgery in 70.6% of cases. The number of early and later complications have considerably decreased (Zuban' et al., 2008).

Bladder TB grade 4 (microcystis) is indicated for cystectomy following by enteroplastic (Kulchavenya and Krasnov, 2012; Kulchavenya et al., 2012). Urinary bladder rehabilitation either by augmentation cystoplasty or orthotopic neobladder reconstruction increases the bladder capacity and storage time and also preserves the upper tracts (Singh et al., 2010). Bladder and ureter reconstruction with ileum is a good option in difficult cases of lack or irreversible damage of the urinary way. Vesico-ureteral reconstruction letting urethral miction improves quality of life (Resina et al., 2009; Singh et al., 2010). Patients after full course of the therapy and, if it was indicated, surgery, should be under surveillance for 3-5 years with annual check-up and anti-relapse therapy, if necessary.

11   Conclusion

UGTB is enough often, but mostly overlooked disease. The main reasons for late diagnosis are lack of alertness on UGTB in urologists and general practitioners relative to patients with UTI, kidney anomalies, renal cysts etc; non-specific variable clinical features, decreasing positive cultures of Mtb due to non-optimal empiric therapy for UTI with prescribing of fluorquinilones and amycacin. Standard chemotherapy is effective only for early diagnosed form of UGTB, in complicated form modified scheme with 5 anti-TB drugs in combination with pathogenetic therapy is indicated. Destructive forms of kidney and male genital TB can't be cured by chemotherapy, the surgery is necessary.

EPTB cases include TB lymphadenitis, pleural TB, TB meningitis, osteoarticular TB, genitourinary TB, abdominal TB, cutaneous TB, ocular TB, TB pericarditis and breast TB, although any organ can be involved. Diagnosis of EPTB can be baffling, compelling a high index of suspicion owing to paucibacillary load in the biological specimens. A negative smear for acid-fast bacilli, lack of granulomas on histopathology and failure to culture Mycobacterium tuberculosis do not exclude the diagnosis of EPTB. Novel diagnostic modalities such as nucleic acid amplification (NAA) can be useful in varied forms of EPTB (Mehta *et al.*, 2012).

References

Abbara, A. & Davidson, R.N. Etiology and management of genitourinary tuberculosis. (2011). Nat Rev Urol. Dec 9;8(12):678-88. doi: 10.1038/nrurol.2011.172.

Ali, A.A. & Abdallah, T.M. (2012). Clinical presentation and epidemiology of female genital tuberculosis in eastern Sudan. Int J Gynaecol Obstet. Sep;118(3):236-8. doi: 10.1016/j.ijgo.2012.04.005. Epub 2012 Jun 20.

Alvarez, S. & McCabe, W.R. (1984). Extrapulmonary tuberculosis revisited: a review of experience at Boston City and other hospitals. Medicine (Baltimore). Jan;63(1):25-55.

Aslan, G., Doruk, E., Emekdaş, G, Serin, M.S., Direkel, S., Bayram, G., & Durmaz, R. (2007). Isolation and identification of Mycobacterium tuberculosis from the urine samples by conventional and molecular methods. Mikrobiyolojy Bulteni. April;41(2):185-192.

Aubry, P., Capdevielle, P., & Durand, G. (1979). Extrapulmonary tuberculosis in Africans. Med Trop (Mars). Mar-Apr;39(2):156-63.

Barry, C.E3rd., Boshoff, H.I., & Dartois, V. (2009). The spectrum of latent tuberculosis: rethinking the biology and intervention strategies. Nature Reviews Microbiology. 7, 845–855.

Batyrov, F.A., Nersesian, A.A., & Merkur'eva, Ia.A. (2004). Urogenital tuberculosis: problems of present-day diagnosis and treatment. Urologiia. September-October;(5):16-24.

Benchekroun, A., Lachkar, A., Soumana, A., Farih, M.H., Belahnech, Z., Marzouk, M., & Faik, M. (1998). Urogenital tuberculosis. 80 cases. Ann Urol (Paris). 32(2):89-94.

Berta, M., Sturm, G., Juri, L., Cosiansi, M.C., Barzón, S., Barnes, A.I., & Rojo, S.C. (2011). Bacteriological diagnosis of renal tuberculosis: an experience at the regional tuberculosis laboratory in Córdoba Province, Argentina. Revista Argentina de Microbiología. Jule-September;43(3):191-194.

Blagodarnyĭla, A., Alimbekova, O.A., & Blonskaia, L.I. (1990). Characteristics of Mycobacteria from patients with genital tuberculosis. Problemy tuberkuleza I bolezneĭ legkikh (1):37-41.

Brühl, P. & Walpert, J. (1989). Epidemiology and current treatment of urogenital tuberculosis. Offentl Gesundheitswes. Dec;51(12):749-55.

Chan, T.H., Ng, K.C., Ho, A., Scheel, O., Lai, C.K, & Leung, R. (1996). Urinary tract infection caused by Mycobacterium terrae complex. International Journal of Tuberculosis and Lung Disease. December; 77(6):555-557.

Chawla, A., Chawla, K., Reddy, S., Arora, N., Bairy, I., Rao, S., Hegde, P., & Thomas, J. (2012). Can tissue PCR augment the diagnostic accuracy in genitourinary tract tuberculosis? Urologia Internationalis. 88(1):34-38.

Colbert, G., Richey, D., & Schwartz, J.C. (2012). Widespread tuberculosis including renal involvement. Proceedings (Baylor University. Medical Center). July;25(3):236-239.

Cremades Romero, M.J., Menéndez Villanueva, R., Santos Durántez, M., Martínez García, M.A., Ferrando García, D., & Perpiñá Tordera, M. (1998). Characteristics of tuberculosis in a tertiary hospital during the years 1993-1996. Influence of the coinfection with HIV. Archivos de bronconeumología. July-August;34(7):333-338.

Daher, Ede. F., da Silva, G.B. Jr., & Barros, E.J. (2013). Renal tuberculosis in the modern era. Am J Trop Med Hyg. Jan;88(1):54-64. doi: 10.4269/ajtmh.2013.12-0413.

Drechsler, A., & Kirch, W. (2010). Urinary bladder tuberculosis and bacillus calmette-guérin instillation: reduced efficacy of bisoprolol in hypertension. Aktuelle Urologie. November;41(6):372-374.

Dumonceaux, G.A., St Leger, J., Olsen, J.H., Burton, M.S., Ashkin, D., & Maslow, J.N. (2011). Genitourinary and pulmonary multidrug resistant Mycobacterium tuberculosis infection in an Asian elephant (Elephasmaximus). Journal of zoo and wildlife medicine. December; 42(4):709-12.

Didilescu, C. & Tănăsescu, M. (2012). Proportion and site distribution of extrarespiratory tuberculosis in 2007-2010 in Romania. Pneumologia. Jan-Mar;61(1):10-4.Dwyer, D.E., McLeod, C., Collignon, P.J., & Sorrell, T.C. (1987). Extrapulmonary tuberculosis—a continuing problem in Australia. Australian and New Zealand journal of medicine. October;17(5):507-11.

el Khader, K., Lrhorfi, M.H., el Fassi, J., Tazi, K., Hachimi, M., & Lakrissa, A. (2001). Urogenital tuberculosis. Experience in 10 years. Prog Urol. Feb;11(1):62-7.

Fekak, H., Rabii, R., Moufid, K., Joual, A., Debbag, A., Bennani, A., Mrini, M. El., & Benjelloun, S. (2003). A rare cause of obstructive acute renal failure: urogenital tuberculosis. Annales d'urologie. 37: 71-74

Figueiredo, A.A., & Lucon, A.M. (2008). Urogenital tuberculosis: update and review of 8961 cases from the world literature. Nature reviews. Urology. Summer; 10(3):207-17.

García-Rodríguez, J.F., Álvarez-Díaz, H., Lorenzo-García, M.V., Mariño-Callejo, A., Fernández-Rial, Á.,& Sesma-Sánchez, P. (2011). Extrapulmonary tuberculosis: epidemiology and risk factors. Enferm Infecc Microbiol Clin. Aug-Sep;29(7):502-9.

Gómez García, I., Gómez Mampaso, E., Burgos Revilla, J., Molina, M.R., Sampietro Crespo, A., Buitrago, L.A., Gómez Rodríguez, A., & Baquero, F. (2010). Tuberculous orchiepididymitis during 1978-2003 period: review of 34 cases and role of 16S rRNA amplification. Urology. October; 76(4):776-81. Epub 2010 Mar 29.

Gunal, S., Yang, Z., Agarwal, M., Koroglu, M., Arıcı, Z.K., & Durmaz, R. (2011). Demographic and microbial characteristics of extrapulmonary tuberculosis cases diagnosed in Malatya, Turkey, 2001-2007. BMC Public Health. Mar 8;11:154. doi: 10.1186/1471-2458-11-154.

Gusmão, L., Galvão, J., & Alfarroba. E. (1998). Tuberculosis and the kidney. Acta médica portuguesa. December;11(12):1107-11.

Hsu, H.L., Lai, C.C., Yu, M.C., Yu, F.L., Lee, J.C., Chou, C.H., Tan, C.K., Yang, P.C., & Hsueh, P.R. (2011). Clinical and microbiological characteristics of urine culture-confirmed genitourinary tuberculosis at medical centers in Taiwan from 1995 to 2007. Eur J Clin Microbiol Infect Dis. Mar;30(3):319-26. doi: 10.1007/s10096-010-1083-z. Epub 2010 Oct 15.

Kao, S.C., Fang, J.T., Tsai, C.J., Chen, K.S., & Huang, C.C. (1996). Urinary tract tuberculosis: a 10-year experience. Chang Gung medical journal. March; 19(1):1-9.

Kim, C.J., Sano, T., & Takimoto, K. (2011). Miliary Tuberculosis Following Transrectal Ultrasonography (TRUS)-Guided Prostate Biopsy. Korean Journal of Urology. 52:425-427

Khanna, A., & Agrawal, A. (2011). Markers of genital tuberculosis in infertility. Singapore medical journal. December; 52(12):864-7.

Korzeniewska, A., Dyła, T., Kosacka, M., & Jankowska, R. (2009). Tuberculosis after renal transplantation. Pneumonologiaialergologiapolska. 77(1):61-5.

Kulchavenya, E. (2009) Tuberculosis of urogenital system in Urology: National Manual. In: Lopatkin N (ed) Geotar-Media, Moscow.pp 584–601

Kulchavenya, E. (2010). Some aspects of Urogenital Tuberculosis. International Journal Nephrology and Urology, 2(2): 351-360

Kul'chavenia, E.V., Azizov, A.P., Brizhatiuk, E.V., Breusov, &A.A., Kholtobin, D.P. (2011). A comparative study of efficacy of 2-, 3- and 4-glass tests in patients with chronic prostatitis. Urologiia. November-December; (6):42-5.

Kulchavenya, E., Kholtobin, D., & Filimonov, P. (2012). Natural and Iatrogenic Bladder Tuberculosis: Two Cases. Mycobacterial Diseases2:110. doi:10.4172/2161-1068.1000110

Kulchavenya, E., & Kim, C.S. (2009). Male genital tuberculosis. In: Naber KG, Schaeffer AJ, Heyns CF, Matsumoto T, Shoskes DA, Bjerklund JohansesTE(eds.) International Consultation on Urogenital Infections. Stockholm, Sweden, March. European Association of Urology - International Consultation on Urological Diseases, Edition 2010, Arnhem, The Netherlands, ISBN: 978-90-79754-41-0, pp. 877-891.

Kulchavenya, E., Kim, C.S., Bulanova, O., & Zhukova, I. (2012). Male genital tuberculosis: epidemiology and diagnostic. World Journal of urology. February ;30(1):15-21. Epub 2011 May21. Review.

Kulchavenya, E.V., & Krasnov, V.A. (2010). Selected Issue of Phthysiourology (monograph.). – Novosibirsk, "Nauka" ("Science") – ISBN 978-5-02-023313-3.

Diseases of urinary bladder /ed. Kulchavenya, E., & Krasnov V. (2012). – Novosibirsk: "Nauka" ("Science"), 187 p. ISBN 978-5-02-019008-5

Kulchavenya, E., & Muzyko, L. (2007). Two cases of tuberculosis after transplantation of the kidney. Urologiia. November-December;(6): 80-82.

Kulchavenya, E., Azizoff, A., Brizhatyuk, E., Khomyakov, V., Kholtobin, D., Breusoff, A. & Naber, K.G. (2012). Improved diagnostics of chronic inflammatory prostatitis. Minerva Urol Nephrol; 64:273-8.

Kulchavenya, E. (2013). Urogenital tuberculosis, an often overlooked infection / E. Kulchavenya // Int J of Antimicrobial Agents, vol.42, suppl.2, s6.

Kulchavenya, E., Koveshnikova, E. & Zhukova, I. Clinical and epidemic peculiarities of current tuberculous spondylitis (2013). Tuberkulez and Bolezni legkih; 1:41-45.

Kulshrestha, V., Kriplani, A., Agarwal, N., Singh, U.B., & Rana, T. (2011). Genital tuberculosis among infertile women and fertility outcome after antitubercular therapy. International journal of gynecology and obstetrics. Jun; 113(3):229-34.

Kumar, V., Jha, V., & Sakhuja, V. (2012). Putty kidney. Iranian journal of kidney diseases. July;6(4):255.

Lee, Y., Huang, W., Huang, J., Wang, J., Yu, C., Jiaan, B., & Huang, J. (2001). Efficacy of chemotherapy for prostatic tuberculosis-a clinical and histologic follow-up study. Urology. May;57(5):872-7.

Lee, J.Y., Park, H.Y., Park, S.Y., Lee, S.W., Moon, H.S., Kim, Y.T., Lee, T.Y., & Park, H.Y. (2011). Clinical Characteristics of Genitourinary Tuberculosis during a Recent 10-Year Period in One Center. Korean journal of urology. 52:200-205

Lenk, S. (2011). Genitourinary tuberculosis in Germany: diagnosis and treatment. Der Urologe. Ausg. A. December; 50(12):1619-27.

Lenk, S., Kalich, R., & Rothkopf, M. (1986). Detection of mycobacteria in tissue in urogenital tuberculosis. Zeitschrift für Urologie und Nephrologie. December;79(12):709-16.39.

Lenk, S., & Schroeder, J. (2001). Genitourinary tuberculosis. Current opinion in urology. January;11(1):93-8.

Lin, J.N., Lai, C.H., Chen, Y.H., Lee, S.S., Tsai, S.S., Huang, C.K., Chung, H.C., Liang, S.H., & Lin, H.H. (2009). Risk factors for extra-pulmonary tuberculosis compared to pulmonary tuberculosis. Int J Tuberc Lung Dis. May;13(5):620-5.

Lima, N.A, Vasconcelos, C.C., Filgueira, P.H., Kretzmann, M., Sindeaux, T.A., FeitosaNeto, B., Silva Junior, G.B., & Daher, E.F. (2012). Review of genitourinary tuberculosis with focus on end-stage renal disease. Revista do Instituto de Medicina Tropical de São Paulo. January-February;54(1):57-60.

Margolis, K., Wranz, P.A., Kruger, T.F., Joubert, J.J., & Odendaal, H.J. (1992). Genital tuberculosis at Tygerberg Hospital--prevalence, clinical presentation and diagnosis. S Afr Med J. Jan 4;81(1):12-5.

Mazza-Stalder, J., Nicod, L., & Janssens, J.P. (2012). Extrapulmonary tuberculosis. Rev Mal Respir. Apr;29(4):566-78. doi: 10.1016/j.rmr.2011.05.021. Epub 2012 Mar 29.

McNaughton-Collins, M., Fowler, F.J., & Elliott, D.B. (2000). Diagnosing and treating chronic prostatitis: do urologists use the four-glass test? Urology 55:403 – 407.

Meares, E.M. Jr., & Stamey, T.A. (1968). Bacteriologic localization patterns in bacterial prostatitis and urethritis.Investigative urology. 5:492

Mehta, P.K., Raj, A., Singh, N., & Khuller, G.K. (2012). Diagnosis of extrapulmonary tuberculosis by PCR. FEMS Immunol Med Microbiol. Oct;66(1):20-36. doi: 10.1111/j.1574-695X.2012.00987.x. Epub 2012 Jun 29.

Miyake, H., & Fujisawa, M. (2011). Tuberculosis in urogenital organs. Rinshō shimyurēshon kenkyū. August;69(8):1417-21.

Mondal, S.K. & Dutta, T.K. (2009). A ten year clinicopathological study of female genital tuberculosis and impact on fertility. JNMA J Nepal Med Assoc. Jan-Mar;48(173):52-7.

Mondal S.K. (2013). Histopathologic analysis of female genital tuberculosis: a fifteen-year retrospective study of 110 cases in eastern India. Turk Patoloji Derg. 29(1):41-5. doi: 10.5146/tjpath.2013.01146.

Muttarak, M., ChiangMai, W.N., & Lojanapiwat, B. (2005). Tuberculosis of the genitourinary tract: imaging features with pathological correlation. Singapore medical journal. October;46(10):568-74; quiz 575.

Nickel, J.C. (2003). Recommendations for the evaluation of patients with prostatitis. World journal of urology. 21(2):75-81.

Nickel, J.C., Shoskes, D., Wang, Y., Alexander, R.B., Fowler, J.E. Jr, Zeitlin, S., O'Leary, M.P., Pontari, M.A., Schaeffer, A.J., Landis, J.R., Nyberg, L., Kusek, J.W., & Propert, K.J. (2006). How does the pre-massage and post-massage 2-glass test compare to the Meares-Stamey 4-glass test in men with chronic prostatitis/chronic pelvic pain syndrome? The Journal of urology;176(1):119-24.

Nickel, J.C. (2000). Prostatitis: lessons from the 20th century. British Journal of Urology International Jan;85(2):179-85.

Nurkić, M. (2006). Frequency of microbiologicaly diagnosed urinary system tuberculosis in Tuzla canton area. Med Arh. 60(6 Suppl 2):66-70.

Patterson, I.Y., Robertus, L.M., Gwynne, R.A., & Gardiner, R.A. (2012). Genitourinary tuberculosis in Australia and New Zealand. BJU international. April;109Suppl 3:27-30.

Peto, H.M., Pratt, R.H., Harrington, T.A., LoBue, P.A., & Armstrong, L.R. (2009). Epidemiology of extrapulmonary tuberculosis in the United States, 1993-2006. Clinical infectious diseases. November 1;49(9):1350-7.

Porter, M. III. (1894). Uro-Genital Tuberculosis in the Male. Annals of surgery. 20(4): 396-405.

Rabbani, M.A, Ahmed, B., & Khan, M.A. (2011). Mycobacterium tuberculosis infection of a native polycystic kidney following renal transplantation. Transplant infectious disease. February;13(1):44-6. Epub 2010 Sep 1.

Resina, R.G., Ruiz, B.C., López, R.A., & Romero, F.J. (2009). Complete vesico-ureteral reconstruction with ileum in a case of genitourinary Tuberculosis. Acta surologica sespañolas. June;33(6):706-11.

Sharma, J.B., Roy, K.K., Pushparaj, M., Kumar, S., Malhotra, N., & Mittal, S. (2008). Laparoscopic findings in female genital tuberculosis. Arch Gynecol Obstet. Oct;278(4):359-64. doi: 10.1007/s00404-008-0586-7. Epub 2008 Feb 14.

Shenoy, V.P., Viswanath, S., D'Souza, A., Bairy, I., &Thomas J. (2012). Isolated tuberculous epididymo-orchitis: an unusual presentation of tuberculosis. J Infect Dev Ctries. Jan 12;6(1):92-4.

Scherban, M. & Kulchavenya, E.V. (2008). Prostate tuberculosis – new sexually transmitted disease. European Journal of Sexology and Sexual Health; Vol. 17 Suppl 1; S 163.

Shcherban', M.N., Kul'chavenia, E.V., Brizhatiuk, E.V., Kaveshnikova, E.Yu., & Sveshnikova, N.N. (2008). Male and female genital tuberculosis. Reproductive function in a patientwith tuberculosis. Problemy tuberkuleza I bolezneĭ legkikh.;(9):3-6. Review. Russian.

Shenoy, V.P., Viswanath, S., D'Souza, A., Bairy, I., & Thomas, J. (2012). Isolated tuberculousepididymo-orchitis: an unusual presentation of tuberculosis. Journal of infection in developing countries. January 12;6(1):92-4.

Silva, G.E., Costa, R.S., & Dantas, M. (2011). Secondary amyloidosis associated with tuberculosis in renal biopsy. Revista da Socieda de Brasileira de Medicina Tropical. November-December;44(6):797.

Singh, D.D., Vogel, M., Müller-Stöver, I., El Scheich, T., Winzer, M., Göbels, S., Hüttig, F., Heinrich, S., Mackenzie, C., Jensen, B., Reuter, S., Häussinger, D., & Richter, J. (2011). TB or not TB? Difficulties in the diagnosis of tuberculosis in HIV-negative immigrants to Germany. European journal of medical research. September 12;16(9):381-4.

Singh, V., Sinha, R.J., Sankhwar, S.N., & Sinha, S.M. (2011). Reconstructive surgery for tuberculosis contracted bladder: experience of a center in northern India. International urology and nephrology. June;43(2):423-30. Epub 2010 August 3.

Singh, J.P., Priyadarshi, V., Kundu, A.K., Vijay, M.K., Bera, M.K., & Pal, D.K. (2013). Genito-urinary tuberculosis revisited--13 years' experience of a single centre. Indian J Tuberc. Jan;60(1):15-22.

Snider, D.E. Jr. (1975). Extrapulmonary tuberculosis in Oklahoma, 1965 to 1973. Am Rev Respir Dis. May;111(5):641-6.

Sreeramareddy, C.T., Panduru, K.V., Verma, S.C., Joshi, H.S., & Bates, M.N. (2008). Comparison of pulmonary and extrapulmonary tuberculosis in Nepal- a hospital-based retrospective study. BMC Infect Dis. Jan 24;8:8. doi: 10.1186/1471-2334-8-8.

Suankwan, U., Larbcharoensub. N., Viseshsindh, W., Wiratkapun, C., & Chalermsanyakorn, P. (2012). A clinicopathologic study of tuberculous epididymo-orchitis in Thailand. Southeast Asian J Trop Med Public Health. Jul;43(4):951-8.

Sun, L., Yuan, Q., Feng, J.M., Yang, C.M., Yao, L., Fan, Q.L., Liu, L.L., Ma, J.F., & Wang, L.N. (2010). Rapid diagnosis in early stage renal tuberculosis by real-time polymerase chain reaction on renal biopsy specimens. The international journal of tuberculosis and lung disease. March;14(3):341-6.

Takeshita, H., Amemiya, M., Chiba, K., Urushibara, M., Satoh,J., & Noro, A. (2012). Disseminated kidney tuberculosis complicating autosomal dominant polycystic kidney disease: a case report. Clinical nephrology. March;77(3):242-5.

Teo, E.Y. & Wee, T.C. (2011). Images in clinical medicine: Renal tuberculosis The New England journal of medicine. September 22;365(12):e26.

Thangappah, R.B., Paramasivan, C.N., & Narayanan, S. (2011). The Indian journal of medical research. July;134:40-6.

Tanthanuch, M., Karnjanawanichkul, W., & Pripatnanont C. (2010). Tuberculosis of the urinary tract in southern Thailand. Journal of the Medical Association of Thailand. August;93(8):916-9.

Türkmen, I.C., Başsüllü, N., Comunoğlu, C., Bağcı, P., Aydın, O., Comunoğlu, N., Gezer, A., Calay, Z., & Ilvan, S. (2012). Female genital system tuberculosis: a retrospective clinicopathological study of 1,548 cases in Turkish women. Arch Gynecol Obstet. Aug;286(2):379-84. doi: 10.1007/s00404-012-2281-y. Epub 2012 Mar 13.

Tzvetkov, D. & Tzvetkova, P. (2006). Tuberculosis of male genital system--myth or reality in 21st century. Archives of andrology. September-October;52(5):375-81.

Vilar, F.C., Neves, F.F., Colares, J.K., & da Fonseca, B.A. (2006). Spinal tuberculosis (Pott's disease) associated to psoas abscess: report of two cases and a literature review. Rev Soc Bras Med Trop. May-Jun;39(3):278-82.

Wildbolz, H. (1937). Ueberurogenicaltuberkulose. Schweizerischemedizinische Wochenschrift. 67: 1125.

Wiler, J.L., Shalev, R., & Filippone, L. (2010). Case report and review: Potts disease and epididymal tuberculosis presenting as back pain and scrotal mass. Am J Emerg Med. Feb;28(2):261.e3-6. doi: 10.1016/j.ajem.2009.06.015.

Wilson G. (1931). The Lubeck disaster. Am J Public Health Nations Health. March; 21(3): 282.

Wise, G.J. & Marella, V.K. (2003). Genitourinary manifestations of tuberculosis. The Urologic clinics of North America. February;30(1):111-21.

Wise, G.J. & Shteynshlyuger, A. (2008). An update on lower urinary tract tuberculosis. Current urology reports. July;9(4):305-13.

Viswaroop, B., Gopalakrishnan, G., Nath, V., & Kekre, N.S. (2006). Role of imaging in predicting salvageability of kidneys in urinary tract tuberculosis. The Journal of the Pakistan Medical Association. December;56(12):587-90.

World Health Organization, Treatment of tuberculosis : guidelines for national programmes. Revision approved by STAG, June 2004. 3rd edition 2004, Geneva: World Health Organization. vii, 43 p.

World Health Organization. Guidelines for the programmatic management of drug resistant tuberculosis— emergency update 2008. Available from: http://www.who.int/tb/publications/2008/programmatic_guidelines_for_mdrtb/en/index.html. Accessed October 22, 2008.

Zarrabi, A.D. & Heyns, C. F. (2009). Clinical Features of Confirmed Versus Suspected Urogenital Tuberculosis in Region With Extremely High Prevalence of Pulmonary Tuberculosis.Urology. July; 74(1):41-5. Epub 2009 May 9.

Zenebe, Y., Anagaw, B., Tesfay, W., Debebe, T., & Gelaw, B. (2013). Smear positive extra pulmonary tuberculosis disease at University of Gondar Hospital, Northwest Ethiopia. BMC Res Notes. Jan 18;6:21. doi: 10.1186/1756-0500-6-21.

Zhuravlev, V.N., Golubev, D.N., Novikov, B.I., Skorniakov, S.N., Medvinskiĭ, I.D., Arkanov, L.V., Cherniaev, I.A., Borodin, É.P., Verbetskiĭ, A.F., & Bobykin, E.N. (2012). Particular features of detection of patients with urogenital tuberculosis and their management. Urologiia. January-February;(1):11-5.

Zuban', O.N., Murav'ev, A.N. & Volkov, A.A. (2008). Surgical treatment of nephrotuberculosis in the present-day epidemiological situation. Vestnik khirurgii imeni I. I. Grekova.; 167(1):92-5.

Sequence Analysis of Mycobacterial PE/PPE Proteins

Veeky Baths
Department of Biological Sciences
Birla Institute of Technology & Science (BITS) Pilani, Goa, India

Utpal Roy
Department of Biological Sciences,
Birla Institute of Technology & Science (BITS) Pilani, Goa, India

1   Background

In bioinformatics, a sequence alignment is a way of arranging the sequences of DNA, RNA, or protein to identify regions of similarity that may be a consequence of functional, structural, or evolutionary relationships between the sequences (Mount, 2004). Aligned sequences of nucleotide or amino acid residues are typically represented as rows within a matrix. Gaps are inserted between the residues so that identical or similar characters are aligned in successive columns.

Pair wise sequence alignment methods are used to find the best-matching piecewise (local) or global alignments of two query sequences. Pair wise alignments can only be used between two sequences at a time, but they are efficient to calculate and are often used for methods that do not require extreme precision (such as searching a database for sequences with high similarity to a query). The three primary methods of producing pair wise alignments are dot-matrix methods, dynamic programming, and word methods, however, multiple sequence alignment techniques can also align pairs of sequences. Although each method has its individual strengths and weaknesses, all three pair wise methods have difficulty with highly repetitive sequences of low information content - especially where the number of repetitions differ in the two sequences to be aligned. One way of quantifying the utility of a given pair wise alignment is the 'maximum unique match', or the longest subsequence that occurs in both query sequence. Longer MUM sequences typically reflect closer relatedness.

The complete genome sequences of *M. tuberculosis* (H37Rv strain) consists of 4,411,529 base pairs and approximately 3,986 proteins (Cole *et al.*, 1998) and the CDC1551 strain consists of 4,403,836 base pairs and approximately 4,187 proteins (Fleischmann *et al.*, 1995). Nearly 10% of the proteins in each of these genomes encode the PPE and PE protein families (Cole *et al* 1998). The names PE and PPE derived from the amino acid sequence motifs Pro-Glu (PE) and Pro-Pro-Glu (PPE) located near the N-terminus in a majority of these proteins. Members of the PE and PPE protein families are characterized by highly conserved N-terminal domains with approximately 110 and 180 amino acid residues, respectively. The C-terminus, however, varies considerably in sequence and the number of amino acid residues. This family of proteins were also identified in the *Mycobacterium leprae* genome (Cole et al., 2001). These two protein groups have been analysed and their phylogenetic analysis has been done.

2   Materials and Methods

2.1   Sequence Alignment and BLAST

Sequence alignment means placing one sequence over other and creating a correspondence between characters or spaces in the first sequence and characters in the second sequence.

Sequence comparison can be done to observe patterns of conservation (or variability), find the common motifs present in both sequences, to assess whether it is likely that two sequences evolved from the same sequence and to find out which sequences from the database are similar to the sequence at hand. Sequence analysis basically includes five biologically relevant topics:

I. Identification of reading frame, ORF, distributions of introns and exons and regulatory elements

II. The comparison of sequence in order to find similar sequence

III. Prediction of protein structures

IV. Genome mapping

V. Comparison of homologous sequences to construct molecular phylogeny

There are two types of sequence alignment: Global and local sequence alignment. Global sequence alignment is the best alignment over the entire length of two sequences suitable when the two sequences are of similar length, with a significant degree of similarity throughout. Local alignment involves stretches that are shorter than the entire sequences, possibly more than one and this is suitable when comparing substantially different sequences, which possibly differ significantly in lengths.

Dynamic programming is used to find alignment between two sequences. Three steps which are used to find the optimal alignment are as as follows:

1. Initialization

2. Matrix fill (scoring)

3. Trace back (alignment)

One possible solution of the matrix fill step finds the maximum global alignment score by starting in the upper left hand corner in the matrix and finding the maximal score $M_{i,j}$ for each position in the matrix (Needleman $et\ al.$, 1970). In order to find $M_{i,j}$ for any i,j it is minimal to know the score for the matrix positions to the left, above and diagonal to i, j. In terms of matrix positions, it is necessary to know $M_{i-1,j}$, $M_{i,j-1}$ and $M_{i-1,j-1}$.

For each position, $M_{i,j}$ is defined to be the maximum score at position i, j; $i.e.$,

$$M_{i,j} = \text{MAXIMUM} \begin{cases} M_{i-1,j-1} + S_{i,j} \text{ (match/mismatch in the diagonal)}, \\ M_{i,j-1} + w \text{ (gap in sequence \#1)}, \\ M_{i-1,j} + w \text{ (gap in sequence \#2)}. \end{cases}$$

Fortunately statistics for the scores of local alignments, unlike those of global alignments, are well understood. This is particularly true for local alignments lacking gaps, which we will consider first. Such alignments were precisely those sought by the original BLAST database search programs (Altschul $et\ al$, 1990). Just as the sum of a large number of independent identically distributed (i.i.d) random variables tends to a normal distribution, the maximum of a large number of i.i.d. random variables tends to an extreme value distribution (Gumbel, 1958).

In the limit of sufficiently large sequence lengths m and n, the statistics of high scoring pairs scores are characterized by two parameters, K and $lambda$. Most simply, the expected number of HSPs:

$$E = Kmne^{-\lambda S}. \tag{1}$$

The statistics described above tend to be somewhat conservative for short sequences. The theory supporting these statistics is an asymptotic one, which assumes an optimal local alignment can begin with any aligned pair of residues. However, a high-scoring alignment must have some length, and therefore cannot begin near to the end of either of two sequences being compared. This "edge effect" may be corrected for by calculating an "effective length" for sequences (Altschul & Gish, 1996); the BLAST programs implement such a correction. For sequences longer than about 200 residues the edge effect correction is usually negligible.

3   Results and Discussion

PPE and PE proteins in *M. tuberculosis* genome were selected for the analysis. Three PPE proteins (Rv1800, Rv3539 and Rv2608) showed sequence similarity corresponding to their C-terminal regions (Adindla & Guruprasad, 2003). BLAST program was used for this analysis. Figure 6.1 shows the amino acid composition in *M. Paratuberculosis.*

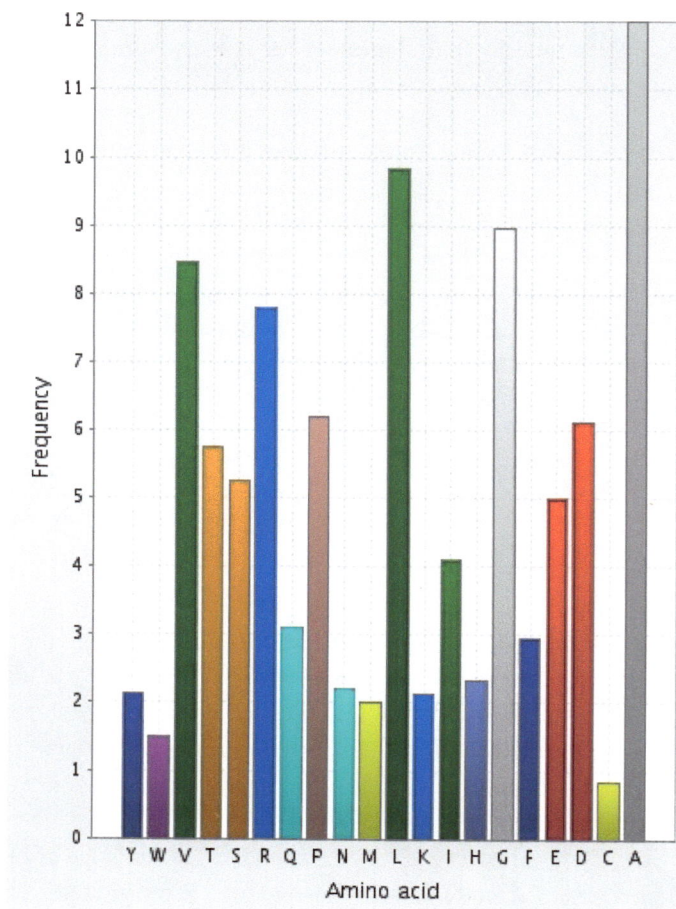

Figure 1: Amino acid compositions in *M. paratuberculosis*

The detailed genome-wide sequence analysis indicated that the PE-PPE domain comprising proteins are present in all mycobacterial genomes. In addition, the PE-PPE domain is also present in hypothetical proteins of some actinobacteria. Further, the presence of ten distinct genes comprising the PE-PPE domain as paralogs in *M. tuberculosis* strain H37Rv is an example of gene duplication. Reconnaissance of the results obtained, indicate that this organism, in order to survive under the selective pressure of the host or environment, the pre-existing genes underwent duplication followed by mutations and rearrangements to cater to the new requirements instead of the synthesizing new genes.

A5WRY5	A5WRY5_MYCTF	unreviewed	Serine/threonine-protein kinase transcriptional regulatory protein pknK	M.tuberculosis (strain F11)	1110	34.00%	86	0.5
A5U795	A5U795_MYCTA	unreviewed	Serine/threonine protein kinase / MalT-related protein	M.tuberculosis (strain ATCC 25177 / H37Ra)	1110	34.00%	86	0.5
A1KN78	A1KN78_MYCBP	unreviewed	Probable serine/threonine-protein kinase transcriptional regulatory protein pknK (EC 2.7.1.-)	Mycobacterium bovis (strain BCG / Pasteur 1173P2)	1110	34.00%	86	0.5
E2WLM5	E2WLM5_MYCTU	unreviewed	Putative uncharacterized protein	M.tuberculosis SUMu012	807	34.00%	86	0.5
E2W9I9	E2W9I9_MYCTU	unreviewed	Serine/threonine-protein kinase transcriptional regulator pknK	M.tuberculosis SUMu011	1110	34.00%	86	0.5
E2W7V3	E2W7V3_MYCTU	unreviewed	Putative PE family protein (Fragment)	M.tuberculosis SUMu011	105	32.00%	86	0.5
E2VYD3	E2VYD3_MYCTU	unreviewed	Serine/threonine-protein kinase transcriptional regulator pknK	M.tuberculosis SUMu010	1110	34.00%	86	0.5
E2VLR1	E2VLR1_MYCTU	unreviewed	Serine/threonine-protein kinase transcriptional regulator pknK	M.tuberculosis SUMu009	1110	34.00%	86	0.5
E2VCP5	E2VCP5_MYCTU	unreviewed	Serine/threonine-protein kinase transcriptional regulator pknK	M.tuberculosis SUMu008	1110	34.00%	86	0.5
E2V1D3	E2V1D3_MYCTU	unreviewed	Serine/threonine-protein kinase transcriptional regulator pknK	M.tuberculosis SUMu007	1110	34.00%	86	0.5
E2UE39	E2UE39_MYCTU	unreviewed	Serine/threonine-protein kinase transcriptional regulator pknK	M.tuberculosis SUMu005	1110	34.00%	86	0.5
E2U2B5	E2U2B5_MYCTU	unreviewed	Serine/threonine-protein kinase transcriptional regulator pknK	M.tuberculosis SUMu004	1110	34.00%	86	0.5
E2TQU1	E2TQU1_MYCTU	unreviewed	Serine/threonine-protein kinase transcriptional regulator pknK	M.tuberculosis SUMu003	1110	34.00%	86	0.5
E2TDN6	E2TDN6_MYCTU	unreviewed	Serine/threonine-protein kinase transcriptional regulator pknK	M.tuberculosis SUMu002	1110	34.00%	86	0.5
E1HDI2	E1HDI2_MYCTU	unreviewed	Serine/threonine-protein kinase transcriptional regulator pknK	M.tuberculosis SUMu001	1110	34.00%	86	0.5
D7ETU6	D7ETU6_MYCTU	unreviewed	Putative uncharacterized protein	M.tuberculosis 94_M4241A	1110	34.00%	86	0.5
D6FQ58	D6FQ58_MYCTU	unreviewed	Serine/threonine-protein kinase transcriptional regulator pknK	M.tuberculosis K85	1110	34.00%	86	0.5
D6FKX7	D6FKX7_MYCTU	unreviewed	Serine/threonine-protein kinase transcriptional regulator pknK	M.tuberculosis CPHL_A	1110	34.00%	86	0.5
D6F961	D6F961_MYCTU	unreviewed	Serine/threonine-protein kinase transcriptional regulator pknK	M.tuberculosis T46	1110	34.00%	86	0.5
D5YW23	D5YW23_MYCTU	unreviewed	Serine/threonine-protein kinase transcriptional regulatory protein	M.tuberculosis 02_1987	1110	34.00%	86	0.5
D5YJ42	D5YJ42_MYCTU	unreviewed	Serine/threonine-protein kinase transcriptional regulatory protein	M.tuberculosis EAS054	1110	34.00%	86	0.5
D5Y7Z7	D5Y7Z7_MYCTU	unreviewed	Serine/threonine-protein	M.tuberculosis	1110	34.00%	86	0.5

			kinase transcriptional regulatory protein	T85				
D5XY80	D5XY80_MYCTU	unreviewed	Serine/threonine-protein kinase transcriptional regulator pknK (Fragment)	*M.tuberculosis* T92	880	34.00%	86	0.5
A7LP28	A7LP28_MYCBP	unreviewed	Serine/threonine protein kinase K	*Mycobacterium bovis* (strain BCG / Pasteur 1173P2)	1110	34.00%	86	0.5
A4KKY1	A4KKY1_MYCTU	unreviewed	Serine/threonine-protein kinase transcriptional regulatory protein pknK	*M.tuberculosis* str. Haarlem	1110	34.00%	86	0.5
A2VNP1	A2VNP1_MYCTU	unreviewed	Serine/threonine-protein kinase transcriptional regulatory protein pknK	*M.tuberculosis* C	1110	34.00%	86	0.5
P95078	PKNK_MYCTU	reviewed	Serine/threonine-protein kinase pknK (EC 2.7.11.1) (Protein kinase K)	*Mycobacterium tuberculosis*	1110	34.00%	86	0.5
Q7TXA9	PKNK_MYCBO	reviewed	Probable serine/threonine-protein kinase pknK (EC 2.7.11.1) (Protein kinase K)	*Mycobacterium bovis*	1110	34.00%	86	0.5
Q79FJ9	Q79FJ9_MYCTU	unreviewed	PE-PGRS FAMILY PROTEIN	*Mycobacterium tuberculosis*	639	32.00%	85	0.65
C6DR80	C6DR80_MYCTK	unreviewed	PE-PGRS family protein	*M.tuberculosis* (strain KZN 1435 / MDR)	650	32.00%	85	0.65
A5WND0	A5WND0_MYCTF	unreviewed	PE-PGRS family protein	*M.tuberculosis* (strain F11)	650	32.00%	85	0.65
A5U3H0	A5U3H0_MYCTA	unreviewed	PE-PGRS family protein	*M.tuberculosis* (strain ATCC 25177 / H37Ra)	650	32.00%	85	0.65
Q8VJW1	Q8VJW1_MYCTU	unreviewed	PE_PGRS family protein	*Mycobacterium tuberculosis*	650	32.00%	85	0.65
E2WHW9	E2WHW9_MYCTU	unreviewed	Putative PE family protein (Fragment)	*M.tuberculosis* SUMu012	507	32.00%	85	0.65
E2W5Y7	E2W5Y7_MYCTU	unreviewed	Putative PE family protein	*M.tuberculosis* SUMu011	275	32.00%	85	0.65
E2VUQ8	E2VUQ8_MYCTU	unreviewed	Putative PE family protein (Fragment)	*M.tuberculosis* SUMu010	558	32.00%	85	0.65
E2UYW2	E2UYW2_MYCTU	unreviewed	Putative PE family protein	*M.tuberculosis* SUMu007	287	32.00%	85	0.65
E2ULK8	E2ULK8_MYCTU	unreviewed	Putative PE family protein (Fragment)	*M.tuberculosis* SUMu006	193	32.00%	85	0.65
E2TYP7	E2TYP7_MYCTU	unreviewed	Putative uncharacterized protein	*M.tuberculosis* SUMu004	650	32.00%	85	0.65
E2T9R7	E2T9R7_MYCTU	unreviewed	Putative uncharacterized protein (Fragment)	*M.tuberculosis* SUMu002	257	32.00%	85	0.65
E1H9W1	E1H9W1_MYCTU	unreviewed	Putative PE family protein	*M.tuberculosis* SUMu001	287	32.00%	85	0.65
D7ERN5	D7ERN5_MYCTU	unreviewed	PE-PGRS family protein	*M.tuberculosis* 94_M4241A	650	32.00%	85	0.65
D6FUB5	D6FUB5_MYCTU	unreviewed	PE-PGRS family protein	*M.tuberculosis* K85	639	32.00%	85	0.65
D5ZHX0	D5ZHX0_MYCTU	unreviewed	PE-PGRS family protein	*M.tuberculosis* T17	639	32.00%	85	0.65
D5YSU9	D5YSU9_MYCTU	unreviewed	Predicted protein	*M.tuberculosis* 02_1987	650	32.00%	85	0.65
D5YFW9	D5YFW9_MYCTU	unreviewed	Predicted protein	*M.tuberculosis* EAS054	639	32.00%	85	0.65
D5Y498	D5Y498_MYCTU	unreviewed	PE-PGRS family protein	*M.tuberculosis* T85	528	32.00%	85	0.65

D5XUA0	D5XUA0_MYCTU	unreviewed	PE-PGRS family protein (Fragment)	*M.tuberculosis* T92	621	32.00%	85	0.65
A4KHV7	A4KHV7_MYCTU	unreviewed	PE-PGRS family protein	*M.tuberculosis* str. Haarlem	650	32.00%	85	0.65
A2VIS5	A2VIS5_MYCTU	unreviewed	PE-PGRS family protein	*M.tuberculosis* C	650	32.00%	85	0.65
Q7TY98	Q7TY98_MYCBO	unreviewed	PE-PGRS FAMILY PROTEIN	*Mycobacterium bovis*	546	30.00%	81	1.9
D0L2D2	D0L2D2_GORB4	unreviewed	PE domain protein	*Gordonia bronchialis* (strain ATCC 25592 / DSM 43247 / JCM 3198 / NCTC 10667) (*Rhodococcus bronchialis*)	101	26.00%	81	1.9
C6DMA3	C6DMA3_MYCTK	unreviewed	PE-PGRS family protein	*M.tuberculosis* (strain KZN 1435 / MDR)	553	30.00%	81	1.9

Table1: Shows BLAST results and E-values of PE proteins of *M. tuberculosis* involved in pathogenesis.

4   Conclusions and Scope

Examination of the amino-acid composition of the *M. tuberculosis* proteome by correspondence analysis (Greenacre, 1984), and comparison with that of other microorganisms whose genome sequences are available, revealed a statistically significant preference for the amino acids Ala, Gly, Pro, Arg and Trp, which are all encoded by G + C-rich codons, and a comparative reduction in the use of amino acids encoded by A + T- rich codons such as Asn, Ile, Lys, Phe and Tyr.The fraction of the proteome that has arisen through gene duplication is similar to that seen in *E. coli* or *B. subtilis* except that the level of sequence conservation is considerably higher, indicating that there may be extensive redundancy or differential production of the corresponding polypeptides. The apparent lack of divergence following gene duplication is consistent with the hypothesis that *M. tuberculosis* is of recent descent.One third of the world population is infected with *M. tuberculosis* and is carried in dormant form. Before entering the dormant form, the bacterium degrades the cell membrane of the host and accumulates the lipids in order to resynthesize complex lipid molecules to suit their survival in the host environment (Daniel *et al.*, 2004). The mycobacteria possess a complex outer cell wall comprising an asymmetric lipid bilayer. The inner layer of the cell wall is a peptidoglycan layer that is linked via phosphodiester bond to the complex carbohydrates and arabinogalactan which are linked to high-molecular weight mycolic acids that forms a glycolipid (Rezwan *et al.*, 2007).

In conclusion, the present study has established that the PE-PPE domain from mycobacteria belongs to the family of serine hydrolase proteins; biochemical characterization would establish the precise function of these proteins.

References

Adindla, S., and L. Guruprasad. (2003). Sequence analysis corresponding tothe PPE and PE proteins in Mycobacterium tuberculosis and other genomes. J. Biosci. 28:169–179.

Altschul, S.F. & Gish, W. (1996). Local alignment statistics. Meth. Enzymol. 266:460-480.

Altschul, S.F., Gish, W., Miller, W., Myers, E.W. & Lipman, D.J. (1990). Basic local alignment search tool. J. Mol. Biol. 215:403-410.

Cole S T, Brosch R, Parkhill J, Garnier T, Churcher C, Harris D, Gordon SV, Eiglmeier K, Gas S, Barry CE 3rd, Tekaia F, Badcock K, Basham D, Brown D, Chillingworth T, Connor R, Davies R, Devlin K, Feltwell T, Gentles S, Hamlin N, Holroyd S, Hornsby T, Jagels K, Krogh A, McLean J, Moule S, Murphy L, Oliver K, Osborne J, Quail MA, Rajandream MA, Rogers J, Rutter S, Seeger K, Skelton J, Squares R, Squares S, Sulston JE, Taylor K, Whitehead S, Barrell BG. (1998). Deciphering the biology of Micobacterium Tuberculosis from the complete genome sequence. Nature. 393:537-544.

Cole ST, Eiglmeier K, Parkhill J, James KD, Thomson NR, Wheeler PR, Honoré N, Garnier T, Churcher C, Harris D, Mungall K, Basham D, Brown D, Chillingworth T, Connor R, Davies RM, Devlin K, Duthoy S, Feltwell T, Fraser A, Hamlin N, Holroyd S, Hornsby T, Jagels K, Lacroix C, Maclean J, Moule S, Murphy L, Oliver K, Quail MA, Rajandream MA, Rutherford KM, Rutter S, Seeger K, Simon S, Simmonds M, Skelton J, Squares R, Squares S, Stevens K, Taylor K, Whitehead S, Woodward JR, Barrell BG. (2001). Massive gene decay in the leprosy bacillus. Nature. 22:409(6823):1007-11

Daniel J, Deb C, Dubey VS, Sirakova TD, Abomoelak B. (2004) Induction of a novel class of diacylglycerol acyltransferases and triacylglycerol accumulation in Mycobacterium tuberculosis as it goes into a dormancy-like state in culture. J Bacteriol 186:5017–5030.

Fleischmann, R. D., Adams MD, White O, Clayton RA, Kirkness EF, Kerlavage AR, Bult CJ, Tomb JF, Dougherty BA, Merrick JM. (1995). Whole-genome random sequencing and assembly of Haemophilus influenzae Rd. Science. 269(5223):496–8, 507–12.

Greenacre, M. (1984). Theory and Application of Correspondence Analysis, Academic, London.

Gumbel, E. J. (1958). Statistics of extremes. Columbia University Press, New York, NY.

Mount DM. (2004) Bioinformatics: Sequence and Genome Analysis, 2nd ed. Cold Spring Harbor Laboratory Press: Cold Spring Harbor, NY. ISBN 0-87969-608-7.

Needleman, Saul B and Wunsch, Christian D. (1970). A general method applicable to the search for similarities in the amino acid sequence of two proteins. Journal of Molecular Biology. 48(3):443–53.

Rezwan M, Lane´elle MA, Sander P, Daffe´ M. (2007). Breaking down the wall: fractionation of mycobacteria. J Microbiol Methods. 68:32–39.

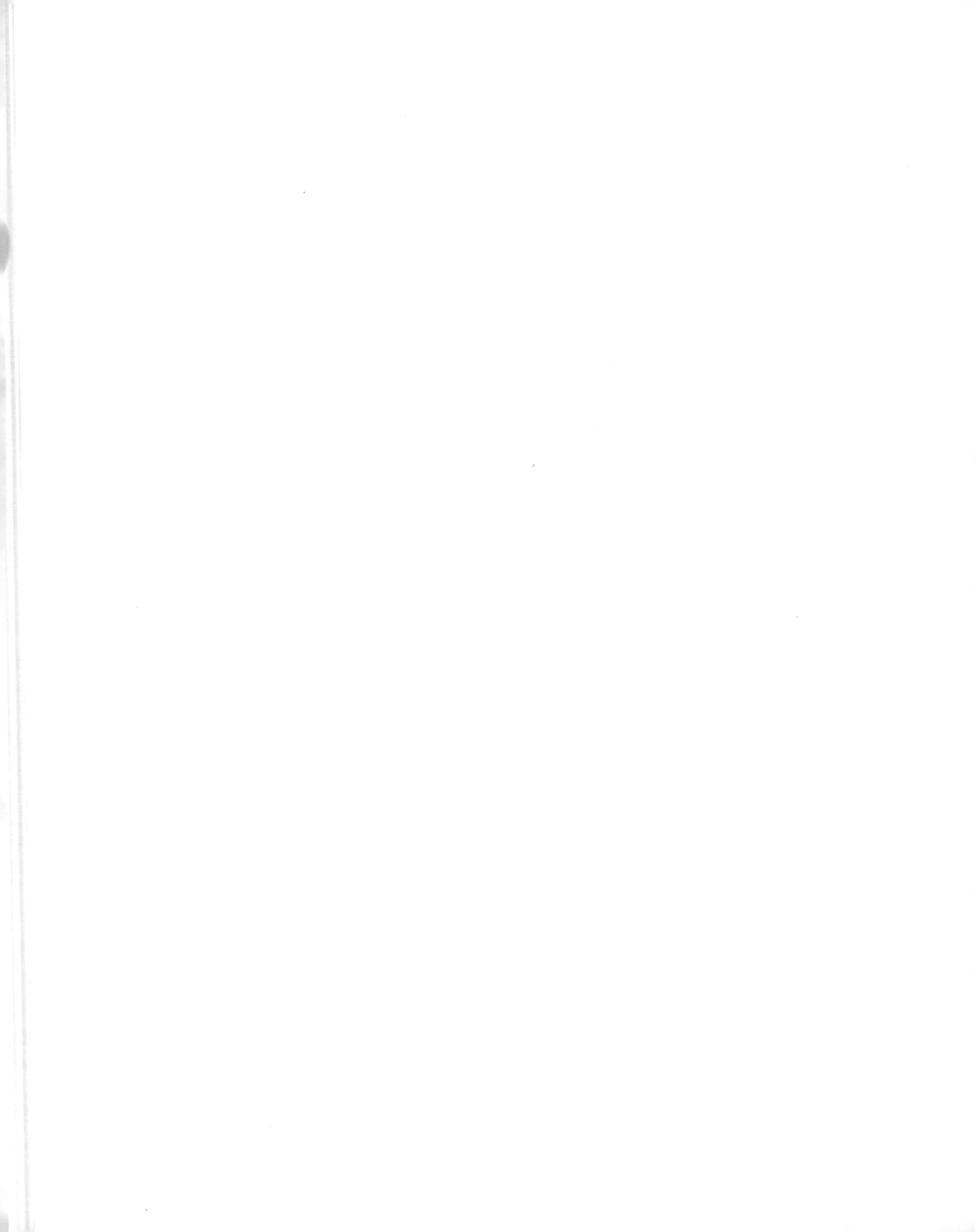

www.ingramcontent.com/pod-product-compliance
Lightning Source LLC
Chambersburg PA
CBHW041705210326
41598CB00007B/534